GENE THERAPY FOR NEUROLOGICAL DISORDERS

Molecular Approaches for Targeted Treatment

GENE THERAPY FOR NEUROLOGICAL DISORDERS

Molecular Approaches for Targeted Treatment

Rishabha Malviya, PhD
Arun Kumar Singh, MPharm
Priyanshi Goyal, MPharm
Sonali Sundram, MPharm

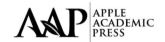

First edition published 2025

Apple Academic Press Inc.
1265 Goldenrod Circle, NE,
Palm Bay, FL 32905 USA

CRC Press
2385 NW Executive Center Drive,
Suite 320, Boca Raton FL 33431

760 Laurentian Drive, Unit 19,
Burlington, ON L7N 0A4, CANADA

4 Park Square, Milton Park,
Abingdon, Oxon, OX14 4RN UK

© 2025 by Apple Academic Press, Inc.

Apple Academic Press exclusively co-publishes with CRC Press, an imprint of Taylor & Francis Group, LLC

Reasonable efforts have been made to publish reliable data and information, but the authors, editors, and publisher cannot assume responsibility for the validity of all materials or the consequences of their use. The authors are solely responsible for all the chapter content, figures, tables, data etc. provided by them. The authors, editors, and publishers have attempted to trace the copyright holders of all material reproduced in this publication and apologize to copyright holders if permission to publish in this form has not been obtained. If any copyright material has not been acknowledged, please write and let us know so we may rectify in any future reprint.

Except as permitted under U.S. Copyright Law, no part of this book may be reprinted, reproduced, transmitted, or utilized in any form by any electronic, mechanical, or other means, now known or hereafter invented, including photocopying, microfilming, and recording, or in any information storage or retrieval system, without written permission from the publishers.

For permission to photocopy or use material electronically from this work, access www.copyright.com or contact the Copyright Clearance Center, Inc. (CCC), 222 Rosewood Drive, Danvers, MA 01923, 978-750-8400. For works that are not available on CCC please contact mpkbookspermissions@tandf.co.uk

Trademark notice: Product or corporate names may be trademarks or registered trademarks and are used only for identification and explanation without intent to infringe.

Library and Archives Canada Cataloguing in Publication

Title: Gene therapy for neurological disorders : molecular approaches for targeted treatment / Rishabha Malviya, PhD, Arun Kumar Singh, PhD, Priyanshi Goyal, MPharm, Sonali Sundram, MPharm.

Names: Malviya, Rishabha, author. | Singh, Arun Kumar, MPharm, author. | Goyal, Priyanshi, author. | Sundram, Sonali, author.

Description: First edition. | Includes bibliographical references and index.

Identifiers: Canadiana (print) 20240444914 | Canadiana (ebook) 20240444949 | ISBN 9781774916780 (hardcover) | ISBN 9781774916797 (softcover) | ISBN 9781003494102 (ebook)

Subjects: LCSH: Nervous system—Diseases—Gene therapy.

Classification: LCC RC350.G45 M35 2025 | DDC 616.8/0442—dc23

Library of Congress Cataloging-in-Publication Data

....

CIP data on file with US Library of Congress

....

ISBN: 978-1-77491-678-0 (hbk)
ISBN: 978-1-77491-679-7 (pbk)
ISBN: 978-1-00349-410-2 (ebk)

Dedication

This book is dedicated to the Honorable CEO of Galgotias University, Dr. Dhruv Galgotia, for creating a research-oriented environment. We express our sincere gratitude for your constant motivation and believing in us that made this book possible.

About the Authors

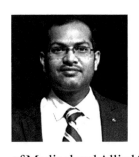

Rishabha Malviya, PhD
Associate Professor, Department of Pharmacy, School of Medical and Allied Sciences, Galgotias University, Greater Noida, Uttar Pradesh, India

Rishabha Malviya, PhD, has 11 years of research experience and is presently working as Associate Professor in the Department of Pharmacy, School of Medical and Allied Sciences, Galgotias University, Greater Noida, Uttar Pradesh, India. His areas of interest include formulation optimization, nanoformulation, targeted drug delivery, localized drug delivery, and characterization of natural polymers as pharmaceutical excipients. He has authored more than 150 research and review papers for national and international journals of repute. He holds over 50 patents and has published many papers in reputed national and international journals, for which he received an outstanding reviewer award from Elsevier. He has edited 13 books (Wiley, Springer Nature, CRC Press/Taylor and Francis, Apple Academic Press, River Publisher, Lambert, and OMICS Publishing Group) and authored 15 book chapters. His name has been included in the World's Top 2% Scientists list by Elsevier BV and Stanford University. He is reviewer, editor, and editorial board member of more than 50 national and international journals. He was an invited author for the magazine *Atlas of Science* as well as a pharma magazine dealing with B2B industry, *Ingredient South Asia*. He completed a BPharm from Uttar Pradesh Technical University and MPharm (Pharmaceutics) from Gautam Buddha Technical University, Lucknow, Uttar Pradesh. His PhD (Pharmacy) work was in novel formulation development techniques.

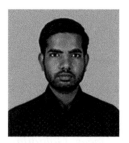

Arun Kumar Singh, PhD
Department of Pharmacy, School of Medical & Allied Sciences, Galgotias University, Greater Noida, Uttar Pradesh, India

Arun Kumar Singh, MPharm, is affiliated with the Department of Pharmacy, School of Medical & Allied Sciences, Galgotias University, Greater Noida, Uttar Pradesh, India. His areas of interest include nanoformulation, blockchain, IoT, machine learning, cancer, artificial intelligence, and big data. He has published three chapters in the field of big data. He has also published two review papers among which one is published in *Biochimica et Biophysica Acta (BBA): Reviews on Cancer*. His strength is his research skill, innovative thinking, leadership qualities, decision-making ability, and positive thinking. He completed his MPharm (pharmaceutics) at Galgotias University, Greater Noida, India.

Priyanshi Goyal, MPharm
Department of Pharmacy, School of Medical and Allied Sciences, Galgotias University, Greater Noida, Uttar Pradesh, India

Priyanshi Goyal, MPharm, is affiliated with the Department of Pharmacy at the School of Medical and Allied Sciences, Galgotias University, Greater Noida, Uttar Pradesh India. She has authored one chapter in a Springer Nature published book (in press). She is the author of one book (authored) published by Apple Academic Press/Taylor and Francis Group. She completed her 10th and 12th years at Krishna International School (CBSE-affiliate), Aligarh, India. She also earned her BPharm from Aligarh College of Pharmacy, Aligarh, affiliated with AKTU, Lucknow, and her MPharm from Galgotias University, Greater Noida, India.

Sonali Sundram, MPharm

Assistant Professor, School of Medical & Allied Sciences,
Galgotias University, Greater Noida, Uttar Pradesh, India

Sonali Sundram, MPharm, is an Assistant Professor in the School of Medical and Allied Sciences at Galgotias University, Greater Noida, Uttar Pradesh, India. Previously, she worked as a research scientist on a project of ICMR at King George's Medical University, Lucknow, India. After that, she joined BBDNIIT (Babu Banarasi Das Northern India Institute of Technology), Lucknow. Her PhD (Pharmacy) work was in neurodegeneration and nanoformulation. Her areas of interest include neurodegeneration, clinical research, and artificial intelligence. She has edited four books (Wiley, CRC Press/Taylor and Francis, River Publisher) and has organized more than 15 national and international seminars, conferences, and workshops. She has more than eight patents, both national and international, to her credit. She completed both BPharm and MPharm (Pharmacology) from Dr. A.P.J. Abdul Kalam Technical University, Lucknow, India.

Contents

Foreword by Brahmeshwar Mishra...*xiii*

Preface ....*xv*

1. **Neurodegenerative Disorders and Their Treatment**............................... 1

2. **Neurodegenerative Disorders: A Mysterious Group of Diseases**.......... 27

3. **Propagation of Neurodegenerative disorders**.. 53

4. **Gene Therapy: A Promising Strategy for the Treatment of Brain Disease** 83

5. **Stem-Cell-Employed Gene Therapy for Neurodegenerative Disorder**.. 113

6. **Current Practice and Prospects in Gene Therapy Based on Genomic DNA**... 129

7. **Targeting Oligodendrocytes with Gene-Silencing Sequences through Vector-Mediated Transgene Delivery** 149

8. **Astrocytes: Genetic Treatment Targets for Alzheimer's Disease**........ 165

9. **Clinical Studies of Gene Therapy for the Treatment of Neurodegenerative Disorders**... 191

Index..*217*

Foreword

Dr. Rishabha Malviya is one of the young and promising researcher and is one of the most motivating and dedicated person to profession of Pharmacy. This unique book entitled as "Gene therapy for neurological disorder- molecular approach for targeted treatment elaborately dealt with various aspects including treatment strategies of neurodegenerative disorders. There are large number of neurodegenerative diseases, and most of them are incurable. Degenerative diseases of the neurological system impose major medical and public health burdens on population throughout the world. Because of the age-related increase in both the prevalence and incidence of these diseases, the number of new cases are likely to rise steadily in coming future .Gene therapy is an important emerging strategy for treating neurodegenerative disorders. Therefore, it is important to carefully examine potential gene-based therapeutic approaches for the treatment of neurodegenerative disorders, including assessment of safety profiles and pharmacological effects that are currently available, as well as identification of individuals who can get benefit .This book comprises the content related to advances in gene therapies including newly emerging RNA and DNA based gene therapies for neurodegenerative disorders.

The contribution by authors is highly appreciable and are of immense use as they highlighted advances in the development and application of gene-based therapies for neurodegenerative diseases and offer a prospective look into this emerging arena. I believe this work will surely become a useful source for readers and also for researchers as it provides the better understanding of the onset and progression of the neurodegenerative disorders that will facilitate prompt diagnosis and target selection and can ensure early treatment of these diseases.

With best wishes
Dr. Brahmeshwar Mishra
Professor (HAG Scale) and Former Head
Department of Pharmaceutical Engineering & Technology
IIT(BHU), Varanasi
Uttar Pradesh, India

Preface

With a significant socioeconomic burden, neurological illnesses pose as one of the biggest hazards to the health care system. The range of pharmacotherapeutics currently available primarily has palliative effects and is ineffective in treating such illnesses. Numerous neurological illnesses have a molecular etiology that is linked to a change in genetic background, which can be inherited or brought on by other environmental variables.

The methods of gene therapy that can be used to treat both inherited and sporadic neurodegenerative diseases are covered in this book. There are nine chapters in this book. The first chapter introduces the idea of neurodegenerative conditions, while the second explains the physiological basis for their occurrence in humans. The third chapter is dedicated to the various proteins, while the fourth discusses many viral applications. The fifth chapter explores how stem cells can be used to learn about the future of gene therapy, which is then discussed in the following chapter. More information on the sequences that silence genes is presented in chapter seven. The eighth chapter discusses the function of astrocytes in the various brain regions, while the ninth discusses in vivo research in gene therapy for neurodegenerative disorder.

Gene therapy for the neurodegenerative disease might be seen as a viable alternative to the few known treatments. In this book, we cover the most significant advances in gene transfer methods as well as the most recent understandings of the mechanisms behind specific neurodegenerative illnesses and place these into the context of gene therapy approaches for the central nervous system. The book provides a thorough overview of state-of-the-art methods for developing gene therapy for neurodegenerative diseases. Uses and applications of gene therapy in the treatment of neurological diseases are explored, and clinical trials of gene therapy on neurodegenerative disorders are studied in this book.

The goal of this book is to encourage the use of gene therapy to treat neurological disorders by providing a thorough examination of the many approaches currently being taken. This book explains the unfathomable mysteries of neurological disease, providing information that is crucial to understanding how gene therapy is being used to treat neurological disorders.

New graduates, pharmacologists, clinical researchers, and anybody else aiming to find a solution to a neurological illness may find this book invaluable. This book has the potential to become one of the most comprehensive resources available because it discusses the most important developments in the field of gene therapy for neurological conditions.

CHAPTER 1

Neurodegenerative Disorders and Their Treatment

ABSTRACT

It is widely acknowledged that neurological diseases [neurodegenerative disorders (NDs)] constitute an important problem in terms of public wellness. According to the WHO, neurological illnesses are among the 10 leading causes of death worldwide. NDs such as Alzheimer's disease (AD), Parkinson's disease (PD), Huntington's disease (HD), amyotrophic lateral sclerosis (ALS), prion disease, brain tumors, spinal cord injuries, and strokes are major health concerns of neurological illnesses in the developed world. There are currently no effective treatments for these conditions since no therapies exist that can effectively transport drugs across to access brain tissue by piercing the blood–brain barrier (BBB) pharmacological impact. Researchers need to find ways to increase the potency of medicines and get beyond BBB. Here, offer a quick overview of treating various neurological illnesses.

1.1 INTRODUCTION

The public health crisis posed by neurodegenerative diseases (NDs) is well documented.[1] NDs are the most difficult and debilitating central nervous system (CNS) disorders. ND is characterized by neuronal dysfunction or dysfunctional neuron loss. Stroke, Alzheimer's disease (AD), Parkinson's disease (PD), Huntington's disease (HD), amyotrophic lateral sclerosis (ALS), and prion disease are only a few of the many causes of ND as

---

Gene Therapy for Neurological Disorders: Molecular Approaches for Targeted Treatment.
Rishabha Malviya, Arun Kumar Singh, Priyanshi Goyal, & Sonali Sundram (Authors)
© 2025 Apple Academic Press, Inc. Co-published with CRC Press (Taylor & Francis)

shown in Figure 1.1. Each illness has its unique pathogenesis. Some NDs cause cognitive and memory decline, while others compromise a person's ability to communicate, act, or even breathe.[2] The WHO reports that strokes, after AD and other forms of dementia, are the second biggest cause of mortality globally in 2019.[3] As life expectancy rises, so does the number of people who suffer from NDs in emerging nations. The origins of most neurological disorders have been established, and the efficacy of various therapies for them has been extensively researched. Diagnosing and treating neurological illnesses can be difficult because of the CNS's fragility and complexity.[4,5] Therapeutic interventions are made more difficult by obstacles whose primary purpose is to control the flow between the bloodstream and the brain of chemicals. Glial and endothelial cells collaborate in the brain to create barriers. The blood–brain barrier (BBB) regulates how drugs are absorbed into the brain and is therefore a crucial part of the system.[6]

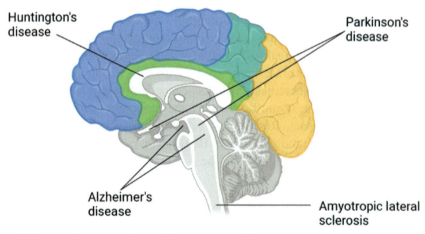

FIGURE 1.1 Representation of different types of ND.

Incurable diseases like NDs are on the rise, and their numbers cannot be ignored. Due to the BBB's impenetrability, no specific therapeutic medicines exist for the vast majority of these disorders, and even fewer pharmaceuticals can be administered in sufficient doses to have any pharmacological effect on the brain. When it comes to treating neurological illnesses, the BBB presents a hurdle, but it is far from the only one. Because of their molecular structure, around 95% of medicines cannot penetrate that BBB. Blood–cerebrospinal fluid and the BBB regulate what can enter the CNS. Drugs that are lipophilic and have a molecular weight of 500 Da or less can pass through the BBB, but conventional medications cannot.[7,8] The BBB's extremely semipermeable nature makes it difficult for therapeutic medications to cross into the CNS; overcoming this barrier is one of the greatest difficulties in developing cutting-edge medicine. Due to its capacity to circumvent the BBB, photothermal and photodynamic treatments are applicable to the management of numerous NDs. On the contrary, these treatments can have unwanted effects such as tissue damage (particularly skin tissue damage) and photosensitization[9,10] To combat these conditions, there is an immediate need for the discovery and development of new medicinal molecules that can traverse the BBB without creating adverse consequences. However, effective therapy of any disease requires a thorough knowledge of the inner workings and root causes.[2,11] Therapeutic techniques that can both bypass the BBB and boost its effectiveness are needed.

1.2   TYPES OF NEURODEGENERATIVE DISEASE

1.2.1   ALZHEIMER'S DISEASE

The long-term repercussions of memory loss and other cognitive issues include AD, an incurable brain condition. It is true that AD often first manifests itself in a decline in short-term memory, but the disease progresses to significant memory failures in later stages[7], leaving patients bedridden with incontinence and recurrent epileptic attacks. cholinergic hypothesis, mitochondrial cascade theory, metabolic hypothesis, vascular hypothesis, amyloidal hypothesis, tau hypothesis, APP trigger tauopathy, and APP trigger tauopathy and the neuroepigenetic modification hypothesis are all part of the molecular mechanism that underpins AD.

1.2.1.1   PATHOPHYSIOLOGY

Amyloid plaques, neurofibrillary tangles (NFT), and neuronal death are hallmarks of AD (particularly cholinergic neurons of the basal forebrain). Dementia is extremely widespread in the United States, although AD is the most frequent form. There are about 120 new cases per 100,000

4 *Gene Therapy for Neurological Disorders*

people each year. In terms of dementia, this is the most frequent type. These structural abnormalities are found at autopsy in the AD brain when neurons in the nucleus basalis (a brain area below the globus pallidus) die off, die, acetylcholine stops being produced. This type of neuron is characteristic of AD because its axons extend far into the brain's cortex and limbic system. Damaged brain areas are characterized by the presence of abnormal protein aggregates called amyloid plaques that accumulate outside of cells and NFTs, which are aberrant clusters of filaments inside cells, are two forms of neurodegeneration.[12] These filaments primarily consist of tau protein that has been hyperphosphorylated. These anomalies and others are caused by a variety of neurotoxic events, such as but not limited to oxidative stress, inflammation, synaptic dysfunction, neurotransmitter depletion, and cell death. Cortical and subcortical neuron loss and atrophy are hallmarks of AD. Excitotoxicity is a word used to describe the damage done to neurons when glutamate levels are too high. In the mammalian brain, glutamate is thought to facilitate most excitatory synaptic communication among numerous neuronal systems.[13] Excess glutamate can cause excitotoxic cell death, even though it is essential for regular brain function. Glutamate receptors, in particular, NMDA glutamate receptors, mediate the neurotoxic effects of glutamate. To a large extent, contemporary attempts at therapeutic intervention are founded on the theorized pathogenic processes underlying AD.[14]

1.2.1.2   MECHANISM OF ACTION

According to the amyloid hypothesis, neuronal dysfunction and cell death in AD[15] may originate from the accumulation of A plaques, which enhances the pathogenic cascade that includes neurite destruction and NFT formation via tau protein. Neurofibrillary tangles NFTs comprised of straight filaments (SFs) or paired helical filaments (PHFs) are a hallmark of tau hyperphosphorylation (SFs). These results imply that tau pathology may be induced by improper sorting of tau, which may in turn influence the AD[16] patients' cognitive decline and metabolic alterations. Dementia can also be caused by problems with APP metabolism, which lead to neuroinflammation and eventually tau pathology.[17] When neurons or synapses die off in the brain's cortex, cholinergic neurotransmission decreases. This in turn reduces the integration of muscarinic M1 receptors into the intracellular signaling pathway which in turn decreases NFT formation, soluble APP secretion, β-amyloid protein

Neurodegenerative Disorders and Their Treatment

production, and glutamate production. These alterations have some bearing on the development of AD's clinical symptoms and the spread of pathology.[18] According to the mitochondrial cascade concept, mitochondria are at the center relating to the beginnings of the Christian era and the development into a ND. However, many researchers have argued that mitochondria do not have a primary role in AD.[19] The intracellular buildup of A is caused by a deficiency in ATP availability as a result of disruptions in the insulin signal transduction cascade. Abnormalities in insulin signal transduction and low ATP[20] levels also exacerbate tau protein hyperphosphorylation and the development of NFT. Acquiring vascular risk factors, which are accountable for the subsequent chronic cerebral hypoperfusion [critically attained threshold of cerebral hypoperfusion (CATCH)], is a crucial stage that transforms natural aging into a whirlwind of mental disorders. Decades may pass before ND and eventually, AD manifests themselves. Dysregulation is a typical AD pathogenic situation, and its participation has been the focus of multiple AD treatment strategies.[21] These enzymes include β-secretase, glycogen synthase kinase-3β, acetylcholinesterase, butyrylcholinesterase, and rho kinase. Neuroepigenetic abnormalities cause neuronal DNA to activate or repress particular genes, hence leading to the onset of pathogenic alterations in NDs such as AD. Distinct areas of the brain shrink, senile plaques (αβ protein deposits), and NFT also appear in advanced stages of AD (composed of highly phosphorylated tau protein) are the typical neuropathological hallmarks of AD.[22] As opposed to addressing the disease's underlying pathophysiological problems, early attempts to treat AD focused instead on alleviating the symptoms of the disease. Drugs such as rivastigmine, donepezil, galantamine, and memantine work effectively to treat AD on this basis. Figure 1.2 systematically represents the mechanism of action of AD.

1.2.1.3 PHARMACOTHERAPY

Treatments for these conditions include those for cholinergic agonists and neurotrophins, antioxidants, anti-inflammatory drugs, the amyloid cascade, effects of food, dietary supplements, steroid deficiency treatment, memantine, and other factors on the condition have all been investigated (low saturated fat diets; moderate alcohol intake). The most advanced treatment for mild-to-severe illness is acetylcholinesterase, a cholinolytic.[23] β-APP levels include the creation of β-amyloid and amyloid-causing

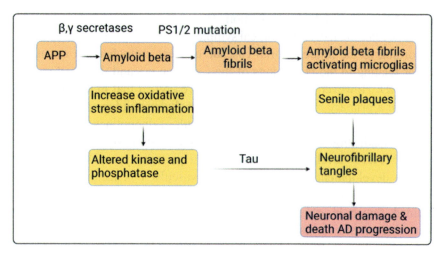

FIGURE 1.2 Flowchart of the mechanism of action of AD.

substances are lowered are hypothesized to be the mechanism through which ACIs decrease disease progression. As an ACI, tacrine was the first to gain widespread use. Donepezil (Aricept®, Eisai Company, and Pfizer, Inc.); galantamine (Hoechst Marion Roussel, Inc., Shire Pharmaceutical Group, and Janssen Pharmaceutical; Reminyl® and Nivalin; U.S. trade name Razadyne); and rivastigmine (Exelon®, Novartis Pharmaceuticals) are some examples of antidepressants used to treat dementia. All around, these medications are safer, more effective, and have longer half-lives. AD incidence and prevalence are reduced when vitamin E is taken alongside vitamin C. Neuroprotective therapies presently AD phase-III clinical trials are testing the following: Atorvastatin, ginkgo Biloba, nonsteroidal anti-inflammatory drugs, docosahexaenoic acid (DHA), ly2062430 solanezumab, ly450139 semagacestat (AZD-103), tamoxifen, xaliproden, valproate, DHA, tarenflurbil, rosiglitazone, simvastatin, and tamoxifen. Recent research has linked the Mediterranean Diet and Protection against AD.[24] A newer study confirms that there's evidence linking the Mediterranean diet to a reduced risk of death from AD and suggests a dosage response relationship between the two. Fish is a staple of this diet, along with moderate amounts of unsaturated fatty acids, fewer dairy products, less meat and poultry, and a modest intake of alcohol. Many of the current vaccine methods being studied are aimed at the humeral response, and many new trials, including immunotherapy, are being conducted

Neurodegenerative Disorders and Their Treatment

to prevent an undesirable T-cell-mediated immune response. Enzyme secretase substrates the protease known as memapsin 2 (β-secretase, BACE1) catalyzes the first step in the conversion of APP into A. Therapy with donepezil, rivastigmine, and glutamate for those with some mild foundation of AD is the outcome of several large clinical investigations.[25] By combining the memory-boosting effects of Rivastigmine and the neuroprotective effects of rasagiline, ladostigil is a molecule with multiple uses. Dimebolin is a medication that can serve multiple purposes and has a wide spectrum of activity on multiple targets to aid in the AD treatment process. It inhibits acetylcholinesterase and butyrylcholinesterase weakly (IC_{50} =7.9 and 42 M, respectively). Some evidence suggests that the acetylcholinesterase inhibitor (AchEI)-acting chemical substance JWS-USC-75-IX (3-[2-(5-dimethylaminomethyl)-2-furanyl]methyl]thio] ethyl]amino]-4-nitropyridazine) can be useful in the treatment of AD.[26] Receptors for the neurotransmitter 5-hydroxytryptamine (5-HT) are abundantly distributed throughout between the brain and the rest of the body, and they take part in a wide range of physiological processes, such as the regulation of the heart rate and digestion, as well as the regulation of body temperature, mood, and memory.[27] Weak: Lecozotan (SRA-333), NAD-299, WAY 100635, and WAY 101405 ameliorate the effects of morphological (fornix and hippocampus) lesions and pharmacological (depression) deficiencies are all 5-HT receptor antagonists. Increasing acetylcholine release and improving some aspects of cognitive function have piqued interest in DAU 6215, granisetron, ondansetron, RS-56812, SEC 579, and WAY 100579 are examples of 5 HT3A receptor antagonists. Research into the effects of phosphodiesterase (PDE) inhibitors (such as papaverine) on cerebral blood flow has revealed promising results for improving metabolic processes and, by extension, cognitive abilities in the aged. Newer studies have focused on how PDE inhibitors affect levels of cAMP and cGMP, two important second messenger chemicals (cGMP). Here are a few more examples of multipurpose compounds Using a two-pronged strategy, researchers were able to combine the AChEI characteristics of caproctamine's polyamine backbone with part of coenzyme Q (CoQ) that scavenges radicals to create memorquin. As time goes on, learn more and more that the disease known as AD is quite complicated with many underlying causes.[28] Understanding how to treat degeneration symptoms can be used to, perhaps, stop the disease in its tracks or at least slow its course. There are several promising new therapeutic options, however, it may be challenging to determine what exactly causes this condition. Nevertheless, research into the mechanisms is progressing.[29]

1.2.2 PARKINSON'S DISEASE

The quality of life for those with PD is significantly diminished, making it the second most common neurological ailment for those who are diagnosed with it, making them dependent on others, and even hastening their deaths. Characteristics include reduced expressiveness, hunched shoulders, a festinating gait, rigidity, and a "pill-rolling" tremor17 are all symptoms of the disease. Some of the most notable pathways, misfolded protein aggregation formation, mitochondrial damage, oxidative stress, excitotoxicity, neuroinflammation, and genetic alterations all play a role in the development of PD.

1.2.2.1 PATHOPHYSIOLOGY

The brain can be broken down into five distinct circuits. Circuits involved in the movement (both voluntary and involuntary movements), vision, memory, emotion, and thought are all severely disrupted. When dopamine levels drop, the result is hypokinesia or a general slowing of movement. Synuclein alpha (SNCA) protein with ubiquitin abnormally accumulates in injured cells. Lewy bodies are clumps of accumulated insoluble protein that can be seen inside neurons. If this is not addressed quickly, it could cause brain cell death. Clusters of protein aggregates are called Lewy bodies. Its random emergence modifies genetics. Synuclein is a protein that is synthesized by the enzyme synuclein, an α-non-A4 component of amyloid precursor. Some mutations are linked to the beginning of PD at a young age. Parkin is a protein that is produced when PD autosomal recessive, juvenile 2 (PARK2) is mutated. In normal circumstances, parkin helps cells degrade proteins for recycling. PARK7, PINK1, and LRRK2 are all mutated. Dementia and other mental health issues typically rule out surgery as an option. Free radicals, unstable chemicals created by the body's routine chemical reactions, are another cause of PD. They can cause harm to tissues such as neurons when they combine with other

Neurodegenerative Disorders and Their Treatment   9

chemicals. Dopamine is lost prematurely dopamine-producing neurons degenerate with age, causing neurons. Severe PD-like symptoms may be brought on by exposure to several poisons, such as MPTP-contaminated illegal substances. MPTP was discovered to be neurotoxic as soon as it entered the brain. Pesticides, herbicides, manganese dust, carbon disulfide, carbon monoxide toxicity, and so on. are all examples of additional toxic substances.[30–32]

1.2.2.2 PHARMACOTHERAPY

Although advancements are being made in PD treatment, there is currently no one-size-fits-all approach due to the idiosyncratic manifestations of the disease's impact on various people. Medications and other treatments including medical procedures and therapies such as physiotherapy, occupational therapy (OT), speech, and cognitive–behavioral therapy (CBT) are often used together to achieve the best possible symptom management. Medication called levodopa, which the body converts into dopamine, is used in chemical treatment to restore normal dopamine levels in the brain. Tablet or capsule form is used for administration. Some medications, such as syndopa, sinemet, tidomet, levodopa and carbidopa (LCD), and madopar (levodopa + benserazide) are all levodopa and carbidopa combinations that lessen the severity of peripheral side effects. Popular antidepressants often contain ropinirole (requip, ropark, and ropiro), pramipexole (pramipex, pramirol, and lisuride), cabergoline (carberlin and cabgol), and bromocriptine (proctinal and parlodel) all examples of dopamine agonists (dopergin). To minimize the risk of adverse effects, they are often administered at a low dose at first. It is recommended to take dopamine agonists with food. Dopaminergic/amantadine has several effects, but it may be most helpful for its ability to increase dopamine release and prolong the neurotransmitter's time at the site of action. As with dopamine, the neurotransmitter acetylcholine appears to maintain a healthy equilibrium with its antagonists, anticholinergics (pacitane, kemadrine, and bexol). Dopamine metabolism is slowed when the enzyme monoamine oxidase type (MAO-B) that typically breaks down dopamine in the brain is blocked. Entacapone (entacom, adcapone, and comtan), and tolcapone (tasmar) are novel drugs that limit the breakdown of levodopa by inhibiting the enzyme catechol-O-methyl transferase (COMT). Pyridoxine, phenothiazine, butyrophenones, antihypertensives, and domperidone are incompatible with levodopa, hence they should not be administered together. PD symptoms are directly tied to low levels of dopamine in the nigrostriatal system and could be alleviated with cell treatment if the cells could survive, migrate, and trigger behavioral recovery.[33] Cell transplantation has the potential to create a homeostatic and reparative milieu in the recipient. Ayurvedic practices such as eating a plant-based diet, getting regular massages with warm oil, and using herbs for purification purposes have been in use for millennia. Atmagupta (Kappikachu) herb has shown promising results in treating PD. Jatamansi and Shanka are two examples of nerve tonics that can help improve the stiffness and poor performance of the nerves that are common in PD patients. The high-fiber foods, legumes, poultry, fish, and low-fat dairy items of the Mediterranean diet also contribute to health and productivity.

1.2.3 PRION DISEASE

A major contributor to the development of various NDs in both humans and animals. Insomnias with a deadly family history, Gerstmann–Straussler syndrome, Creutzfeldt–Jakob disease, and kuru are the main categories used to classify human prion diseases, they can be broken down into three groups based on where they originated: genetic, random, and learned (transmitted between animals or people). A disease with so many potential causes has never before been dominated by a single protein.[34] Prion illnesses in humans are extremely deadly, and there is currently no treatment. Prion disorders are treated with various medications, which have shown some promise in tissue culture and whole animal models.[35] Given the current status of the treatment plan, there is a compelling need to create pharmaceutical or alternative treatments for prion disorders. Therefore, Michal Mizrahi et al. looked into whether clinical worsening, neurodegenerative pathological characteristics, and prions are all mitigated by pomegranate seed oil (PSO) in its NE form when administered to TgMHu2ME1990K animals. The E200K PrP mutation has been linked to this specific strain of mice. In a mouse model of ND therapy, PSO injection was found to postpone the drug's action.[36] Preventing and treating a genetic prion disease model using nano-success PSOs suggests that compounds that limit lipid oxidation could be effective in relieving a wide variety of NDs.[37]

Neurodegenerative Disorders and Their Treatment 11

1.2.4 HUNTINGTON'S DISEASE

Choreoathetoid and dystonic movements, incoordination, and cognitive and behavioral changes are all hallmarks of HD, a progressive ND. Although the condition typically manifests in midlife after childbearing years, it can manifest at any age.[38] Caused by a high concentration of cytosine, adenine, and guanine (CAG) trinucleotide repeats in the HTT gene (of varied length). Epigenetic alterations have been associated with HD progression. One of the primary pathogenic mechanisms in HD is transcriptional dysregulation, which links food availability to cellular activities. Reduced histone acetylation, which is linked to neuronal damage and death (in HD),[39] perhaps what happens when mutated HTTs clump together.

1.2.5 AMYOTROPHIC LATERAL SCLEROSIS

Motor neuron death is a hallmark of ALS, which affects the CNS. There are some similarities between the pathobiology of this neurodegenerative illness and that of frontotemporal dementia, and many people show signs of both disorders. Because the disease is caused by a wide variety of genes and pathophysiological mechanisms, effective treatments will require an understanding of this variation.[40] Extensive studies have gone into the improvement of diagnostic methods that have allowed as a means of speedy diagnosis and treatment for a wide range of illnesses. In recent years, some development, but only a little. However, the BBB continues to be a significant barrier to therapeutic medications and diagnostic tools reaching the brain, which is a major reason why more effective treatments haven't been developed yet. Nearly finished methods of treating NDs include stem cell therapy, antitoxins directed superoxide dismutase (SOD1), copper and zinc mutants, nanotechnology, and other forms of molecular engineering.[41] Cerium oxide nanoparticles (CeNPs) containing the superoxide dismutase 1 (SOD1) enzyme are a potentially effective therapy for ALS in humans' widespread belief to a significant extent, oxidative stress is responsible for the development of the disease. Since oxidative stress has been associated with ALS, CeNPs were tested in the SOD1 G93A mouse model and in humans with ALS in an attempt to extend their lifespan and reduce the severity of the disease. CeNPs protected muscle function and prolonged lifespan in male and female SOD1 G93A mice when treated twice weekly at the onset of muscular weakening.[42]

1.2.6 SPINAL CORD INJURY (SCI)

SCIs are neurological conditions caused by trauma or disease that have negative effects on motor control and sensation as well as the autonomic nervous system, which has repercussions on the body's ability to control breathing, heart rate, blood pressure, digestion, and urination. Common psychological concerns for those with SCIs include sexual dysfunction, obesity, disturbed sleep, impaired mental performance, and persistent discomfort are just a few of the negative effects of this disorder.[43] Other issues include relationship stress and breakdown, social prejudice, and fewer employment opportunities. Although SCI is not as common as other injuries, the effects on a person's body and mind are just as devastating. Very few people fully recover from a SCI.[44] Attempts have been made to use neuroprotective approaches in SCI models to preserve drug-mediated protective effects on populations of neuronal and glial cells, aiming for a certain secondary injury event described above. There have been very few pharmaceutical treatments that have been proven therapeutically useful in actual patients.[45]

1.2.7 STROKE

Stroke is a major global killer and disabler. The two most common kinds of stroke are ischemic stroke and hemorrhagic stroke.[46] Hypoperfused, electrically-inactive brain regions known as the ischemic penumbra are in a state of hibernation and were found to be the cause of early clinical insufficiency in stroke patients by pioneering experiments undertaken in the 1970s.[47] Stroke is a worldwide epidemic that poses serious challenges to public health. After suffering a stroke, one in three people will die within a year, and another third will be permanently incapacitated.[48] Over a period of decades, researchers have tried and failed to adapt more than a thousand potential medicines from the study of cells and animals for use in humans.[49,50] Improved treatment for brain and spinal cord injuries may one day be possible because of therapeutic and reconstructive uses of nanotechnology in regenerative medicine and cell biology. Because they

Neurodegenerative Disorders and Their Treatment 13

migrate to and repair damaged tissue stem cells contribute in functional restoration in the brain and spinal cord.[51]

1.2.8 BRAIN TUMOR

Several distinct brain tumors can develop from several different kinds of cells,[52,53] and they can afflict people of any age. As a heterogeneous collection of neoplasms, brain tumors are often categorized as either benign or malignant. Researchers believe that exposure to toxic chemicals, radiation, or biological organisms contributes significantly to the growth of cancerous brain tumors.[54] There are 1–5 new cases of CNS tumors per 100,000 persons every year,[55] making them the most frequent solid tumor and the leading cause of cancer-related mortality among young adults. Surgery, radiation therapy, and systemic chemotherapy are all often used to treat brain tumors, but they have all been linked to poor patient outcomes and prolonged suffering a high mortality rate. Alternatives to intravenous and oral administration of anti-cancer medications, such as intra-arterial administration, have been explored in recent decades.[54]

1.3 STRATEGY OF TREATMENT

1.3.1 GENE THERAPY

Gene therapy for NDs has made steady development over the past several decades. Finding fresh vectors for the delivery of treatments and new treatment targets[56] are two examples of the many breakthroughs in essential technologies made possible by a deeper comprehension pertaining to the underlying pathogenetic mechanisms of various disorders. With this newfound information, researchers have been able to successfully tackle the underlying genetic origins remarkable progress in the treatment of neurodegenerative illnesses of both single-gene and multifactorial origin. Gene therapy is long-lasting for compartmentalized organs such as the eye, cochlea, or CNS (BBB), even permanent therapeutic effects are especially appealing because most agents cannot cross physiological barriers such as the blood–cerebrospinal fluid barrier (BCSFB), the blood–retina barrier (BRB), and the BBB.[57–59] Any kind of mutation, whether it is a gain of function or loss of function, is amenable to treatment via gene therapy making it a promising option for treating genetic targets that have not responded to conventional treatments.

Therapeutic transgenes expressing both viral and nonviral vectors can be used to transport therapeutic proteins, antibodies, Cas9/gRNA for gene editing, microRNAs, or small interfering RNAs (siRNAs) to diseased tissues in people and animals. The most common vector for treating neurodegenerative illnesses is adeno-associated virus (AAV), a subtype of adenovirus.[60] Multiple CNS cells and tissues, such as oligodendrocytes, astrocytes, and neurons, can be targeted favorably by using a wide variety of capsids that can be used between species.[61–68]

Important progress has been made in designing efficient delivery pathways, particularly for the CNS and the eye. Subpial, intracerebroventricular, intrathecal, intraparenchymal, intravitreal, and subretinal injections have all been shown in preclinical investigations to deliver sufficient gene amounts to sick tissues.[69–72] A benefit of intravenous injection is that it is minimally intrusive, although the BBB and BRB present challenging barriers to the entry of medicines into the CNS or optic nerve.[73] The intramuscular injection is a reliable method for the administration and generation of antibodies, and it can provide a supply of antibodies at therapeutically effective levels for crossing these physiological barriers.[74]After systemic injection, certain vectors have been shown to transport genes to the brain according to recent studies. It is clear that these vectors are superior to AAV9, and they may increase their capacity to treat various neurological disorders.[75,76]

Numerous gene therapy for ND clinical studies have been conducted (Table 1.1). A lack of adequate biodistribution to the necessary tissues may have played a role in the lackluster treatment outcomes shown in certain earlier clinical trials. Gene treatments have improved transgene expression and therapeutic safety as Both AAVs and methods of nonviral administration have seen significant development. Reports of functional improvements in animal models of neurodegenerative illnesses such as AD, HD, aromatic l-amino acid decarboxylase (AADC) impairment, and PD after treatment with this drug have emerged in recent years.[77–80] Here, summarize recent developments when dealing with NDs using gene therapy based on a review of clinical and preclinical investigations. Zero in on the most important aspects of the research and improvement of vectors, transgenic methods, and administration methods that aid in effective gene therapy. Further, give your own perspectives and observations on the current state of genAe therapy as well as its potential future developments.

Neurodegenerative Disorders and Their Treatment 15

TABLE 1.1 Gene Therapy Trials in Humans for Neurodegenerative Illnesses.

Disease	Trial code	Route of administration	Gene therapy	Phase
Huntington's disease	NCT02519036	Intrathecal injection	ASOs to HTT messenger RNA	Phase III
Huntington's disease	NCT03225833 NCT03225846	Intrathecal injection	ASOs to HTT messenger RNA	Phase I
Alzheimer's disease	NCT00876863	Direct basal forebrain injection	AAV2-NGF	Phase II
Parkinson's disease	NCT03065192 NCT01793543	Intraputaminal injection	AAV2-AADC	Phase I
Parkinson's disease	NCT01621581	Intraputaminal injection	AAV2-GDNF	Phase I
Parkinson's disease	NCT01621581	Intraputaminal injection	AAV2-AADC	Phase II
Amyotrophic lateral sclerosis	NCT01041222	Intrathecal injection	ASOs to SOD1	Phase I

1.3.2 STEM CELL THERAPY

Dementia stem cell therapy increases the intriguing possibility that neuro-degeneration and regeneration coexist in mature humans in a dynamic balance.[81] Despite recent doubts about adult neurogenesis in humans, Animal models of NDs show that stem cell therapy can boost neurogenesis's effectiveness.[82–85] Deterioration in cognitive abilities is often linked to the degeneration of synapses even though the etiology of many neuro-degenerative illnesses varies. Consequently, stem cell transplantation as a form of regenerative or replacement therapy may slow mental loss shown in many forms of degenerative disease.[86] Most current research is focusing on the following four types of stem cells: Neural, embryonic, induced pluripotent, and mesenchymal for stem cell therapy (Figure 1.3). Each of he stem cell is elaborated as follows:

1.3.2.1 NEURAL STEM CELLS

Somatic cells from a patient can be coaxed into becoming neural stem cells (NSCs).[87,88] Embryonic brain tissue can also be used to extract NSCs. Their uniqueness lies in their capacity to specialize as either astrocytes, oligodendrocytes, or neurons.[89] Careful regulation of NSC cell destiny in vitro and in vivo is now possible thanks to extensive research into the regulation of NSC differentiation by signaling pathways.[88] Exogenous transplantation of NSCs is currently the focus of clinical investigations, as the spinal injections of embryonic NSCs for ALS in Phase-I trials (clinical study NCT01640067) have shown some promise in delaying the progression of the disease.[90] Furthermore, NSC treatment of positive results has been seen with the use of human NSCs in animal models of AD. Animal models of AD showed an improvement in cognitive function when the HuCNS-SC human NSCs line was used to stimulate endogenous synaptogenesis. Transplanted cells upregulated synaptic markers like synaptophysin, synapsin, and growth-associated protein-43, indicating successful differentiation into juvenile neurons and glia (GAP-43). According to the results, the neurogenic capacity of NSCs may help slow the brain atrophy associated with AD and it enhanced cognitive function in two separate AD mice models without reducing Aβ or tau pathology.

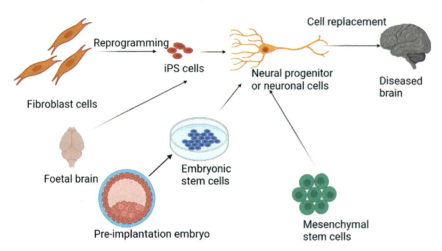

FIGURE 1.3 Different types of stem cells that work on ND.

1.3.2.2 EMBRYONIC STEM CELLS

In addition to their impressive embryonic stem cells (ESCs) have the capacity for both self-renewal and differentiation. also famous for their near-total versatility as a differentiation source. However, the use of ESCs

Neurodegenerative Disorders and Their Treatment 17

to treat NDs has been constrained by ethical and medical issues. Because of their ability to divide and spread quickly, ESCs pose a substantial threat to tumor development and cancer.[91,92] The host patient's immune system can have a significant reaction when exposed to ESCs from an allogenic source.[93] While adult dopaminergic neurons cannot be made from NSCs in mouse models, ESCs have shown promising results. how well-transplanted cells interact with the host brain network is unknown, although the restoration of dopaminergic neurons is essential to help with PD symptoms.[85] Even more, ESC therapy migrated into the afflicted tissues (the parenchyma and the spinal cord) and enhanced motor function in rats with SCI.[94] This is promising progress toward stopping the progression of motor impairment in PD.

1.3.2.3 INDUCED PLURIPOTENT STEM CELLS

Since it was found in 2006 that somatic cells have undergone terminal Recent years have seen significant development in the research of induced pluripotency, the process by which differentiated cells can be transformed into pluripotent stem cells with properties comparable to those of embryos.[95] Reprogrammed cells from a patient can be mass-produced and then transplanted back into the patient in an autologous fashion this method alleviates fears of immunological rejection. The ethical dilemmas associated with ESC harvesting are avoided when induced pluripotent stem cells (iPSCs) are used for cell therapy.[96] Human iPSCs, like ESCs, can develop into dopaminergic neurons, making them a promising therapeutic option for treating PD. However, unlike ESCs, it is necessary to first cultivate iPSCs to a progenitor stage before they can be transplanted because they do not create DA neurons on their own after implantation. High risk of teratoma formation from transplanted iPSCs in undifferentiated settings continues to impede clinical applications and FDA approval for iPSC therapy.[96] Because common retroviral or lentiviral vectors can cause chromosomal aberrations and mutations in iPSCs during reprogramming, this technique is crucial for ensuring clinical safety. Use of nonviral vectors, such as plasmid DNA, RNA, miRNAs, proteins, or small molecules, has improved the efficiency and safety of reprogramming.[97] Oct4, Sox2, c-Myc, and Klf4 plasmids are required for the successful generation of iPSCs—the four necessary pluripotency factors—have been delivered using calcium phosphate nanoparticles as carriers.[98]

1.3.2.4 MESENCHYMAL STEM CELLS

In vitro, MSCs have been shown to differentiate into neuronal and glial cells; in vivo, adult MSC cells; have been found to differentiate into bone, cartilage, fat, and epithelial cells Tissues from the bone marrow, umbilical cord, fat, and spleen all provide simple access points for collecting them from human patients. Cells that become MSCs can be cultured in a lab after which they are implanted in the nervous system (either the brain or the spinal cord). The fundamental function of MSCs in neuroregeneration is to increase the clearance of Aβ plaques[93] through the activation of microglia following the release of neurotrophic substances such as brain-derived neurotrophic factor (BDNF) and glial cell line-derived neurotrophic factor (GDNF). Angiogenic cytokines, stromal-derived factor 1 (SDF1), angiopoietin-1, and ECM components released by MSCs all work together to stimulate new blood vessel formation and brain progenitor proliferation cell recruitment.[101]

1.3.3 INTEGRATIVE MEDICINE

The morbidity and mortality rates of neurodegenerative illnesses both sudden and long-term are extremely high.[102,103] Such diseases include prion disease, FTD, Pick's disease, progressive supranuclear palsy, spinocerebellar ataxias, brain trauma, ALS, HD, AD, and PD. Symptomatic of many NDs is the loss of nerve cells due to aging or injury.[104] Over the past decade, researchers have made significant strides in their understanding of apoptosis.[105] Due to their unique processes of cell death, these diseases manifest and progress in very distinct ways, and can be treated in very different ways.

Degenerative illnesses have no cure at present, although there are several therapies available to alleviate their symptoms. Dopaminergic treatments for PD and other advantages of Western medicine for these conditions include the treatment of movement disorders,[106,107] drugs such as cholinesterase inhibitors,[108,109] antipsychotics,[108,110] analgesics,[109,111] anti-inflammatories,[112,113] and even deep brain stimulation[111] for tremor and refractory movement disorders. NSAIDs for AD (114), caffein A2A receptor antagonists, and CERE-120 all show promise as neuroprotectants for PD (AAV serotype 2-neurturin),[115,116] and other medicines have all been developed to slow the progression of various diseases. Researchers have not come very far yet; there are still too many obstacles to overcome to manage the chronic and debilitating symptoms of these disorders.[106]

1.4 CONCLUSION

Unfortunately, there is currently no cure for neurodegenerative illnesses. This results in difficulties with mobility (known as ataxia) and cognitive abilities (called dementia). Among the several dementias, AD is by far the most prevalent. There is now no treatment available for this disease, which only worsens with time and ultimately proves fatal. The condition cannot be cured at this time. However, for a short period of time, some medications may help prevent symptoms from worsening. They can be managed to a limited extent by a variety of physical and chemical treatments. However, there are only a select number of medications that are now in the stage of development involving clinical trials. Additionally, being developed and investigated for use in the treatment of some disorders are gene and stem cell therapies.

KEYWORDS

- **neurodegenerative disease**
- **Alzheimer's disease**
- **Parkinson's disease**
- **prion disease**
- **brain tumor**

REFERENCES

1. Re, F.; Gregori, M.; Masserini, M. Nanotechnology for Neurodegenerative Disorders. *Maturitas* **2012**, *73*, 45–51.
2. Gitler, A. D.; Dhillon, P.; Shorter, J. *Neurodegenerative Disease: Models, Mechanisms, and a New Hope*, Vol. 10; The Company of Biologists Ltd.: Cambridge, 2017; pp 499–502.

3. WHO. The Top 10 Causes of Death-WHO|World Health Organization; WHO: Geneva, Switzerland, 2020. https://www.who.int/news-room/fact-sheets/detail/the-top-10-causes-of-death (accessed on 12 Jan 2022).

4. Ramos-Cabrer, P.; Agulla, J.; Argibay, B.; Pérez-Mato, M.; Castillo, J. Serial MRI Study of the Enhanced Therapeutic Effects of Liposome-Encapsulated Citicoline in Cerebral Ischemia. *Int. J. Pharm.* **2011**, *405*, 228–233.

5. El-aziz, E. A. E.-d.A.; Elgayar, S. F.; Mady, F. M.; Abourehab, M. A.; Hasan, O. A.; Reda, L. M.; Alaaeldin, E. The Potential of Optimized Liposomes in Enhancement of Cytotoxicity and Apoptosis of Encapsulated Egyptian Propolis on Hep-2 Cell Line. *Pharmaceutics* **2021**, *13*, 2184.

6. Abbott, N. J.; Patabendige, A. A.; Dolman, D. E.; Yusof, S. R.; Begley, D. J. Structure and Function of the Blood–Brain Barrier. *Neurobiol. Dis.* **2010**, *37*, 13–25.

7. Tosi, G.; Costantino, L.; Ruozi, B.; Forni, F.; Vandelli, M. A. Polymeric Nanoparticles for the Drug Delivery to the Central Nervous System. *Expert Opin. Drug Deliv.* **2008**, *5*, 155–174.

8. Cano, A.; Sánchez-López, E.; Ettcheto, M.; López-Machado, A.; Espina, M.; Souto, E. B.; Galindo, R.; Camins, A.; García, M. L.; Turowski, P. Current Advances in the Development of Novel Polymeric Nanoparticles for the Treatment of Neurodegenerative Diseases. *Nanomedicine* **2020**, 15, 1239–1261.

9. Zhang, W.; Sigdel, G.; Mintz, K. J.; Seven, E. S.; Zhou, Y.; Wang, C.; Leblanc, R. M. Carbon dots: A future Blood–Brain Barrier Penetrating Nanomedicine and Drug Nanocarrier. *Int. J. Nanomed.* **2021**, *16*, 5003.

10. Ashrafizadeh, M.; Mohammadinejad, R.; Kailasa, S. K.; Ahmadi, Z.; Afshar, E. G.; Pardakhty, A. Carbon dots as Versatile Nanoarchitectures for the Treatment of Neurological Disorders and Their Theranostic Applications: A Review. *Adv. Colloid Interface Sci.* **2020**, *278*, 102123.

11. Sim, T. M.; Tarini, D.; Dheen, S. T.; Bay, B. H.; Srinivasan, D. K. Nanoparticle-Based Technology Approaches to the Management of Neurological Disorders. *Int. J. Mol. Sci.* **2020**, *21*, 6070.

12. Seitz, D. P.; Reimer, C. L. and Siddiqui, N.; A Review of Epidemiological Evidence for General Anesthesia as a Risk Factor for Alzheimer's Disease. *Progress Neuro-Psychopharmacol. Biol. Psychiatry* **2013**, *47*, 122–127.

13. Palmer, A. M.; Neuroprotective Therapeutics for Alzheimer's Disease: Progress and Prospects. *Trends in pharmacological sciences*, **2011**, *32*(3), 141–147.

14. Terry, A. V. Jr.; Callahan, P. M. et al. Alzheimer Disease and Age Related Memory Decline (Preclinical). *Pharmacol. Biochem. Behav.* **2011**, *99*, 356–365.

15. Scholl, M.; Hansson, O.; Zetterberg, H.; Blennow, K.; Mattsson, N. Amyloid Biomarkers in Alzheimer's Disease. *Trends Pharmacol. Sci.* **2015**, 36, 297–209.

16. Zempel, H.; Mandelkow, E. Lost After Translation: Missorting of Tau Protein and Consequences for Alzheimer Disease. *Trends Neurosci.* **2014**, *37*, 721–732.

17. Cheryl Leyns, E. G.; David Holtzman, M. Glial Contributions to Neurodegeneration in Tauopathies. *Mol. Neurodegen.* **2017**, *12*(1). DOI: 10.1186/s13024–017–0192-x; 151–153

18. Nitsch, R. M. From Acetylcholine to Amyloid: Neurotransmitters and the Pathology of Alzheimer's Disease. *Neurodegeneration* **1996**, *5*, 477–482.

19. Swerdlow, R. H.; Khan, S. M. A "Mitochondrial Cascade Hypothesis" for Sporadic Alzheimer's Disease. *Med. Hypotheses* **2004**, *63*, 8–20.

20. Duarte, A.; Moreira, P. An Integrative View of the Role of Oxidative Stress, Mitochondria and Insulin in Alzheimer's Disease. *J. Alzheimer's Dis.* **2009**, *16* (4), 741–761.
21. Faghihi, M. A.; Modarresi, F.; Khalil, A. M.; Wood, D. E.; et al, Expression of a noncoding RNA is elevated in Alzheimers disease and drives rapid feed-forward regulation of betasecretase. Nature Medicine 2008; 14: 723–730.
22. Rani, V.; Deshmukh, R.; Jaswal, P.; Kumar, P.; Bariwal J. Alzheimers disease: Is this a brain specific diabetic condition? *Physiol. Behav.* **2016**, *164*, 259–267.
23. Hogan, D. B.; Biley, P. et al. Management of Mild to Moderate Alzheimer Disease and Dementia. *Rev. Article* **2007**, *3*, 355–384.
24. Chen, W.; Song, X. Advances in Perfusion Magnetic Resonance Imaging in Alzheimer. *Review article, Alzheimer Dementia* **2011**, *7*, 185–196.
25. Chaurasia, B. D. *Human Anatomy*; CBS Publishers, 1999.
26. Say Kin Andrew, J.; Li, S. et al. Alzheimer Disease Neuroimaging Initiative: A Review of Paper Published Since Its Inception. *Alzheimer Dementia* **2012**, *8*, Si–S68.
27. Ranganathan, T. S. *A Textbook of Human Anatomy*; Published by S. Chand, 1982.
28. Salloway, S.; Mintzer, J. et al. Disease- Modifying Therapies in Alzheimer Disease. *Rev. Article Alzheimer Dementia* **2008**, *4*, 65–114.
29. Antioxidant Neuroprotection in Alzheimer disease as Preventive and Therapeutic Approach. *Original Res. Article Free Radical Biol. Med.* **2002**, *33*, 182–191.
30. Giasson, B. I.; Ischiropoules, H et al. The Relationship between Oxidative/Nitrative Stress and Pathological inclusions in Alzheimer and Parkinson Disease, We Now and Where Are We Headed? Review Article the American. *J. Geriartric Pharmacol.* **2009**, *7*, 167–185.
31. Satoskar, R.S.; Bhandarkar, S.D. *Pharmacology and Pharmacotherapeutics*; Mumbai Popular Prakashan, 1999.
32. Rang, H. P.; Dale, M. M.; *Pharmacology*; Churchill Livingstone Elsevier, 2007.
33. Tripathi, K. D. *Essentials of Medical Pharmacology*; Jaypee Publishers, 2010.
34. Mead, S. Prion Disease Genetics. *Eur. J. Hum. Genet.* **2006**, *14*, 273–281.
35. Skinner, P. J.; Kim, H. O.; Bryant, D.; Kinzel, N. J.; Reilly, C.; Priola, S. A.; Ward, A. E.; Goodman, P. A.; Olson, K.; Seelig, D. M. Treatment of Prion Disease with Heterologous Prion Proteins. *PLoS ONE* **2015**, *10*, e0131993.
36. Nirale, P.; Paul, A.; Yadav, K. S. Nanoemulsions for Targeting the Neurodegenerative Diseases: Alzheimer's, Parkinson's and Prion's. *Life Sci.* **2020**, *245*, 117394.
37. Chountoulesi, M.; Demetzos, C. Promising Nanotechnology Approaches in Treatment of Autoimmune Diseases of Central Nervous System. *Brain Sci.* **2020**, *10*, 338.
38. Walker, F. O. *Huntington's Disease. Lancet* **2007**, *369*, 218–228.
39. Cong, W.; Bai, R.; Li, Y.-F.; Wang, L.; Chen, C. Selenium Nanoparticles as an Efficient Nanomedicine for the Therapy of Huntington's Disease. *ACS Appl. Mater. Interfaces* **2019**, *11*, 34725–34735.
40. Van Es, M. A.; Hardiman, O.; Chio, A.; Al-Chalabi, A.; Pasterkamp, R. J.; Veldink, J. H.; Van den Berg, L. H. Amyotrophic Lateral Sclerosis. *Lancet* **2017**, *390*, 2084–2098.
41. Mazibuko, Z.; Choonara, Y. E.; Kumar, P.; Du Toit, L. C.; Modi, G.; Naidoo, D.; Pillay, V. A Review of the Potential Role of Nanoenabled Drug Delivery Technologies in Amyotrophic Lateral Sclerosis: Lessons Learned from Other Neurodegenerative Disorders. *J. Pharm. Sci.* **2015**, *104*, 1213–1229.

42. Bondì, M. L.; Craparo, E. F.; Giammona, G.; Drago, F. Brain-Targeted Solid Lipid Nanoparticles Containing Riluzole: Preparation, Characterization and Biodistribution. *Nanomedicine* **2010,** *5,* 25–32.
43. Li, J.; Cai, S.; Zeng, C.; Chen, L.; Zhao, C.; Huang, Y.; Cai, W. Urinary Exosomal Vitronectin Predicts Vesicoureteral Reflux in Patients with Neurogenic Bladders and Spinal Cord Injuries. *Exp. Ther. Med.* **2022,** *23,* 65.
44. Chen, Y.; Tang, Y.; Vogel, L.; DeVivo, M. Causes of Spinal Cord Injury. *Top. Spinal Cord Inj. Rehabil.* **2013,** *19,* 1–8.
45. Zimmermann, R.; Vieira Alves, Y.; Sperling, L. E.; Pranke, P. Nanotechnology for the Treatment of Spinal Cord Injury. *Tissue Eng. Part B Rev.* **2021,** *27,* 353–365.
46. Astrup, J.; Siesjö, B. K.; Symon, L. Thresholds in Cerebral Ischemia-the Ischemic Penumbra. *Stroke* **1981,** *12,* 723–725.
47. Cook, D. J.; Teves, L.; Tymianski, M. Treatment of Stroke with a PSD-95 Inhibitor in the Gyrencephalic Primate Brain. *Nature* **2012,** *483,* 213–217.
48. Sacchetti, M. L. Is It Time to Definitely Abandon Neuroprotection in Acute Ischemic Stroke? *Am. Heart Assoc.* **2008,** *39,* 1659–1660.
49. Kubinová, Š.; Syková, E. Nanotechnology for Treatment of Stroke and Spinal Cord Injury. *Nanomedicine* **2010,** *5,* 99–108.
50. Sarmah, D.; Banerjee, M.; Datta, A.; Kalia, K.; Dhar, S.; Yavagal, D. R.; Bhattacharya, P. Nanotechnology in the diagnosis and treatment of stroke. Drug Discov. Today **2021,** 26, 585–592.
51. Mohan, A.; Narayanan, S.; Balasubramanian, G.; Sethuraman, S.; Krishnan, U. M. Dual Drug Loaded Nanoliposomal Chemotherapy: A Promising Strategy for Treatment of Head and Neck Squamous Cell Carcinoma. *Eur. J. Pharm. Biopharm.* **2016,** *99,* 73–83.
52. Huang, R.; Boltze, J.; Li, S. Strategies for Improved Intra-Arterial Treatments Targeting Brain Tumors: A Systematic Review. *Front. Oncol.* **2020,** *10,* 1443.
53. Beccaria, K.; Canney, M.; Bouchoux, G.; Puget, S.; Grill, J.; Carpentier, A. Blood-Brain Barrier Disruption with Low-Intensity Pulsed Ultrasound for the Treatment of Pediatric Brain Tumors: A Review and Perspectives. *Neurosurg. Focus* **2020,** *48,* E10.
54. Reese, T.; Karnovsky, M. J. Fine Structural Localization of a Blood-Brain Barrier to Exogenous Peroxidase. *J. Cell Biol.* **1967,** *34,* 207–217.
55. Chen, E. M.; Quijano, A. R.; Seo, Y.-E.; Jackson, C.; Josowitz, A. D.; Noorbakhsh, S.; Merlettini, A.; Sundaram, R. K.; Focarete, M. L.; Jiang, Z. Biodegradable PEG-poly (ω-Pentadecalactone-co-p-dioxanone) Nanoparticles for Enhanced and Sustained Drug Delivery to Treat Brain Tumors. *Biomaterials* **2018,** *178,* 193–203.
56. Dunbar, C. E.; High, K. A.; Joung, J. K.; Kohn, D. B.; Ozawa, K.; Sadelain M. Gene Therapy Comes of Age. *Science* **2018,** *59,* eaan4672.
57. Hudry, E.; Vandenberghe LH. Therapeutic AAV Gene Transfer to the Nervous System: A Clinical Reality. *Neuron* **2019,** *101,* 839e62.
58. Wang, D.; Tai, P. W. L.; Gao, G. Adeno-Associated Virus Vector as a Platform for Gene Therapy Delivery. *Nat. Rev. Drug Discov.* **2019,** *18,* 358e78.
59. Lee, J. H.; Wang, J. H.; Chen, J.; Li, F.; Edwards, T. L.; Hewitt, A. W. et al. Gene Therapy for Visual Loss: Opportunities and Concerns. *Prog Retin Eye Res* **2019,** *68,* 31e53.
60. Weinberg, M. S.; Samulski, R. J.; McCown TJ. Adeno-Associated Virus (AAV) Gene Therapy for Neurological Disease. *Neuropharmacology* **2013,** *69,* 82e8.

Neurodegenerative Disorders and Their Treatment   23

61. Samaranch, L.; Salegio, E. A.; San Sebastian, W.; Kells, A. P.; Bringas, J. R.; Forsayeth, J. et al. Strong cortical and spinal cord transduction after AAV7 and AAV9 Delivery into the CSF of Non-Human Primates. *Hum. Gene Ther.* 2013. *24*, 526e32.

62. Xiang, C.; Zhang, Y.; Guo, W.; Liang, X. J. Biomimetic Carbon Nanotubes for Neurological Disease Therapeutics as Inherent Medication. *Acta Pharm Sin B* **2020**, *10*, 239e48.

63. Cearley, C. N.; Vandenberghe, L. H.; Parente, M. K.; Carnish, E. R.; Wilson, J. M.; Wolfe, J. H. Expanded Repertoire of AAV Vector Serotypes Mediate Unique Patterns of Transduction in Mouse Brain. *Mol. Ther.* **2008**, *16*, 1710e8.

64. Bartlett, J. S.; Samulski, R. J.; McCown TJ. Selective and Rapid Uptake of Adeno-Associated Virus Type 2 in Brain. *Hum. Gene Ther.* **1998**, *9*, 1181e6.

65. Hutson, T. H.; Verhaagen, J.; Ya´n~ez-Mun~oz, R. J.; Moon LD. Corticospinal Tract Transduction: A Comparison of Seven Adeno-Associated Viral Vector Serotypes and a Non-Integrating Lentiviral Vector. *Gene Ther.* **2012**, *19*, 49e60.

66. Katz, M. L.; Tecedor, L.; Chen, Y.; Williamson, B. G.; Lysenko, E.; Wininger, F. A. et al. AAV gene transfer delays disease onset in a TPP1-Deficient Canine Model of the Late Infantile Form of Batten Disease. *Sci. Transl. Med.* **2015**, *7*, 313ra180.

67. Federici, T.; Taub, J. S.; Baum, G. R.; Gray, S. J.; Grieger, J. C.; Matthews, K. A. et al. Robust Spinal Motor Neuron Transduction Following Intrathecal Delivery of AAV9 in pigs. *Gene Ther*. **2012**, *19*, 852e9.

68. Passini, M. A.; Watson, D. J.; Vite, C. H.; Landsburg, D. J.; Feigenbaum, A. L.; Wolfe, J. H. Intraventricular Brain Injection of Adeno-Associated Virus Type 1 (AAV1) in Neonatal Mice Results in Complementary Patterns of Neuronal Transduction to AAV2 and Total Long-Term Correction of Storage Lesions in the Brains of b-glucuronidase Deficient Mice. *J Virol* **2003**, *77*, 7034e40.

69. Richardson, R. M.; Gimenez, F.; Salegio, E. A.; Su, X.; Bringas, J.; Berger, M. S. et al. T2 Imaging in Monitoring of Intraparenchymal Real-Time Convection-Enhanced Delivery. *Neurosurgery* **2011**, *69*, 154e63.

70. Miyanohara, A.; Kamizato, K.; Juhas, S.; Juhasova, J.; Navarro, M.; Marsala, S. et al. Potent Spinal Parenchymal AAV9-Mediated Gene Delivery by Subpial Injection in Adult Rats and Pigs. *Mol. Ther. Methods Clin. Dev.* **2016**, *3*, 16046.

71. Morabito, G.; Giannelli, S. G.; Ordazzo, G.; Bido, S.; Castoldi, V.; Indrigo, M. et al. AAV-PHP.B-Mediated Global-Scale Expression in the Mouse Nervous System Enables GBA1 Gene Therapy for Wide Protection from Synucleinopathy. *Mol. Ther.* **2017**, *25*, 2727e42.

72. Passini, M. A.; Bu, J.; Richards, A. M.; Treleaven, C. M.; Sullivan, J. A.; O'Riordan, C. R. et al. Translational Fidelity of Intrathecal Delivery of Self-Complementary AAV9-Survival Motor Neuron 1 for Spinal Muscular Atrophy. *Hum Gene Ther* **2014**, *25*, 619e30.

73. Challis, R. C.; Ravindra Kumar, S.; Chan, K. Y.; Challis, C.; Beadle, K.; Jang, M. J. et al. Systemic AAV Vectors for Widespread and Targeted Gene Delivery in Rodents. *Nat Protoc* **2019**, *14*, 379e414.

74. Balazs, A. B.; Bloom, J. D.; Hong, C. M.; Rao, D. S.; Baltimore D. Broad Protection Against Influenza Infection by Vectored Immunoprophylaxis in Mice. *Nat Biotechnol* **2013**, *31*, 647e52.

75. Deverman, B. E.; Pravdo, P. L.; Simpson, B. P.; Kumar, S. R.; Chan, K. Y.; Banerjee, A. et al. Cre-Dependent Selection Yields AAV Variants for Widespread Gene Transfer to the Adult Brain. *Nat Biotechnol.* **2016,** *34,* 204e9.
76. Duque, S.; Joussemet, B.; Riviere, C.; Marais, T.; Dubreil, L.; Douar, A. M. et al. Intravenous Administration Of Self-Complementary AAV9 Enables Transgene Delivery to Adult Motor Neurons. *Mol. Ther.* **2009,** *17,* 1187e96.
77. Hwu, W. L.; Muramatsu, S.; Tseng, S. H.; Tzen, K. Y.; Lee, N. C.; Chien, Y. H. et al. Gene Therapy for Aromatic L-Amino Acid Decarboxylase Deficiency. *Sci. Transl. Med.* 2012;4:134ra61.
78. Sehara, Y.; Fujimoto, K. I.; Ikeguchi, K.; Katakai, Y.; Ono, F.; Takino, N. et al. Persistent Expression of Dopamine-Synthesizing Enzymes 15 Years After Gene Transfer in a Primate Model of Parkinson's Disease. *Hum. Gene Ther. Clin. Dev.* 2017;28:74e9.
79. Mittermeyer, G.; Christine, C. W.; Rosenbluth, K. H.; Baker, S. L.; Starr, P.; Larson, P. et al. Long-Term Evaluation of a Phase 1 Study of AADC Gene Therapy for Parkinson's Disease. *Hum. Gene Ther.* **2012,** *23,* 377e81.
80. Murphy, S. R.; Chang, C. C.; Dogbevia, G.; Bryleva, E. Y.; Bowen, Z.; Hasan, M. T. et al. Acat1 Knockdown Gene Therapy Decreases Amyloidbeta in a Mouse Model of Alzheimer's Disease. *Mol. Ther.* **2013,** *21* 1497e506.
81. Armstrong, R. J.; Barker, R. A. Neurodegeneration: A Failure of Neuroregeneration? *Lancet* **2001,** *358* (9288), 1174–1176.
82. Snyder, J. S. Questioning Human Neurogenesis. *Nature* **2018,** *555* (7696), 315–316.
83. Sorrells, S. F. et al. Human Hippocampal Neurogenesis Drops Sharply in Children to Undetectable Levels in Adults. *Nature* **2018,** *555* (7696), 377–381.
84. Boldrini, M. et al.; Human Hippocampal Neurogenesis Persists Throughout Aging. *Cell Stem Cell* **2018,** *22* (4), 589–599 (e5).
85. Lindvall, O.; Kokaia, Z.; Martinez-Serrano, A. Stem Cell Therapy for Human Neurodegenerative Disorders-How to Make It Work. *Nat. Med.* **2004,** *10,* S42–S50.
86. Ager, R. R. et al. Human Neural Stem Cells Improve Cognition and Promote Synaptic Growth in Two Complementary Transgenic Models of Alzheimer's Disease and Neuronal Loss. *Hippocampus* **2015,** *25* (7), 813–826.
87. Thier, M. et al. Direct Conversion of Fibroblasts into Stably Expandable Neural Stem Cells. *Cell Stem Cell* **2012,** *10* (4), 473–479.
88. Carradori, D. et al. The Therapeutic Contribution of Nanomedicine to Treat Neurodegenerative Diseases via Neural Stem Cell Differentiation. *Biomaterials* **2017,** *123,* 77–91.
89. Murrell, W. et al. Expansion of Multipotent Stem Cells from the Adult Human Brain. *PLoS ONE* **2013,** *8* (8), e71334.
90. Mazzini, L. et al. Human Neural Stem Cell Transplantation in ALS: Initial Results from a Phase I Trial. *J. Transl. Med.* **2015,** *13,* 17.
91. Carson, C. T.; Aigner, S.; Gage, F. H. Stem Cells: The Good, Bad and Barely in Control. *Nat. Med.* **2006,** *12* (11), 1237–1248.
92. Kazmerova, Z. et al. Can We Teach Old Dogs New Tricks? Neuroprotective Cell Therapy in Alzheimer's and Parkinson's Disease. *J. Alzheimers Dis.* **2013,** *37* (2), 251–272.
93. Wang, Y. et al. Stem Cell Therapies in Age-Related Neurodegenerative Diseases and Stroke. *Ageing Res. Rev.* **2017,** *34,* 39–50.

Neurodegenerative Disorders and Their Treatment

94. Kerr, D. A. et al. Human Embryonic Germ Cell Derivatives Facilitate Motor Recovery of Rats with Diffuse Motor Neuron Injury. *J. Neurosci.* **2003,** *23* (12), 5131–5140.

95. Takahashi, K.; Yamanaka, S. Induction of Pluripotent Stem Cells from Mouse Embryonic and Adult Fibroblast Cultures by Defined Factors. *Cell* **2006,** *126* (4), 663–676.

96. Sonntag, K. C. et al. Pluripotent Stem Cell-Based Therapy for Parkinson's Disease: Current Status and Future Prospects. *Prog. Neurobiol.* **2018,** *168,* 1–20.

97. Feng, B. et al. Molecules That Promote or Enhance Reprogramming of Somatic Cells to Induced Pluripotent Stem Cells. *Cell Stem Cell* **2009,** *4* (4), 301–312.

98. Sohn, Y. D. et al. Induction of Pluripotency in Bone Marrow Mononuclear Cells via Polyketal Nanoparticle-Mediated Delivery of mature microRNAs. *Biomaterials* **2013,** *34* (17), 4235–4241.

99. Sanchez-Ramos, J. R. Neural Cells Derived from Adult Bone Marrow and Umbilical Cord Blood. *J. Neurosci. Res.* **2002,** *69* (6), 880–893.

100. Glat, M. J.; Offen, D. Cell and Gene Therapy in Alzheimer's Disease. *Stem Cells Dev.* **2013,** *22* (10), 1490–1496.

101. Chierchia, A. et al. Secretome Released from Hydrogel-Embedded Adipose Mesenchymal Stem Cells Protects Against the Parkinson's Disease Related Toxin 6-Hydroxydopamine. *Eur. J. Pharm. Biopharm.* **2017,** *121,* 113–120.

102. Prusiner, S. B. Shattuck Lecture—Neurodegenerative Diseases and Prions. *N. Engl. J. Med.* **2001,** *344,* 1516–1526.

103. Friedlander, R. M: Apoptosis and Caspases in Neurodegenerative Diseases. *N. Engl. J. Med.* **2003,** *348,* 1365–1375.

104. Yuan, J.; Yankner, B. A. Apoptosis in the Nervous System. *Nature* **2000,** *407,* 802–809.

105. Hengartner, M. O. The Biochemistry of Apoptosis. *Nature* **2000,** *407,* 770–776.

106. Mizuno, Y. Recent Research Progress in and Future Perspective on Treatment of Parkinson's Disease. *Integr. Med. Int.* 2014. *1,* 67–79.

107. Crane, P. K.; Doody, R. S. Donepezil Treatment of Patients with MCI: A 48-week Randomized, Placebo-Controlled Trial. *Neurology* **2009,** *73,* 1514–1515.

108. Desai, A. K.; Grossberg, G. T. Diagnosis and Treatment of Alzheimer's Disease. *Neurology* **2005,** *64* (suppl 3), S34–S39.

109. Chaudhuri, K. R.; Schapira AHV: Non-Motor Symptoms of Parkinson's Disease: Dopaminergic Pathophysiology and Treatment. *Lancet Neurol* **2009,** *8,* 464–474.

110. Tizabi, Y.; Hurley, L. L.; Qualls, Z.; Akinfiresoye L: Relevance of the Anti-Inflammatory Properties of Curcumin in Neurodegenerative Diseases and Depression. *Molecules* **2014,** *19,* 20864–20879.

111. Okun, M. S. Deep-Brain Stimulation—Entering the Era of Human Neural-Network Modulation. *N. Engl. J. Med.* **2014,** *371,* 1369–1373.

112. Traynor, B. J.; Bruijn, L.; Conwit, R. et al. Neuroprotective Agents for Clinical Trials in ALS: A Systematic Assessment. *Neurology* **2006,** *67,* 20–27.

113. Ristori, G.; Romano, S.; Visconti, A. et al. Riluzole in Cerebellar Ataxia: A Randomized, Double-Blind, Placebo-Controlled Pilot Trial. *Neurology* **2010,** *74,* 839–845.

114. Stewart, W. F.; Kawas, C.; Corrada, M.; Metter, E. J. Risk of Alzheimer's Disease and Duration of NSAID Use. *Neurology* **1997,** *48,* 626–632.

115. Schwarzschild, M. A.; Xu, K.; Oztas, E.; Petzer, J. P. Neuroprotection by Caffeine and More Specific A2A Receptor Antagonists in Animal Models of Parkinson's Disease. *Neurology* **2003**, *61* (suppl 6), S55–S61.

116. Marks WJ Jr, Ostrem, J. L.; Verhagen, L. et al. Safety and Tolerability of Intraputaminal Delivery of CERE-120 (Adeno-Associated Virus Serotype 2-Neurturin) to Patients with Idiopathic Parkinson's Disease: An Open-Label, Phase I Trial. *Lancet Neurol.* **2008**, *7*, 400–408.

CHAPTER 2

Neurodegenerative Disorders: A Mysterious Group of Diseases

ABSTRACT

The prevalence of neurodegenerative diseases is on the rise across the world's population. Many genetic mutations and proteins related to family neurodegenerative illness have been identified, but no effective treatments for any neurodegenerative illness have yet been developed. Research into the cellular and molecular mechanisms that underlie neurodegeneration has been sparked by these results. Commonalities among these ailments include protein misfolding and aggregation, reduced protein clearance, mitochondrial malfunction, altered energy metabolism, disturbed axonal transport, neuroinflammation, and RNA-mediated toxicity. Transsynaptic seed transmission is also emerging as a common motif that has relevance for creating treatments. As postmitotic neurons' specific shape and function make them particularly sensitive to age-related disruptions of cellular homeostasis, aging itself is a risk factor for neurodegenerative disorders. It is possible to test theories regarding pathogenic processes and potential therapies using a broad range of animal models, particularly transgenic mice. By the time symptoms appear, considerable neurodegeneration has already taken place; therefore, the only method to prevent further damage is to identify at-risk individuals and test them through breakthroughs in diagnostics. To develop new and effective therapies for these debilitating illnesses, need to fill in information gaps, reexamine preconceived notions about disease processes, and dedicate ourselves in investigating a wide range of potential targets.

Gene Therapy for Neurological Disorders: Molecular Approaches for Targeted Treatment.
Rishabha Malviya, Arun Kumar Singh, Priyanshi Goyal, & Sonali Sundram (Authors)
© 2025 Apple Academic Press, Inc. Co-published with CRC Press (Taylor & Francis)

2.1 INTRODUCTION

Biomedical research on neurodegenerative illnesses is among the most challenging. Debilitating and fatal illnesses such as Alzheimer's disease (AD), Parkinson's disease (PD), frontotemporal dementia (FTD), amyotrophic lateral sclerosis (ALS), Huntington's disease (HD), and prion disorders are still incurable despite the efforts of various laboratories throughout the world, both academic and industrial.[1–5]

At best, all currently approved therapeutics work to alleviate symptoms; degeneration of neurons and synapses is an inevitable consequence of aging, and these treatments do nothing to mitigate this process.[6] Despite significant advancements in the understanding of neurodegenerative illnesses, this research has not yet resulted in effective treatments. Researchers still do not know enough about what causes diseases, as evidenced by the fact that so many potential medications have failed in clinical trials.[7]

Solving these issues is urgently required. The number of persons with a neurodegenerative disease is staggering 50 million worldwide, including 6 million in the United States. Invariably, these illnesses are progressive, debilitating, and ultimately fatal. It may be difficult for patients, their families, and caregivers to cope as the victim becomes more and more incapacitated. Increasing healthcare costs and an aging population that makes neurodegenerative diseases more likely suggest that if the current demographic trends continue, future societies will be severely taxed.[8]

As neurons are postmitotic and generally do not regenerate after death, treating neurodegenerative diseases has proven to be a difficult task. Although new neurons can be created in the adult human brain, most of the brain's 100 billion neurons are present by the time a baby is born. Axons of neurons are more vulnerable to illness than other cells due to their long-distance communication capabilities.[9–11] Certain motor neurons, for example, have projections that can span several meters. Transport systems are required in both axons and dendrites to deliver biomolecules and organelles to distal synapses. Synaptic failure may result if these processes are disrupted or blocked, and strong synaptic connections are essential to the health of neurons. Neuronal death may result from synaptic dysfunction.[12]

Neurons are particularly vulnerable because of their postmitotic nature and reliance on proper connections, as well as the fact that they are virtually irreplaceable and undergo lengthy processes. Kill neurons, one can do so in numerous ways.[13] Proteotoxicity, the accumulation of toxic proteins as a result of excessive production or ineffective clearance, is one possible route. Most neurodegenerative diseases are characterized by abnormal protein accumulation in the brain.[14] AD is characterized by the buildup of tau protein-induced neurofibrillary tangles inside the cell and the deposition of amyloid β-protein in extracellular plaques.[15] Tau deposition identical to that seen in AD is present in diseases such as FTD, which are categorized as tauopathies, although there are no amyloid plaques. PD causes the α-synuclein to collect in the dopaminergic neurons of the substantia nigra. While TAR DNA-binding protein 43 (TDP-43) is deposited in motor neurons in ALS, huntingtin (Htt) protein is localized in the basal ganglia of HD neurons.[16]

For instance, the prion protein is present in Creutzfeldt–Jakob disease (CJD) patients (PrP) plaques are diagnostic. In rare genetic cases, the disease-associated protein is overproduced, which leads to protein aggregation.[17] Most of the time, however, these proteins are misfolded because molecular chaperones have failed to ensure the proper folding of the proteins. They are not cleared fast enough because the ubiquitin-proteasome system and autophagic processes cannot keep up. Toxin-induced neurodegeneration can also be caused by other mechanisms such as the accumulation of toxic and nontoxic proteins, which can lead to neuronal dysfunction or even death.[17]

In addition to the noncell autonomous actions of support cells such as astrocytes and brain immune cells like microglia, neuroinflammation offers yet another pathway to neurotoxicity.[18]

In this field of research, the fundamental question of why some neurons or brain networks are more prone to abnormal protein and RNA accumulation remains unanswered.[19] This selective neurotoxicity is clearly linked to a particular disease's emergence. Neurons in the subthalamic nucleus, which control movement, are especially vulnerable to damage from misfolded or aggregated "-synuclein," which is why PD develops.[20]

Due to neurons' enhanced sensitivity to these anomalies, aberrant tau aggregates in the frontotemporal lobe cause specific cognitive and behavioral symptoms of FTD.[21] Injuries to neurons and brain networks at the molecular level may shed light on what causes neurodegenerative diseases. Researchers hope to find novel treatment targets for neurodegenerative diseases by elucidating the cellular and molecular basis of these conditions. A basic summary of these disorders, current ideas and data about disease processes, key unresolved problems, and prospective strategies for resolving these perplexing problems and developing useful medicines are discussed.[22]

2.2 BACTERIAL INFECTION AND BIOMEDICAL PRESENTATION

Over 6 million people in the United States and 35 million people worldwide suffer from AD. AD primarily affects persons over the age of 65 and is characterized by memory and cognitive impairment; however, early-onset hereditary forms of the illness are present in 1–2% of cases.[23] The average duration for the disease to advance is 8 years from the commencement of the initial symptoms until death, though this time period can extend to as long as 20 years in some cases.[24] As a result of its widespread prevalence and progressive character, AD has a high economic cost to society. Involuntary linguistic, motor, and psychological changes are all possible manifestations of FTD, a term used to define a collection of illnesses that share similar symptoms.[25]

The frontal and temporal lobes are the areas of the brain most affected, as the name implies. When it comes to dementia, FTD is by far the most common kind among people under 65, typically appearing between the ages of 45 and 64 years.

Mendelian genetic inheritance accounts for at least 15% of FTD cases, and some estimates put the figure as high as 40%.

Just 1% of people over 65 have PD.[26] Postural instability, slowness of movement, limb and trunk stiffness, and resting tremors of the limbs and face are all symptoms of this illness.[27] The absence of neurons in the substantia nigra pars compacta of the midbrain, which are related to circuits that control the parts of the basal ganglia responsible for voluntary movement, may be the cause of these signs and symptoms. Dopaminergic neuron loss symptoms have long been treated with L-DOPA, a dopamine precursor.[28–32] However, this treatment is not effective because it does not stop the underlying neurodegenerative process. PD patients typically have a life expectancy of 7–11 years after diagnosis. In the brain and spinal cord, the illness results in a gradual, cumulative loss of motor neurons. Muscle atrophy appears to be the result of damage to the spinal cord's lateral axons brought on by inadequate innervation of muscles (so-called "amyotrophic").[33] Around 20,000–30,000 Americans are affected by ALS right now. Death often occurs within 35 years after diagnosis, however, in exceptional cases, it may take decades for the disease to proceed.[34] Mild

Neurodegenerative Disorders: A Mysterious Group of Diseases 31

cramping or weakened muscles in the limbs or in the muscles involved in speaking and swallowing are the earliest symptoms of the disease, and they typically appear between the ages of 55 and 60 years. The majority of the body's skeletal muscles become paralyzed as a result of the illness. Researchers are more aware than ever before that HD is a devastating neurological condition that is solely inherited.[35,36]

The signs and symptoms of HD are comparable to those of ALS, PD, and AD. Huntington's chorea refers to involuntary limb motions and was inspired by dance. Slurred speech, trouble swallowing, and irritability or depression are further symptoms of dementia. Even though it can strike at any age, the disease typically manifests itself around middle age. Like other progressive neurodegenerative diseases, this one has a lethal 10–20-year course.[37] Despite its widespread effects, dementia initially manifests in the striatum, a region of the basal ganglia critical for motor coordination, cognition, motivation, and reward. Aside from the hippocampus and cerebral cortex, the substantia Nigra is affected.[38]

The protein agent that causes prion disease manifests in a variety of forms, each with its own distinct set of symptoms and neuropathology but all are ultimately traced back to the same source.

Prion illness can appear for no apparent reason, develop into an infection, or be passed down through families. Human prion illnesses include CJD, kuru, Gerstmann–Straussler–Scheinker syndrome, and fatal familial insomnia.[39] After researching kuru, scientists realized these fatal brain diseases spread easily from person to person. High in the Papua New Guinean mountains, the Fore ethnic group practices ritual cannibalism in which members of the community consume the brains of deceased family members. All forms of prion disease are characterized by long incubation periods and rapid disease development once symptoms first appear. Postmortem examination revealed spongiform pathology and abundant PrP plaque deposition. Common examples of prions are mad cow disease, also referred to as scrapie, chronic wasting illness (CWD), and bovine spongiform encephalopathy (BSE) in deer and elk.[40]

2.3 THEORY OF CELLULAR DISEASE

These illnesses' postmortem pathological characteristics were initially used to understand the underlying molecular pathways. The development of neurofibrillary tangles and the buildup of plaques are symptoms of AD.[41] Proteins A and tau were shown to be the main building blocks of plaques and tangles, respectively, according to biochemical analysis of samples of brain tissue. As much as 25 years prior to the expected symptom onset, a deposition appears to constitute the first pathogenic alteration. On the contrary, even if it occurs later, tau deposition is linked to neuronal loss both geographically and temporally.[42] As demonstrated by this work, aberrant A may serve as a pathogenic initiator, but it is more likely that downstream pathological abnormalities in tau are responsible for neurodegenerative disorders. Also potentially contributing to neuronal dysfunction or death is neuroinflammation, which can arise as a result of a number of pathogenic events.[43]

There are fewer neurons in the pars compacta area of the substantia nigra in dementia patients, and these neurons also have Lewy bodies. The dopaminergic neurons that are lost in Lewy bodies are essential for motor function and contain a protein called synuclein. When PD patients do not also have dementia, tau deposition is not typically observed.[44–48]

However, in roughly 50% of FTD cases, tau tangles are seen. However, a deposition is not. According to research published this week in the journal Neurology, abnormal A in AD may be one of the multiple ways in which dangerous tau may be created.[49]

Nearly half of those with FTD, though, have neuronal deposits of a protein that is neither tau nor ubiquitin. These deposits frequently contain TDP-43, a protein that binds to RNA. TDP-43, which typically resides in the nucleus, is overproduced in neurons affected by FTD.[50]

This and other data point to FTD and ALS as two conditions at opposite ends of the TDP-43 proteinopathies spectrum.

Superoxide dismutase 1 (SOD1) and TDP-43, a protein linked to the fused in the sarcoma virus, are two examples of unusual hereditary variants of ALS that have neuronal deposits of other proteins [FUsed in Sarcoma (FUS)].[51] Many people with ALS have been shown to have an enlarged hexanucleotide repeat sequence in a gene called c9orf72.

A key and widespread HD pathogenic characteristic is the presence of cytoplasmic and nuclear aggregates and inclusions throughout the brain.[52] The Htt protein variation discovered in these deposits is mutant in that it has an extra polyglutamate extension at its N-terminus. Htt ensnares a wide variety of other proteins, including those engaged in protein quality control and transcription. Prion illnesses are characterized by the development of plaques and spongiform pathology.[53] PrP, a protein

Neurodegenerative Disorders: A Mysterious Group of Diseases 33

that may change its structure and glycosylation pattern, is the primary component of these plaques and is responsible for their spread throughout the brain. The results of this work suggest that the ability of PrP to infect a wide variety of species is due, at least in part, to its ability to adopt a wide range of conformations and glycosylation patterns. A single protein can transmit disease and even encode various harmful strains, according to Dr. Stanley Prusiner, who received the 1997 Nobel Prize for his research.[54]

The growing understanding of how molecular illness spreads from neuron to neuron in a networked manner via synaptic transmission may be the most intriguing and pervasive pathogenic discovery in neurodegeneration in recent years.[55] The emergence and spread of PrP illnesses have been linked to this mechanism. Only PrP has been proven to be contagious; other proteins' prion-like characteristics seem to be restricted to the molecular and cellular levels, despite the fact that many proteins have been related to neurodegenerative disorders. Despite this, a key emerging topic in the research is the idea of prion-like synaptic transmission and assembly. We will get into the specifics of this issue later.[56]

2.4 GENETICS

The study of families with Mendelian inheritance patterns in genetics has led to important discoveries on the origins of diseases.[57–59] Several forms of neurodegeneration may be traced back to mutations in a variety of genes in different families, each of which may point to a unique cellular mechanism, pathway, or function. Autosomal-dominant missense mutations in the genes for presenilin-1 (PSEN1), presenilin-2 (PSEN2), and the precursor to amyloid (APP) are what cause familial early-onset AD (PSEN2). Presenilin is the catalytic component of secretase, one of two proteases that produce a peptide that builds up in the AD brain.[60] A is implicated significantly in the etiology of AD, according to genetic information from families, clinical observations, and biochemical study. One of the main causes of sporadic, late-onset AD is the APOE gene, which produces the cholesterol transporter protein. A factor of 34 is added to the risk associated with one allele of this gene, a factor of 1215 is subtracted from the risk associated with the other allele, and the risk associated with the E3 allele is unaltered. An elevated risk of late-onset AD is linked to uncommon missense mutations in TREM2, which codes for an immune cell receptor (triggering receptor expressed on myeloid cells 2).[61-64] This raises the possibility that neuroinflammation has a role in the progression of the disease. A mutation in the gene encoding the microtubule-associate protein tau (MAPT) was discovered as a result of research into the genetic causes of dominantly inherited forms of FTD. Mutations in the protein's coding area are mostly responsible for its increased propensity to build up in the body, but mutations in the noncoding region, called intronic regions, can also result in tau isoforms that are abnormal and more likely to assemble.[65]

The evidence supporting tau's involvement in both AD and its milder version, mild tauomania, was strengthened by the discovery of tau mutations that cause FTD. Like MAPT, the PRG gene is found on chromosome 17. It is interesting to note that there are FTD instances in families where there is no tau pathology but there are deposits that are ubiquitin-positive because of PRG gene mutations. FTD is caused by dominantly inherited mutations in the c9orf72 gene's promoter, which lends credence to the notion that the RNA transcript has neurotoxic properties. Recurrent expansion of c9orf72 affects 25% of families and 10% of people with ALS.[66]

2.5 MOLECULE-BASED CLUES TO THE MECHANISMS OF DISEASE PROGRESSION

These studies were made possible by earlier studies that assessed the typical and abnormal functions of proteins found in pathological deposits as well as by the identification of genes linked to family types of neurodegenerative disorders.[67]

In prion diseases, PrP has an undeniable pathological role that cannot be ignored. The "protein-only" disease caused by introducing PrP from diseased brains is prevented by silencing the gene responsible for producing PrP.[68] Amyloid plaques form in the brain as a result of dominant mutations in the PrP gene that cause inherited illnesses. Mutations in PrP can be inherited in a recessive pattern, but they can also occur naturally or be acquired from environmental infection. PrP is a glycoprotein that is embedded in membranes, although its normal function has not been determined. The most widely accepted explanation for PrP's pathogenic mechanism is that it exists as an ensemble of PrP conformations, some of which are able to proliferate and serve as a template for the conversion to a lethal PrP form.[69]

Infectious forms may spread independently of PrP expression levels over a long enough incubation time to spread the disease. Illness develops more quickly in transgenic mice due to overexpression of PrP compared to wild-type mice, whereas disease development is slowed in animals lacking PrP heterozygous in the genome.[70–74] Amyloid plaques form in the brain as a result of dominant mutations in the PrP gene that cause inherited illnesses. These kinetic analyses suggest that the velocity of prion spread and the toxicity of the protein are two distinct properties of the prions themselves. The identities of the infectious and fatal forms of PrP, as well as the mechanisms of neurotoxicity, remain a mystery despite the evident advancement and understanding of PrP's relevance in prion illnesses. Although the evidence for A's harmful effects in AD is considerable, it does not compare to the evidence for PrP in prion diseases. Autosomal-dominant familial AD is mostly brought on by missense mutations in the A region of the APP and the catalytic subunit of the protease that generates A.[75] The single-pass membrane protein APP undergoes two different proteolytic steps to produce A. The transmembrane domain of the APP is first removed by secretase from its C terminus.[76–79] The length of the peptides secreted by the body ranges from 38 to 43 amino acids, with the 40-residue peptide being the most common (A40). The longer A42 peptide (A42), which has a greater proportion of the hydrophobic transmembrane region and is more prone to aggregation, makes up the majority of the amyloid plaques in AD. Mutations in the APP N-terminus that cause FAD production in middle age also promote cleavage by secretase, leading to elevated levels of production for the rest of the organism's existence. Another way to phrase it is that a protective mutation, likewise present at the N-terminus of A, inhibits the same proteolytic pathway, hence reducing a synthesis. The likelihood of A aggregating is increased by mutations in the APP's A region.[80–84]

Aggregation-prone peptides are produced in greater quantities when mutations in the C-terminal region of APP alter their cleavage by secretase.

Mutations in PSEN1 and PSEN2 also impact peptide aggregation.

The protein complex known as secretase is found in membranes and hydrolyzes lipids within the lipid bilayer's hydrophobic environment.[85] The complex's catalytic component is presenilin. Mutations in presenilins that cause AD to alter proteolysis of the APP transmembrane domain, leading to A peptides that are longer and more prone to aggregation.[86]

Similar to prion illnesses, the AD pathogenic organism has yet to be identified. As far as can tell, amyloid plaques are not directly linked to neurodegeneration, and the most widely held view is that only oligomeric forms of A42 are synaptotoxic.[87] However, oligomers of all sizes have been heralded as the principal pathogenic species due to their great variability. This includes dimers, trimers, dodecamers, and beyond. It's probable that a toxic cocktail, or "Soup," is at blame. Furthermore, the mechanism by which pathogenic a leads to abnormal tau and neurofibrillary tangles is not well understood.[88] Both the involvement of the risk factors APOE and TREM2 in A clearance and the role of these proteins are unclear. The degree of cognitive impairment in AD is more significantly correlated with tau pathology than with a pathology.[89] These findings imply that tau is downstream and closer to pathogenic trigger A than tau is to neuronal cell death in both time and space. The tau gene (MAPT) has not been shown to be mutated, however, families with familial AD have been found to have mutations in the substrate and the enzyme that produce it.[90] Familial forms of FTD have been linked to changes in the tau protein, proving that this change alone is sufficient to produce dementia and neurodegeneration. Together, these results suggest that tau plays a significant role in the genesis of AD. There is growing evidence that a number of neurodegenerative disorders have tau pathology, CTE included. Pathogenic A is just one potential cause of neurodegeneration, and abnormal tau appears to play a role as a mediator in many cases. Another candidate gene for familial FTD is the PRG gene, which is located in close proximity to MAPT. These changes lead to nonsense-mediated delays in the form of truncated transcripts.[91]

There is currently no understanding of the molecular basis via which PRG heterozygous deletion results in FTD. To clarify, these mutations do not cause tau disorder, but rather the RNA-binding protein TDP-43's deposition in neurons.[92] TDP-43 proteinopathies include a wide range of illnesses, from FTD with an early beginning to ALS with a late onset, that are defined by TDP-43 deposits in neurons. TDP43 shortened, hyperphosphorylated, and ubiquitinated abnormal type nuclear translocation. The pathophysiology of TDP-43 may be caused by abnormal RNA processing rather than toxic TDP-43 protein aggregates. FTD-ALS Mutations in the TARPBP gene, which produces TDP-43, as well as the elongation of an intronic region in the c9orf72 gene, have been linked to TDP-43 disease. It has been proposed that a variety of mechanisms, including haploinsufficiency, aggregation, and non-ATG translation of the repeat-expanded mRNA, contribute to neurodegeneration caused by c9orf72 repeat expansion.[93]

Misfolded or aggregated proteins are a typical sign of ALS in people with a mutation in the SOD1 gene.

Dopaminergic neurons of the substantia nigra appear to be particularly sensitive to a variety of chemical insults, which is supported by the fact that multiple distinct genes are linked to familial PD.[94] Mutations in the synuclein gene as well as the doubling or triple of the homologous gene can cause the production of misfolded or aggregated synuclein. The inclusion of synuclein, which is frequently linked to synaptic vesicles, may also occur in sporadic PD. Mitochondrial dysfunction is caused by further mutations. In response to malfunctioning mitochondria, Parkin and PINK1 often coordinate signals to initiate mitophagy.[95] The E3 ubiquitin ligase Parkin is recruited and activated by PINK1 buildup on the surface of damaged mitochondria. To process the organelle, parkin ubiquitylates proteins in the outer mitochondrial membrane. Additionally, a number of PD-related gene products have critical roles in vesicle trafficking, particularly to lysosomal organelles; deficiencies in these proteins may prevent the removal of aggregated and misfolded proteins from the cell as well as damaged mitochondria.[96]

HD is a neurodegenerative disorder with a single recognized origin, however, it is complicated by a number of processes. The polyglutamine-expanded Htt protein has a broad interactome that links it to numerous unique cellular activities.[97] Mutant Htt (mHtt) has been shown to interact with and disrupt many transcription-related proteins, providing more evidence that mHtt dramatically alters the transcriptome. Important regulators of gene expression such as histone acetyltransferases are rendered inactive.[98] By interacting with chaperones and obstructing correct proteasome degradation, the mutant protein has an impact on proteostasis. Consequently, the mechanism for managing protein waste as a whole might experience stress. Due to mHtt inhibiting mitochondrial activity, biosynthesis, and mitophagy, it may result in a decrease in energy output. Exactly how mHtt causes such a profound change in medium spiny neurons in the striatum remains a mystery, but one theory is that it raises the excitotoxicity of glutaminergic neurons.[99]

RNA toxicity is a new hypothesis on how HD develops. Nucleolar stress and disruption of nuclear export may result from an accumulation of CAG triplet repeats, which could lead to the formation of hairpin structures that bind nuclear proteins. It is not easy to disentangle the role of the mHTT mRNA from that of polyglutamine-expanded polypeptides in pathogenicity.[100] Degenerative diseases such as myotonic dystrophy 1, HD-like 2, and spinocerebellar ataxia 8 can be brought on by CTG expansion in the noncoding regions of other genes, such as the DMPK, JPH3, and ATXN8 genes. Experiments with human neural cell lines have established that mRNA-mediated neurotoxicity is caused by the prolonged CAG tract in mHtt exon 1. According to Drosophila research, replacing a CAG codon with a CAA codon may stop neurodegeneration.[101]

2.6 NEURODEGENERATION CONCEPTS AND DISPUTES

Researchers may start to establish some general theories about the molecular and cellular bases of causation and progression in neurodegenerative illnesses in light of these discoveries. The scientific community as a whole is not in agreement on all of these points. The most revolutionary idea is probably that pathogenic protein seeds propagate like prions in a variety of neurological diseases. Prion illnesses are a paradigm change since they are so rare and spread only by protein transmission from one animal to another. The formation of normal cellular PrP from a seed of misfolded and aggregated PrP protein can increase the amount of infectious particles in the brain. The dynamics of titer development and illness progression show that infectious and lethal PrP forms may be distinguished, and misfolded and/or aggregated PrP eventually functions as a template for the transformation of cellular PrP into a fatal form.[102] Figure 2.1 diagrammatic representation of neurodegenerative processes at the cellular and molecular levels.

Transsynaptic processes allow pathogenic proteins implicated in the etiology and course of disorders like AD and PD to spread from one cell to the next. This theory proposes that the specific manifestation of the disease is tied to the integration of neurons into neural circuits and the precise anatomical location of the instigating pathogenic seed. This concept could have far-reaching implications for the investigation of disease mechanisms and the formulation of fresh strategies for the search for and development of effective therapeutic drugs for the prevention and treatment of illness.[103] Although PrP and other proteins associated with neurodegenerative illnesses such as AD, FTD, and PD have some properties, classifying these other proteins as "prion-like" is challenging. The word "transmission" is borrowed from the field of infectious illness and refers to the potential spread of pathogens from one neuron to another.[104] It is more accurate to refer to the spread from neuron to neuron as synaptic transmission in neural signaling.

Neurodegenerative Disorders: A Mysterious Group of Diseases

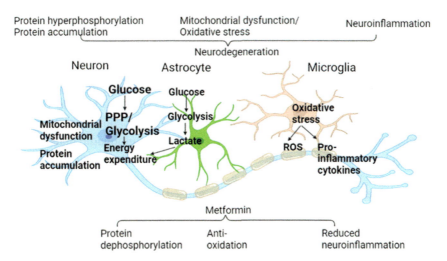

FIGURE 2.1 Diagrammatic representation of neurodegenerative processes at the cellular and molecular levels.

This behavior is better described by the term "trans-synaptic propagation." Remarkably, pathogenic PrP does not appear to spread unambiguously from one brain cell to the next.[105] Transsynaptic transmission has been linked to the spread of several pathogenic proteins, most notably tau and synuclein. Some pathogenic proteins misfold and aggregate into discrete forms that can be reproduced, and this has led to speculation about the existence of diverse strains. Because it is unclear whether or not these various aggregated states will be referred to as "strains," the phrase may be deceptive in the same way that the term "PrP" is in reference to the prion disorders. Misfolded and/or aggregated proteins, regardless of their origin, are to blame for the spread of protein diseases.[106–109] Can this anomaly be explained in any way? It is possible that the disease-related protein is too large for the protein folding mechanism to handle. Protein aggregation and neurodegeneration can be mitigated, for instance, by overexpressing molecular chaperones and foldases in animal models of illness. Proteins associated with disease can build up and eventually overwhelm protein disposal mechanisms if they are not folded properly. The ability of the ubiquitin-proteasome system to degrade proteins declines when misfolded proteins build up in the neuron. These interactions may lead to a proteotoxic accumulation. Similarly, autophagic machinery must use more energy to dispose of disease-associated protein aggregates, impeding its ability to remove other trash, such as malfunctioning mitochondria. Due to their unique makeup, neurons are especially susceptible to cellular stress, including proteotoxic stress. Because of protein buildup, macromolecules and organelles may not make it from the cell body to the synaptic termini.[110] Loss of synaptic function could be another consequence of protein aggregation, which in turn could contribute to neurodegeneration. Neurons rely heavily on the energy provided by functioning mitochondria to carry out their essential operations. Aggregated proteins can overwhelm the autophagic machinery, which can prevent mitophagy from maintaining mitochondrial quality control. As an added complication, mitochondrial delivery to synapses can be impeded by an axonal blockage caused by aggregated proteins.[111] Neuronal health and function can be negatively impacted by mitochondrial dysfunction, as mitochondria have their own cellular stress response mechanism. Mitochondria may be damaged by methods other than protein aggregation. For instance, defective mitophagy can result from PD-related mutations in Parkin and PINK1, two proteins crucial to the regulation of mitophagy. Mitochondria contain their own DNA, and mitochondrial malfunction and altered energy metabolism may result from cumulative mutations as age.[112]

It turns out that errant proteins are not the only cause of neurodegenerative illness; RNA-mediated pathways may play a role as well. When the RNA-binding protein TDP-43 aggregates, it can cause stress granules to develop that rich in cognate mRNA, a hallmark of FTD and ALS. The sabotage prevents mRNA from being digested and translated into functional proteins, rendering the mRNA useless.[113] Critical nuclear proteins can be silenced by hairpin-like structures in the mRNA of triplet repeat diseases including HD and several ataxia conditions. Multiple sclerosis is just one of many neurodegenerative disorders associated with an enlarged C9orf72 gene caused by a hexanucleotide repeat expansion (MS).[114]

2.7 CONSIDERATIONS FOR THE FUTURE OF THERAPEUTICS

There is currently no cure for neurodegenerative disorders. Symptoms can be managed, but the disease itself and the deterioration of neurons cannot be stopped. The incomplete knowledge of the disease's fundamental mechanisms is a major contributor.[115] For quite some time, it has been understood that AD and other tauopathies are characterized by the hyperphosphorylation of pathogenic tau filaments; hence, many efforts have been made to develop particular kinase inhibitors for these diseases. However, the exact tau kinases and phosphorylation sites that may be involved in pathogenicity remain to be found. Sometimes, inhibiting just one kinase is not enough when there are several involved. The issue is compounded by the lack of understanding of how hyperphosphorylation contributes to the accumulation of tau in neurons. The exact causes of neuronal death, as well as the pathogenic agents and pathways involved, are unclear in every form of neurodegenerative disease. When it comes to HD, it is not yet known which types of PrP or Htt lead to neurotoxicity, but RNA-mediated neurotoxicity is a possibility.[116]

Using natural human macromolecules is a major hurdle in the treatment of neurodegenerative diseases.

However, while deletion of APP and PrP-encoding genes may be manageable, loss of Htt and TDP-43 is usually lethal.[117]

Therefore, it is not reasonable to look for small-molecule medicines, immunotherapies, or gene treatments that interfere with the normal activity of these proteins.[118] Targeting secretase to stop APP from generating A may demonstrate the risks of interfering with a crucial macromolecule's normal function. Notch receptors are among the membrane proteins that are cleaved by secretase. Notch undergoes proteolysis, which releases its intracellular domain. This region is then shuttled to the nucleus, where it promotes the transcription of genes that ultimately decide a cell's fate. Notch signaling has been connected to the failure of several secretase inhibitors in clinical studies for the treatment of AD.[119]

Neurodegenerative diseases exacerbate the difficulty of drug delivery to the brain [central nervous system (CNS)].

Substances with a dilution coefficient greater than 500 are usually filtered out by the brain's molecular weight (Da). An efflux pump for P-glycoprotein efficiently expels tiny lipophilic molecules from the brain through the blood–brain barrier.[120] Keeping drug candidate molecular weight low while preserving efficacy and specificity for the target macromolecule is a formidable challenge. Because of the size of the surfaces on which protein–protein interactions occur, larger pharmacological molecules are typically used to effectively inhibit smaller compounds that are designed to disrupt interactions Between proteins (e.g., self-assembly of aggregation-prone proteins). Early diagnosis is essential for the effective treatment of neurodegenerative disorders. By the time AD or another kind of dementia shows any symptoms, neurodegeneration has already occurred in the brain. Neither now nor in the foreseeable future do have a reliable method for restoring function by replacing destroyed neurons with functionally equivalent neuronal subtypes and interneuronal connections.[121] In any case, avoiding problems entirely is ideal. Changes in cerebrospinal fluid (CSF) A levels can be detected in AD up to 25 years before the start of symptoms is predicted, and plaque development can begin as early as 15 years before that. Patients' fears that the pathogenic process has shifted from A to tau by the time of diagnosis are not unfounded.[122] Because those taking part in clinical studies already showed symptoms of AD, all anti-A methods to treating the condition have failed. Those who are likely to develop AD can now be identified before the disease even manifests, thanks to the development of an amyloid imaging agent.[123] New imaging agents finally make it possible to conduct more selective trials, excluding those with other types of dementia and keeping just those with type-A disease. Anti-A medicines (including monoclonal antibodies) can be used to prove target engagement by removing amyloid deposits after therapy.[124] Clinical investigations will need to be extensive and large even if only a small number of people participate. Neurodegenerative illnesses typically present with a gradual onset. Due to the variability in the onset and progression of illness among high-risk populations, large sample sizes, and prolonged trial durations are required to demonstrate the efficacy of a given pharmacological treatment. Biomarkers in the CSF and plasma will be valuable stand-ins for determining whether or not a treatment is having its intended effect and, if so, how much to administer.[125–129] Patients may be good candidates for early clinical trials if they have a family history of the disease, a mutation with known disease onset and progression, or other important clues to pathogenic pathways. With the current understanding of neurodegenerative diseases, a specialized treatment plan along the lines of that utilized for cancer patients should be feasible.

If efficacy can be demonstrated in Mendelian genetic diseases, then trials in sporadic cases could be conducted with more certainty.

2.8   CONCLUSION

The mechanisms of several neurodegenerative illnesses have been successfully elucidated. Through the study of pathological lesions and genetics, scientists have been able to generate more nuanced hypotheses on the neurodegenerative molecular and cellular processes. Among the many recurring topics in the scientific literature are RNA-mediated toxicity and neuroinflammation, as well as protein misfolding and aggregation. In addition, protein diseases that spread like prions are becoming more common, which could lead to novel therapeutic opportunities. The increasing prevalence of disease with age provides a connecting thread. Neurons are postmitotic, making them especially susceptible to the accumulation of misfolded proteins and overall homeostasis as they age. The understanding of illness causes and evaluating possible treatment medicines has been greatly aided by the use of animal models that resemble disease phenotypes in molecular, pathological, and behavioral terms. Despite recent advancements in understanding the etiology of neurodegenerative disorders and the development of fresh tools and approaches for drug discovery, there are currently no disease-modifying drugs available for any neurodegenerative ailment.

KEYWORDS

- **Creutzfeldt–Jakob disease**
- **neurodegenerative disorder**
- **frontotemporal dementia**
- **Parkinson's disease**
- **Huntington's disease**
- **amyotrophic lateral sclerosis**
- **prion disorders**

REFERENCES

1. Jellinger, K. A. Recent Advances in Our Understanding of Neurodegeneration. *J. Neural Transm.* **2009,** *116*, 1111–1162.
2. Skovronsky, D. M.; Lee VM-Y, Trojanowski, J. Q. Neurodegenerative Diseases: New Concepts of Pathogenesis and Their Therapeutic Implications. *Annu. Rev. Pathol. Mech. Dis.* **2006,** *1*, 151–170.
3. Golde, T. E.; Miller, V. M. Proteinopathy-Induced Neuronal Senescence: A Hypothesis for Brain Failure in Alzheimer's and Other Neurodegenerative Diseases. *Alzheimers Res. Ther.* **2009,** *1*, 5.

4. Uversky, V. N. Intrinsic Disorder in Proteins Associated with Neurodegenerative Diseases. *Front. Biosci.* **2009**, *14*, 5188–238.
5. Herczenik, E.; Gebbink, M. F. Molecular and Cellular Aspects of Protein Misfolding and Disease. *FASEB J.* **2008**, *22*, 2115–2133.
6. Ovádi, J.; Orosz, F. *Protein Folding and Misfolding: Neurodegenerative Diseases*; Netherlands: Springer; 2009; p 274.
7. Dickson, D. W. Neuropathology of Non-Alzheimer Degenerative Disorders. *Int. J. Clin. Exp. Pathol.* **2010**, *3*, 1–22.
8. Kovacs, G. G.; Budka, H. Protein-Based Neuropathology and Molecular Classification of Human Neurodegenerative Diseases. In: *Protein Folding and Misfolding: Neurodegenerative Diseases*; Ovádi, J., Orosz, F., Eds.; Netherlands: Springer; 2009; pp 251–272.
9. Migliore, L.; Coppede, F. Genetics, Environmental Factors and the Emerging Role of Epigenetics in Neurodegenerative Diseases. *Mutat. Res.* **2009**, *667*, 82–97.
10. Palop, J. J.; Chin, J.; Mucke, L. A Network Dysfunction Perspective on Neurodegenerative Diseases. *Nature* **2006**, *443*, 768–773.
11. Seeley, W. W.; Crawford, R. K.; Zhou, J. et al. Neurodegenerative Diseases Target Large-Scale Human Brain Networks. *Neuron.* **2009**, *62*, 42–52.
12. Ecroyd, H.; Carver, J. A. Unraveling the Mysteries of Protein Folding and Misfolding. *IUBMB Life.* **2008**, *60*, 769–774.
13. Morris, A. M.; Watzky, M. A.; Finke, R. G. Protein Aggregation Kinetics, Mechanism, and Curve-Fitting: A Review of the Literature. *Biochim. Biophys. Acta.* **2009**, *1794*, 375–397.
14. Israeli, E.; Sharon, R. Beta-Synuclein Occurs In Vivo in Lipid-Associated Oligomers and Forms Hetero-Oligomers with Alpha-Synuclein. *J. Neurochem.* **2009**, *108*, 465–74.
15. Selkoe, D. J. Soluble Oligomers of the Amyloid Beta-Protein Impair Synaptic Plasticity and Behavior. *Behav Brain Res.* **2008**, *192*, 106–113.
16. Soto, C.; Estrada, L. D. Protein Misfolding and Neurodegeneration. *Arch. Neurol.* **2008**, *65*, 184–189.
17. Aguzzi, A.; Sigurdson, C.; Heikenwaelder, M. Molecular Mechanisms of Prion Pathogenesis. *Annu. Rev. Pathol.* **2008**, *3*, 11–40.
18. Lafaye, P.; Achour, I.; England, P. et al. Single-Domain Antibodies Recognize Selectively Small Oligomeric Forms of Amyloid Beta, Prevent Abeta-Induced Neurotoxicity and Inhibit Fibril Formation. *Mol. Immunol.* **2009**, *46*, 695–704.
19. Moore, R. A.; Taubner, L. M.; Priola, S. A. Prion Protein Misfolding and Disease. *Curr. Opin. Struct. Biol.* **2009**, *19*, 14–22.
20. Williams, A. J.; Paulson, H. L. Polyglutamine Neurodegeneration: Protein Misfolding Revisited. *Trends Neurosci.* **2008**, *31*, 521–528.
21. Xia, W.; Yang, T.; Shankar, G. et al. A Specific Enzyme-Linked Immunosorbent Assay for Measuring Beta-Amyloid Protein Oligomers in Human Plasma and Brain Tissue of Patients with Alzheimer Disease. *Arch. Neurol.* **2009**, *66*, 190–199.
22. Tomic, J. L.; Pensalfini, A.; Head, E. et al. Soluble Fibrillar Oligomer Levels Are Elevated in Alzheimer's Disease Brain and Correlate with Cognitive Dysfunction. *Neurobiol. Dis.* **2009**, *35*, 352–358.
23. Harmeier, A.; Wozny, C.; Rost, B. R. et al. Role of Amyloid-Beta Glycine 33 in Oligomerization, Toxicity, and Neuronal Plasticity. *J. Neurosci.* **2009**, *29*, 7582–7590.

24. Kim, J.; Onstead, L.; Randle, S. et al. Abeta40 Inhibits Amyloid Deposition In Vivo. *J. Neurosci.* **2007**, *27*, 627–633.
25. Schmidt, M.; Sachse, C.; Richter, W. et al. Comparison of Alzheimer Abeta(1–40) and Abeta(1–42) Amyloid Fibrils Reveals Similar Protofilament Structures. *Proc. Natl. Acad. Sci. USA.* **2009**, *106*, 19813–19818.
26. Lauren, J.; Gimbel, D. A.; Nygaard, H. B. et al. Cellular Prion Protein Mediates Impairment of Synaptic Plasticity by Amyloid-Beta Oligomers. *Nature* **2009**, *457*, 1128–32.
27. Shankar, G. M.; Li, S.; Mehta, T. H. et al. Amyloid-Beta Protein Dimers Isolated Directly from Alzheimer's Brains Impair Synaptic Plasticity and Memory. *Nat Med.* **2008**, *14*, 837–842.
28. Abramov, E.; Dolev, I.; Fogel, H. et al. Amyloid-beta as a positive endogenous regulator of Release Probability at Hippocampal Synapses. *Nat. Neurosci.* **2009**, *12*, 1567–1576.
29. Nygaard, H. B.; Strittmatter, S. M. Cellular Prion Protein Mediates the Toxicity of Beta-Amyloid Oligomers: Implications for Alzheimer Disease. *Arch. Neurol.* **2009**, *66*, 1325–8.
30. Nimmrich, V.; Ebert, U. Is Alzheimer's Disease a Result of Presynaptic Failure? Synaptic Dysfunctions Induced by Oligomeric Beta-Amyloid. *Rev. Neurosci.* **2009**, *20*, 1–12.
31. Dinamarca, M. C.; Colombres, M.; Cerpa, W. et al. Beta-Amyloid Oligomers Affect the Structure and Function of the Postsynaptic Region: Role of the Wnt Signaling Pathway. *Neurodegener Dis.* **2008**, *5*, 149–152.
32. Moreno, H.; Yu, E.; Pigino, G. et al. Synaptic Transmission Block by Presynaptic Injection of Oligomeric Amyloid Beta. *Proc. Natl. Acad. Sci. USA* **2009**, *106*, 5901–5906.
33. Deshpande, A.; Kawai, H.; Metherate, R. et al. A role for synaptic zinc in Activity-Dependent Abeta Oligomer Formation and Accumulation at Excitatory Synapses. *J. Neurosci.* **2009**, *29*, 4004–4015.
34. Wang, Z.; Wang, B.; Yang, L. et al. Presynaptic and Postsynaptic Interaction of the Amyloid Precursor Protein Promotes Peripheral and Central Synaptogenesis. *J. Neurosci.* **2009**, *29*, 10788–10801.
35. Hoe, H. S.; Fu, Z.; Makarova, A. et al. The Effects of Amyloid Precursor Protein on Postsynaptic Composition and Activity. *J. Biol. Chem.* **2009**, *284*, 8495–506.
36. Dahlstroem, A.; Fuxe, K.; Olson, L.; Ungerstedt, U. Ascending Systems of Catecholamine Neurons from the Lower Brain Stem. *Acta. Physiol. Scand.* **1964**, *62*, 485–486.
37. Davies, P. Biochemical Changes in Alzheimer's Disease-Senile Dementia: Neurotransmitters in Senile Dementia of the Alzheimer's Type. *Res. Publ. Assoc. Res. Nerv. Ment. Dis.* **1979**, *57*, 153–166.
38. Davies, P.; Maloney, A. J. Selective Loss of Central Cholinergic Neurons in Alzheimer's Disease. *Lancet* **1976**, *2*, 1403.
39. Davis, G. C.; Williams, A. C.; Markey, S. P.; Ebert, M. H.; Caine, E. D.; Reichert, C. M.; Kopin, I. J. Chronic Parkinsonism Secondary to Intravenous Injection of Meperidine Analogues. *Psychiatry Res.* **1979**, *1*, 249–254.

40. de Leon, M. J.; Ferris, S. H.; George, A. E.; Christman, D. R.; Fowler, J. S.; Gentes, C.; Reisberg, B.; Gee, B.; Emmerich, M.; Yonekura, Y.; Brodie, J.; Kricheff, I. I.; Wolf, A. P. Positron Emission Tomographic Studies of Aging and Alzheimer Disease. *AJNR Am. J. Neuroradiol.* **1983**, *4*, 568–571.

41. DeLong, M. R. Primate models of movement disorders of basal ganglia origin. Trends Neurosci. **1990**, *13*, 281–285.

42. Eccles, J. C. The Electrophysiological Properties of the Motoneurone. *Cold Spring Harb. Symp. Quant. Biol.* **1952**, *17*, 175–183.

43. Eckert, T.; Tang, C.; Eidelberg, D. Assessment of the Progression of Parkinson's Disease: A Metabolic Network Approach. *Lancet Neurol.* **2007**, *6*, 926–932.

44. Ehringer, H.; Hornykiewicz, O. [Distribution of Noradrenaline and Dopamine (3-Hydroxytyramine) in the Human Brain and Their Behavior in Diseases of the Extrapyramidal System.] *Klin Wochenschr.* **1960**, *38*, 1236–1239.

45. Feigin, A.; Tang, C.; Ma, Y.; Mattis, P.; Zgaljardic, D.; Guttman, M.; Paulsen, J. S.; Dhawan, V.; Eidelberg, D. Thalamic Metabolism and Symptom Onset in Preclinical Huntington's Disease. *Brain* **2007**, *130*, 2858–2867.

46. Fink, R. P.; Heimer, L. Two Methods for Selective Silver Impregnation of Degenerating Axons and Their Synaptic Endings in the Central Nervous System. *Brain Res.* **1967**, *4*, 369–374.

47. Foster, N. L.; Heidebrink, J. L.; Clark, C. M.; Jagust, W. J.; Arnold, S. E.; Barbas, N. R.; DeCarli, C. S.; Turner, R. S.; Koeppe, R. A.; Higdon, R.; Minoshima, S. FDG-PET Improves Accuracy in Distinguishing Frontotemporal Dementia and Alzheimer's Disease. *Brain* **2007**, *130*, 2616–2635.

48. Fuxe, K.; Goldstein, M.; Hökfelt, T.; Joh, T. H. Immunohistochemical Localization of Dopamine–Hydroxylase in the Peripheral and Central Nervous System. *Res. Commun. Chem. Pathol. Pharmacol.* **1970**, *1*, 627–636.

49. Gasser, T. Update on the Genetics of Parkinson's Disease. *Mov Disord.* **2007**, *22*, S343–S350.

50. Glenner, G. G.; Wong, C. W. Alzheimer's Disease: Initial Report of the Purification and Characterization of a Novel Cerebrovascular Amyloid Protein. *Biochem. Biophys. Res. Commun.* **1984**, *120*, 885–890.

51. Goldberg, A. L. Protein Degradation and Protection Against Misfolded or Damaged Proteins. *Nature* **2003**, *426*, 895–899.

52. Goldberg, A. L. Functions of the Proteasome: from Protein Degradation and Immune Surveillance to Cancer Therapy. *Biochem. Soc. Trans.* **2007**, *35*, 12–17.

53. Graybiel, A. M.; Devor, M. A Microelectrophoretic Delivery Technique for Use with Horseradish Peroxidase. *Brain Res.* **1974**, *68*, 167–173.

54. Gusella, J. F.; Wexler, N. S.; Conneally, P. M.; Naylor, S. L.; Anderson, M. A.; Tanzi, R. E.; Watkins, P. C.; Ottina, K.; Wallace, M. R.; Sakaguchi, A. Y.; Young, A. B.; Shoulson, I.; Bonilla, E.; Martin, J. B. A polymorphic DNA Marker Genetically Linked to Huntington's Disease. *Nature* **1983**, *306*, 234–238.

55. Hullay, J. Subthalamotomy in Parkinson's Disease. Analysis of Responses to Electrostimulation. *Acta Med. Acad. Sci. Hung.* **1971**, *28*, 57–68.

56. Javitch, J. A.; Snyder, S. H. Uptake of MPP(+) by Dopamine Neurons Explains Selectivity of Parkinsonism-Inducing Neurotoxin, *MPTP. Eur. J. Pharmacol.* **1984**, *106*, 455–456.

57. Karch, C. M.; Prudencio, M.; Winkler, D. D.; Hart, P. J.; Borchelt, D. R. Role of Mutant SOD1 Disulfide Oxidation and Aggregation in the Pathogenesis of Familial ALS. *Proc. Natl. Acad. Sci. USA* **2009,** *106,* 7774–7779.

58. Kindt, M. V.; Heikkila, R. E.; Nicklas, W. J. Mitochondrial and Metabolic Toxicity of 1-Methyl-4-(2'-Methylphenyl)-1,2,3,6-Tetrahydropyridine. *J. Pharmacol. Exp. Ther.* **1987,** *242,* 858–863.

59. Kish, S. J.; Rajput, A.; Gilbert, J.; Rozdilsky, B.; Chang, L. J.; Shannak, K.; Hornykiewicz, O. Elevated Gamma-Aminobutyric Acid Level in Striatal But Not Extrastriatal Brain Regions in Parkinson's Disease: Correlation with Striatal Dopamine Loss. *Ann Neurol.* **1986,** *20,* 26–31.

60. Kish, S. J.; Shannak, K.; Hornykiewicz, O. Elevated Serotonin and Reduced Dopamine in Subregionally Divided Huntington's Disease Striatum. *Ann Neurol.* **1987,** *22,* 386–389.

61. Klucken, J.; Shin, Y.; Masliah, E.; Hyman, B. T.; McLean, P. J. Hsp70 Reduces Alpha-Synuclein Aggregation and Toxicity. *J Biol Chem.* **2004,** *279,* 25497–25502.

62. Kordower, J. H.; Chu, Y.; Hauser, R. A.; Freeman, T. B.; Olanow, C. W. Lewy Body-Like Pathology in Long-Term Embryonic Nigral Transplants in Parkinson's Disease. *Nat Med.* **2008,** *14,* 504–506.

63. Laitinen, L. V.; Bergenheim, A. T.; Hariz, M. I. Leksell's Posteroventral Pallidotomy in the Treatment of Parkinson's Disease. *J. Neurosurg.* **1992,** *76,* 53–61.

64. Langston, J. W.; Ballard, P.; Tetrud, J. W.; Irwin, I. Chronic Parkinsonism in Humans Due to a Product of Meperidine-Analog Synthesis. *Science* **1983,** *219,* 979–980.

65. Langston, J. W.; Irwin, I.; Langston, E. B.; Forno, L. S. 1-Methyl-4-Phenylpyridinium Ion (MPP+): Identification of a Metabolite of MPTP, a Toxin Selective to the substantia nigra. *Neurosci Lett.* **1984,** *48,* 87–92.

66. La Spada, A. R.; Wilson, E. M.; Lubahn, D. B.; Harding, A. E.; Fischbeck, K. H. Androgen Receptor Gene Mutations in X-Linked Spinal and Bulbar Muscular Atrophy. *Nature* **1991,** *352,* 77–79.

67. LaVail, J. H.; LaVail, M. M. The Retrograde Intraaxonal Transport of Horseradish Peroxidase in the Chick Visual System: A Light and Electron Microscopic Study. *J. Comp. Neurol.* **1974,** *157,* 303–357.

68. Levine, B.; Kroemer, G. Autophagy in the Pathogenesis of Disease. *Cell* **2008,** *132,* 27–42

69. Limousin, P.; Pollak, P.; Benazzouz, A.; Hoffmann, D.; Broussolle, E.; Perret, J. E.; Benabid, A. L. Bilateral Subthalamic Nucleus Stimulation for Severe Parkinson's Disease. *Mov Disord.* **1995,** *10,* 672–674.

70. Limousin, P.; Pollak, P.; Benazzouz, A.; Hoffmann, D.; Le Bas, J. F.; Broussolle, E.; Perret, J. E.; Benabid, A. L. Effect of Parkinsonian Signs and Symptoms of Bilateral Subthalamic Nucleus Stimulation. *Lancet* **1995,;** *345,* 91–95.

71. Maire, J. C.; Wurtman, R. J. Choline Production from Choline-Containing Phospholipids: A Hypothetical Role in Alzheimer's Disease and Aging. *Prog. Neuropsychopharmacol. Biol. Psychiatry* **1984,** *8,* 637–642.

72. Mattis, V. B.; Ebert, A. D.; Fosso, M. Y.; Chang, C. W.; Lorson, C. L. Delivery of a Read-Through Inducing Compound, TC007, Lessens the Severity of a SMA Animal Model. *Hum Mol Genet.* 2009. DOI: 10.1093/hmg/ddp333

73. McGeer, P. L.; McGeer, E. G. Enzymes Associated with the Metabolism of Catecholamines, Acetylcholine and GABA in Human Controls and Patients with Parkinson's Disease and Huntington's Chorea. *J. Neurochem.* **1976,** *26,* 65–76.

74. McGeer, P. L.; McGeer, E. G.; Fibiger, H. C. Glutamic-Acid Decarboxylase and Choline Acetylase in Huntington's Chorea and Parkinson's Disease. *Lancet* **1973,** *2,* 622–623.

75. McLaughlin, B. J.; Wood, J. G.; Saito, K.; Barber, R.; Vaughn, J. E.; Roberts, E.; Wu, J. Y. The Fine Structural Localization of Glutamate Decarboxylase in Synaptic Terminals of Rodent Cerebellum. *Brain Res.* **1974,** *76,* 377–391.

76. Medicherla, B.; Goldberg, A. L. Heat Shock and Oxygen Radicals Stimulate Ubiquitin-Dependent Degradation Mainly of Newly Synthesized Proteins. *J. Cell Biol.* **2008,** *182,* 663–673.

77. Meyer-Luehmann, M.; Spires-Jones, T. L.; Prada, C.; Garcia-Alloza, M.; de Calignon, A.; Rozkalne, A.; Koenigsknecht-Talboo, J.; Holtzman, D. M.; Bacskai, B. J.; Hyman, B. T. Rapid Appearance and Local Toxicity of Amyloid-Beta Plaques in a Mouse Model of Alzheimer's Disease. *Nature* **2008,** *451,* 720–724.

78. Kubota, H. Quality Control Against Misfolded Proteins in the Cytosol: A Network for Cell Survival. *J. Biochem.* **2009,** *146,* 609–616.

79. Scheper, W.; Hoozemans, J. J. Endoplasmic Reticulum Protein Quality Control in Neurodegenerative Disease: The Good, the Bad and the Therapy. *Curr Med Chem.* **2009,** *16,* 615–26.

80. Eliezer, D. Biophysical Characterization of Intrinsically Disordered Proteins. *Curr Opin Struct Biol.* **2009,** *19,* 23–30.

81. Mendoza-Espinosa, P.; Garcia-Gonzalez, V.; Moreno, A. et al. Disorder-to-Order Conformational Transitions in Protein Structure and Its Relationship to Disease. *Mol Cell Biochem.* **2009,** *330,* 105–20.

82. Balch, W. E.; Morimoto, R. I.; Dillin, A. et al. Adapting Proteostasis for Disease Intervention. *Science* **2008,** *319,* 916–919.

83. Winklhofer, K. F.; Tatzelt, J.; Haass, C. The Two Faces of Protein Misfolding: Gain- and Loss-of-Function in Neurodegenerative Diseases. *EMBO J.* **2008,** *27,* 336–349.

84. Mirzaei, H.; Regnier, F. Protein: Protein Aggregation Induced by Protein Oxidation. *J. Chromatogr. B Analyt Technol. Biomed. Life Sci.* **2008,** *873,* 8–14.

85. Hutt, D. M.; Powers, E. T.; Balch, W. E. The Proteostasis Boundary in Misfolding Diseases of Membrane Traffic. *FEBS Lett.* **2009,** *583,* 2639–2646.

86. Powers, E. T.; Morimoto, R. I.; Dillin, A. et al. Biological and Chemical Approaches to Diseases of Proteostasis Deficiency. *Annu Rev Biochem.* **2009,** *78,* 959–991.

87. Arndt, V.; Rogon, C.; Hohfeld, J. To be, or Not to be–Molecular Chaperones in Protein Degradation. *Cell Mol. Life Sci.* **2007,** *64,* 2525–2541.

88. Broadley, S. A.; Hartl, F. U. The role of Molecular Chaperones in Human Misfolding Diseases. *FEBS Lett.* **2009,** *583,* 2647–2653.

89. Roelofs, J.; Park, S.; Haas, W. et al. Chaperone-Mediated Pathway of Proteasome Regulatory Particle Assembly. *Nature* **2009,** *459,* 861–865.

90. Kalmar, B.; Greensmith, L. Induction of Heat Shock Proteins for Protection Against Oxidative Stress. *Adv. Drug Deliv Rev.* **2009,** *61,* 310–318.

91. Calderwood, S. K.; Murshid, A.; Prince, T. The Shock of Aging: Molecular Chaperones and the Heat Shock Response in Longevity and Aging–A Mini-Review. *Gerontology.* **2009,** *55,* 550–558.

Neurodegenerative Disorders: A Mysterious Group of Diseases 49

92. Goldbaum, O.; Riedel, M.; Stahnke, T. et al. The Small Heat Shock Protein HSP25 Protects Astrocytes Against Stress Induced by Proteasomal Inhibition. *Glia* **2009,** *57,* 1566–1577.

93. Roodveldt, C.; Bertoncini, C. W.; Andersson, A. et al. Chaperone Proteostasis in Parkinson's Disease: Stabilization of the Hsp70/alpha-Synuclein Complex by Hip. *EMBO J.* **2009,** *28,* 3758–3770.

94. Malhotra, J. D.; Kaufman, R. J. The Endoplasmic Reticulum and the Unfolded Protein Response. *Semin. Cell. Dev. Biol.* **2007,** *18,* 716–731.

95. Lindholm, D.; Wootz, H.; Korhonen, L. ER Stress and Neurodegenerative Diseases. *Cell Death Differ.* **2006,** *13,* 385–392.

96. Uversky, V. N. Alpha-Synuclein Misfolding and Neurodegenerative Diseases. *Curr. Protein Pept. Sci.* **2008,** *9,* 507–540.

97. Tan, J. M.; Wong, E. S.; Lim, K. L. Protein Misfolding and Aggregation in Parkinson Disease. *Antioxid Redox Signal.* **2009,** *11,* 2119–2134.

98. Mondragon-Rodriguez, S.; Basurto-Islas, G.; Binder, L. I. et al. Conformational Changes and Cleavage; Are These Responsible for the Tau Aggregation in Alzheimers Disease. *Future Neurol.* **2009,** *4,* 39–53.

99. Takashima, A. Hyperphosphorylated Tau Is a Cause of Neuronal Dysfunction in Tauopathy. *J Alzheimers Dis.* **2008,** *14,* 371–375.

100. Rabins, P. V.; Lyketsos, C. G. Cholinesterase Inhibitors and Memantine Have a Role in the Treatment of Alzheimer's Disease. *Nat. Clin. Pract. Neurol.* **2006,** *2,* 578–579.

101. Roberts, E. Disinhibition as an Organizing Principle in the Nervous System: The role of Gamma-Aminobutyric Acid. *Adv Neurol.* **1974,** *5,* 127–143.

102. Rosen, D. R. Mutations in Cu/Zn Superoxide Dismutase Gene Are Associated with Familial Amyotrophic Lateral Sclerosis. *Nature* **1993,** *364,* 362.

103. Saito, K.; Barber, R.; Wu, J.; Matsuda, T.; Roberts, E.; Vaughn, J. E. Immunohistochemical Localization of Glutamate Decarboxylase in Rat Cerebellum. *Proc. Natl. Acad. Sci. USA* **1974,** *71,* 269–273.

104. Schwarcz, R.; Coyle, J. T. Striatal Lesions with Kainic Acid: Neurochemical Characteristics. *Brain Res.* **1977,** *127,* 235–249.

105. Schwarcz, R.; Köhler, C. Differential Vulnerability of Central Neurons of the Rat to Quinolinic Acid. *Neurosci Lett.* **1983,** *38,* 85–90.

106. Selkoe, D. J. Soluble Oligomers of the Amyloid Beta-Protein Impair Synaptic Plasticity and Behavior. *Behav. Brain Res.* **2008,** *192,* 106–113.

107. Sherrington, R.; Rogaev, E. I.; Liang, Y.; Rogaeva, E. A.; Levesque, G.; Ikeda, M.; Chi, H.; Lin, C.; Li, G.; Holman, K.; Tsuda, T.; Mar, L.; Foncin J-F, Bruni, A. C.; Montesi, M. P.; Sorbi, S.; Rainero, I.; Pinessi, L.; Nee, L.; Chumakov, I. et al. Cloning of a Gene Bearing Missense Mutations in Early-Onset Familial Alzheimer's Disease. *Nature* **1995,** *375,* 754–760.

108. Spillantini, M. G.; Goedert, M. Tau Protein Pathology in Neurodegenerative Diseases. *Trends Neurosci.* **1998,** *21,* 428–433.

109. Spires-Jones, T. L.; Stoothoff, W. H.; de Calignon, A.; Jones, P. B.; Hyman, B. T. Tau Pathophysiology in Neurodegeneration: A Tangled Issue. *Trends Neurosci.* **2009,** *32,* 150–159.

110. Spires-Jones, T. L.; Mielke, M. L.; Rozkalne, A.; Meyer-Luehmann, M.; de Calignon, A.; Bacskai, B. J.; Schenk, D.; Hyman, B. T. Passive Immunotherapy Rapidly

Increases Structural Plasticity in a Mouse Model of Alzheimer Disease. Neurobiol Dis. **2009**, *33*, 213–220.

111. Stoessl, A. J. Positron Emission Tomography in Premotor Parkinson's Disease. *Parkinsonism Relat. Disord.* **2007**, *13* (Suppl 3), S421–S424.

112. Tanzi, R. E. Molecular Genetics of Alzheimer's Disease and the Amyloid Beta Peptide Precursor Gene. *Ann Med.* **1989**, *21*, 91–94.

113. Tanzi, R. E.; Gusella, J. F.; Watkins, P. C.; Bruns, G. A.; St George-Hyslop, P.; Van Keuren, M. L.; Patterson, D.; Pagan, S.; Kurnit, D. M.; Neve, R. L. Amyloid Beta Protein Gene: cDNA, mRNA Distribution, and Genetic Linkage Near the Alzheimer Locus. *Science* **1987**, *235*, 880–884.

114. The Huntington's Disease Collaborative Research Group. A Novel Gene Containing a Trinucleotide Repeat That Is Expanded and Unstable on Huntington's Disease Chromosomes. *Cell* **1993**, *72*, 971–983.

115. Trojanowski, J. Q. Tauists, Baptists, Syners, Apostates, and New Data. *Ann. Neurol.* **2002**, *52*, 263–265.

116. Trojanowski, J. Q.; Lee, V. M. Brain Degeneration Linked to "Fatal Attractions" of Proteins in Alzheimer's Disease and Related Disorders. *J. Alzheimers Dis.* **2001**, *3*, 117–119.

117. Tsien, R. Y. Constructing and Exploiting the Fluorescent Protein Paintbox (Nobel Lecture). *Angew. Chem. Int. Ed. Engl.* **2009**, *48*, 5612–5626.

118. Ungerstedt, U. 6-Hydroxy-Dopamine Induced Degeneration OF Central Monoamine Neurons. *Eur. J. Pharmacol.* **1968**, *5*, 107–110.

119. Valdmanis, P. N.; Rouleau, G. A. Genetics of Familial Amyotrophic Lateral Sclerosis. *Neurology.* **2008**, *70*, 144–152.

120. van Oostrom, J. C.; Maguire, R. P.; Verschuuren-Bemelmans, C. C.; Veenma-van der Duin, L.; Pruim, J.; Roos, R. A.; Leenders, K. L. Striatal Dopamine D2 Receptors, Metabolism, and volume in preclinical Huntington disease. Neurology. **2005**, *65*, 941–943.

121. Vingerhoets, F. J.; Snow, B. J.; Tetrud, J. W.; Langston, J. W.; Schulzer, M.; Calne, D. B. Positron Emission Tomographic Evidence for Progression of Human MPTP-Induced Dopaminergic Lesions. *Ann. Neurol.* **1994**, *36*, 765–770.

122. Watson, J. D.; Crick, F. H. Genetical Implications of the Structure of Deoxyribonucleic Acid. *Nature* **1953**, *171*, 964–967.

123. Wexler, N. S.; Lorimer, J.; Porter, J.; Gomez, F.; Moskowitz, C.; Shackell, E.; Marder, K.; Penchaszadeh, G.; Roberts, S. A.; Gayán, J.; Brocklebank, D.; Cherny, S. S.; Cardon, L. R.; Gray, J.; Dlouhy, S. R.; Wiktorski, S.; Hodes, M. E.; Conneally, P. M.; Penney, J. B.; Gusella, J. et al. Venezuelan Kindreds Reveal That Genetic and Environmental Factors Modulate Huntington's Disease Age of Onset. *Proc. Natl. Acad. Sci. USA* **2004**, *101*, 3498–3503.

124. Whitehouse, P. J.; Price, D. L.; Clark, A. W.; Coyle, J. T.; DeLong, M. R. Alzheimer Disease: Evidence for Selective Loss of Cholinergic Neurons in the Nucleus Basalis. *Ann. Neurol.* **1981**, *10*, 122–126.

125. Williams, A. J.; Paulson, H. L. Polyglutamine Neurodegeneration: Protein Misfolding Revisited. *Trends Neurosci.* **2008**, *31*, 521–528.

126. Williams, J. H.; Schray, R. C.; Patterson, C. A.; Ayitey, S. O.; Tallent, M. K.; Lutz, G. J. Oligonucleotide-Mediated Survival of Motor Neuron Protein Expression in CNS

Improves Phenotype in a Mouse Model of Spinal Muscular Atrophy. *J. Neurosci.* **2009,** *29*, 7633–7638.

127. Yahr, M. D.; Duvoisin, R. C.; Hoehn, M. M.; Schear, M. J.; Barrett, R. E. L-Dopa (L-3,4-dihydroxyphenylanine)—Its Clinical Effects in Parkinsonism. *Trans Am Neurol Assoc.* **1968,** *93*, 56–63.

128. Yamamoto, A.; Lucas, J. J.; Hen, R. Reversal of Neuropathology and Motor Dysfunction in a Conditional Model of Huntington's Disease. *Cell* **2000,** *101*, 57–66.

129. Young, A. B.; Penney, J. B.; Dauth, G. W.; Bromberg, M. B.; Gilman, S. Glutamate or Aspartate as a Possible Neurotransmitter of Cerebral Corticofugal Fibers in the Monkey. *Neurology* **1983,** *33*, 1513–1516.

CHAPTER 3

Propagation of Neurodegenerative disorders

ABSTRACT

Protein aggregates play a role in some forms of neurodegeneration. These disorders have been linked to transmissible spongiform encephalopathies (TSEs), according to new study. Proteins in TSEs or prion disorders take on a specific shape that is infectious and causes illness. In many degenerative diseases associated with aging, including Alzheimer's, Parkinson's, and Huntington's, the prion-like theory postulates that specific proteins have biochemical and biological properties with prions. Different disease-related proteins physically migrate from cell to cell inside the central nervous system, resulting in the progression of illness. Targeting the production of prion-like proteins could lead to novel diagnostic and therapeutic methods according to these findings.

3.1 INTRODUCTION

All biological systems rely on a complicated mechanism to ensure proper protein folding. In order to avoid improper protein folding and keep proteins in their functional condition, maintaining protein homeostasis and a healthy cellular metabolism is essential.[1–5] The aggregation of proteins in nonphysiological conformations is a characteristic of many neurodegenerative diseases. It is interesting to see how, after they have misfolded, the proteins implicated in various neurodegenerative illnesses seem to have a commonality despite their varying biochemical, functional, and

---

Gene Therapy for Neurological Disorders: Molecular Approaches for Targeted Treatment.
Rishabha Malviya, Arun Kumar Singh, Priyanshi Goyal, & Sonali Sundram (Authors)
© 2025 Apple Academic Press, Inc. Co-published with CRC Press (Taylor & Francis)

biological characteristics.[6] A molecular template may be transmitted and used to initiate and promote illness when aggregated proteins implicated in neurodegenerative disease are present.

A new picture emerging from the last ten years of study reveals that various progressive neurodegenerative disorders share specific molecular traits that include "prionlike" activity of protein aggregation-prone aggregates.[7] The development of symptoms may be aided by the cell-to-cell transfer of misfolded protein complexes. Researchers are still trying to figure out exactly how amyloid proteins contribute to disease etiology despite overwhelming evidence that they do so. Experimental evidence for prion-like activity in protein aggregates has been established in a wide range of neurodegenerative illnesses that will be discussed in this chapter. Experimentation models and clinical circumstances are discussed in detail. New molecular processes driving replication and transmission of disease-causing proteins in a prion-like fashion are discussed here, as well as promising avenues of investigation to pursue.[8] Highlighting both similarities and differences, also briefly explore how prion-like neurodegenerative disorders might be dissected to offer new avenues for the development of innovative therapeutics that can halt the course of the disease. According to this prion-like theory of illness, proteins might be used to cause disease by mimicking infectious particles like live bacteria and viruses. Determining the precise function of prion-like proteins in spreading infection has proved challenging in recent years, and the resulting semantic arguments continue to be intense.[9] They need to grasp the prion-like concept's historical roots in order to frame it. Since the prion-like notion has been the topic of a continually changing and expanding area of study, we will first address it in its social scientific context.[10]

3.2 HISTORICALLY SPEAKING, PRION-LIKE FEATURES IN NEURODEGENERATIVE DISORDERS

3.2.1 VIRULENCE ACCORDING TO KOCH'S POSTULATES

Upon the publication of Koch's postulates in 1882, German physicians Robert Koch and Friedrich Loeffler developed the first definitions and tests to describe and evaluate infectiousness and the function of infectious live organisms in TB pathogenesis.[11]

Propagation of Neurodegenerative disorders 55

Koch's postulates have been used since the late 19th century to determine the role of a certain microorganism in the pathogenesis of a disease. Koch's postulates did not prevent new and important discoveries, but they did make it harder to identify viruses because viruses could not be isolated and grown in a pure culture that could be used to infect other species.[12] Since this was the case, it was quite some time before viruses were identified and infectiousness was understood to be a universal occurrence. The discovery of viruses revised Koch's postulates of infectivity.[13]

Another question arose when virologists Gajdusek and Zigas (1957) discovered that sickness may be spread between people during tribal practices of cannibalism. Kuru is a disease with a short incubation period (B4-40 years) and rapid progression. Neurological symptoms were present, but there was no evidence of fever or inflammation. Since these symptoms are not present in cases of bacterial or viral infections, various theories were put up to explain Kuru, but the illness was still mysterious. It took almost a decade for researchers to notice that Kuru was very similar to scrapie, another neurodegenerative illness.[14–18] Scrapie is a type of transmissible spongiform encephalopathy (TSE) found in animals. Because of an interesting connection to scrapie, Gajdusek chose bigger animals and conducted further transmission tests on chimpanzees after his previous efforts to develop and disseminate the attempt to transmit Kuru from humans to rodents in the lab had failed. Humans may be able to "cultivate" Kuru in chimpanzees, causing the primate to develop tremors and ataxias after one to three years. His research suggested that an unidentified infectious pathogen was responsible for Kuru. Scrapie was thought to be caused by a slow-moving virus until it was successfully transmitted from goats to mice in an experiment.[19] Although prior experiments demonstrated that infectivity could be isolated and maintained after filtration of diseased brain, the fact that infectivity was maintained even in the absence of nucleic acids was remarkable. Amyloid-rich prion protein (PrP) emerged as a possible culprit after two decades of conjecture and several efforts to locate an infectious agent.[20] A protein-only theory was eventually proven in 2010 when pure versions of synthetic PrP were found to be able to self-propagate and transmit illness following exogenous application. Koch's notion of infectivity had to be reworked with the discovery of the PrP's infectivity and ability to cause illness.[21]

It is evident that Koch and Loeffler's original definition of infectivity has undergone such radical transformation that it is now nearly a priceless piece of history. In light of current developments in neurodegenerative research, we must reexamine the idea of infectiousness in light of the protein-only theory.[22] It seems that the involvement of proteins as "nucleating" or "infectious" agents in neurodegenerative disorders is broader than previously thought. Despite their apparent similarities to PrP, these pathogenic proteins exhibit slight changes in their method of action.[23]

3.2.2 SEEDS OF INFECTIOUSNESS CONTINUALLY PROLIFERATE

For many years, it has been known that viral illnesses and neurodegenerative diseases have many similarities. Thus, several of the world's leading experts have suggested that infectious-like processes play a role.[24]

Initial theories included those based on medical accounts from more than a century ago. Small groups of psychiatrists in the early 20th century documented the existence of aberrant protein deposits in individuals diagnosed with memory loss. A case study of presenile dementia based on an autopsy by German psychiatrist Alois Alzheimer was given at the Tu Bingen conference in 1906 by members of the Southwest German Psychiatrists (SWGP).[25–30] Auguste Deter, a female patient who had been brought to Frankfurt's mental institution a few years previously with growing memory loss, hallucinations, and delusions, was examined clinically and histopathologically.[31]

"In the middle of an otherwise nearly normal cell, there stands out one or more fibrils owing to their unique thickness and unusual impregnability," he wrote in his postmortem study of his patient's brain.[32]

Tau neurofibrillary tangles (NFTs), as they are now called, were first described by Alois Alzheimer. NFTs and miliary foci, often known as senile plaques, were also seen. Even though extracellular plaques were not discovered until 1882, the work of neurologists Paul Blocq and Georges Marinesco in Martin Charcot's Paris ward at Salpetrie're Clinic, were the first to see them. These senile plaques in an epileptic patient's brain were characterized by both neurologists as "round piles".[33] The more patients Alzheimer saw who had symptoms that matched those of infectious disorders, particularly syphilitic dementia, and the sooner he was able to narrow down his differential diagnosis.

Syphilitic dementia, as a result of these findings, became one of the criteria for diagnosing dementia in the beginning of the 20th century. Another common neurodegenerative condition, Parkinson's disease (PD),

Propagation of Neurodegenerative disorders 57

was used as a comparison point.[34–36] Scientist Fritz Jacob Heinrich Lewy of Germany, who collaborated with Alois Alzheimer at the Munich Royal Psychiatric Clinic, examined brain tissue from more than half a dozen persons who had died from Parkinson's disease after their bodies had been examined postmortem. Inclusions that were eosinophilic and insoluble in alcohol, benzene, and chlorform were discovered in the vagus nerve, the nucleus basalis of Meynert, and several thalamic nuclei in 1912. This indicated that these inclusions were primarily constituted of proteins.[37]

When James Parkinson proposed that PD progresses over time, Lewy made the similarity between the transmission of a virus and the course of PD pathogenesis clear.[38] The recently discovered proteinaceous inclusions were studied alongside the inclusions (or negri bodies) caused by rabies virus infection. In the substantia nigra of those with Parkinson's disease, Russian-trained neuropathologist Konstantin Tretiakoff discovered the same kind of inclusion (PD). Six of his patients with paralysis agitans or parkinsonism exhibited inclusions in their nigral neurons that he dubbed "corps de Lewy" or "Lewy Bodies" due to Lewy's contribution to the field.[39]

Clearly, the discovery of Alzheimer and Lewy has significant clinical and historical consequences. To their surprise, their findings not only indicated the importance of proteinaceous inclusions but also pointed to a pattern of protein deposits extending throughout the central nervous system (CNS). Scientists felt obliged to investigate the link between the worsening of clinical symptoms and the accumulation of protein deposits after noticing this pattern.[40] The spatial and temporal pattern of tau inclusions in Alzheimer's disease (AD) was first investigated in depth by Braak et al. Clinical pathological examination of the brains of dementia patients who died at different stages of the disease provided evidence linking one of AD's pathological characteristics to disease development.[41] Neurofibrillary tangles (NFTs), which are made of hyperphosphorylated tau protein, are located in the transentorhinal cortex, which is part of the temporal lobe, and not all over the brain. At this point, deposits may be discovered in additional parts of the brain, such as limbic areas (such as the hippocampus and insular cortex), as well as in almost every neocortical subdivision.

This pattern suggests that inclusions are disseminated through neural anatomical connections. Research into Alzheimer's disease initially concentrated on NFTs in the pyramidal neurons of the isocortex, which exhibit the disease's signature radiating fibrillar filaments. It is unclear why he did not investigate the allocortical regions hit hardest by tau illness.[41–44] Later on, Braak et al. discovered a spatiotemporal progression of protein deposits following neural tracts, providing a framework for disease staging correlating with clinical symptoms: early episodic memory loss followed by associated cognitive deficits, leading to executive dysfunction, which includes motor tasks, visuospatial and perceptual deficits, and semantic dysfunction, and finally overt full-blown dementia. Plaques are spreading to new regions of the brain at the opposite rate that tau is.

There is a trend, but it is difficult to anticipate. As a consequence, many stage systems for extracellular A deposits have been suggested.[45]

Extracellular A plaques typically manifest in the isocortex, move to allocortical regions like the entorhinal cortex, hippocampus, and amygdala, and then to subcortical nuclei in the brainstem. Although A accumulates extracellularly, the anatomical connections between the affected brain regions point to a transneuronal spread of the disease.[46] In Alzheimer's disease, A and tau pathology show strikingly different anatomical patterns, and it is unclear why this happens. There is evidence that A and tau may impact each other's toxicity in both in vitro and in vivo studies. Both viruses operate together to cause neuronal damage and cell death when their spreading patterns meet and merge from opposing directions.[47] The number of inclusions in A and tau aggregates expands with time, and the aggregates get larger.

Certain neurons and areas may be more or less prone to neurodegeneration in Alzheimer's disease (AD) based on the proteinaceous distribution of A and tau and their anatomical linkages. The apparent progression of disease via these neuroanatomical routes cannot be explained by a theory based on the deposit of harmful proteins.[48] The selective susceptibility of sensitive neurons, as an alternate theory, might thereby explain why specific groups of neurons are more vulnerable to toxic shocks.

Progressive changes in the deposit patterns of -synuclein (Syn) are characteristic of Parkinson's disease (PD) and other synucleinopathies. Inclusions in distinct brain areas may be linked to clinical symptoms and indicators, according to Braak. This may be due to a disease that may infect bodies and spread to brains through physically related areas, such the spread of a neurotropic virus, which can infect bodies and transmit to the brain via transsynaptic transmission. Perhaps, "Such a virus might have unusual traits and could consist of misfolded Syn fragments," important

Propagation of Neurodegenerative disorders 59

because no previous studies had reported prion-related characteristics of misfolded Syn.[49] Initially, Braak stages were described as having synpathy that originated in the vagus nerve's dorsal motor nucleus.

3.2.3 THE PRION-LIKE HYPOTHESIS

Gajdusek's initial attempts to determine the heritability of Alzheimer's disease and other neurodegenerative illnesses failed. The possibility of transmitting Alzheimer's disease from human brain tissue to monkeys was examined by Gajdusek et al. (1980); however, they discovered no indication of the disease.[50] Studies like this were carried out long before A and tau were found to be the structural causes of Alzheimer's disease (AD). For a long time, the scientific consensus held that Alzheimer's disease (AD) is not contagious. However, prion disease pioneers Prusiner (1984) and Gajdusek (1994) have long hypothesized that certain neurological diseases may be contagious and have prion-like traits under specific circumstances.

Alzheimer's disease pathology can indeed be transmitted to marmosets via brain homogenates, as demonstrated by subsequent attempts to transfer AD pathology via brain homogenates.

Kuru had a major flaw: A pathology only developed after lengthy incubation periods of up to seven years.

Amyotrophic lateral sclerosis (ALS) was first described as a neurodegenerative disease in the early 1960s (ALS). ALS-like pathology was observed in monkeys after spinal cord homogenate from a deceased ALS patient was injected into their brains.[51]

Unlike other laboratory animals, monkeys were able to pass this infectious agent multiple times. More than five years of incubation were required. This suggests that ALS may be a virus-related disease. Cell transplantation in therapy provided additional evidence supporting the hypothesis of a prion-like mechanism. In Parkinson's disease, fetal mesencephalic cells, which replenish the striatum's supply of dopamine, are grafted into the brain in an attempt to replace the dopamine that has been lost and alleviate the disease's crippling motor symptoms.[52]

Autopsies of patients who underwent cell replacement therapy revealed Lewy bodies in their graft brains that had been studied using morphological markers more than a decade after the procedure.

The transplanted fetal cells described in the first two descriptions of Lewy bodies were 10–16 years old. The subject of whether aggregated protein may grow within transplanted fetal transplantation in HD patients after death, which can be interpreted as evidence of cell-to-cell transfer of misfolded protein, was also investigated.[53] Due to a polyglutamine (poly Q) repeat expansion that runs through the hunter's family (Htt), HD patients have a variety of symptoms, including abnormalities in their motor, cognitive, and psychological functions. There have been mixed findings from morphological investigations on grafts in HD. Initial observations suggested that there are not any Htt aggregates within the transplanted cells; nevertheless, a subsequent publication found Htt aggregates inside grafts in there were three patients who had surgery and then died ten years later.[54] The conventional view of HD holds that the illness process is cellular, but that there is a long lag time (years to decades) between the production of aggregation-prone protein and the emergence of pathology and symptoms in the brain. Based on these findings, it is possible that the progression of HD in three patients whose transplanted cells also showed protein aggregates is due to the spread of aggregated Htt from one cell to the next. The reason is the prion-like idea is relevant to more diseases than just those where environmental factors are assumed to initiate the illness in genetically vulnerable persons, like Parkinson's. It has been postulated that in HD, a genetic disorder, aggregates may spread from one cell to another and induce neurodegeneration in a nonautonomous fashion.[55]

3.3 PRIONS IN NEURODEGENERATIVE DISORDERS

Prion proteins are formed by endogenous proteins that change their shape and self-replicate. GSS syndrome and FFI are examples of prion illnesses that are inherited and are caused by gene mutations, deletions, or multiplications. For the most prevalent form of prion disease, Creutzfeldt Jacob's disease (CJD), the wild-type protein produces toxic aggregates that induce illness. Most neurodegenerative disorders with prion characteristics are likewise rare (90%), but polyQ diseases (like HD) are caused by an expanded glutamine repeat in the original sequence.[56] Many of the key components in neurodegenerative illnesses like Alzheimer's and Parkinson's can, like prions, adopt a different conformation, interact with other protein molecules, and fold into nonphysiological assemblies with a characteristic-sheet structure. Infectious amplification of disease transmission and pathogenesis may result from these insoluble assemblies "seeding" further aggregation processes, as shown experimentally below.

Propagation of Neurodegenerative disorders 61

It is hypothesized that prions may spread and multiply in a spatiotemporal way, leading to particular disease phenotypes such as Alzheimer's and Parkinson's syndromes, as well as other forms of motor dysfunction.[57] Figure 3.1 represents the types of prion's in neurodegenerative disorder dysfunction.

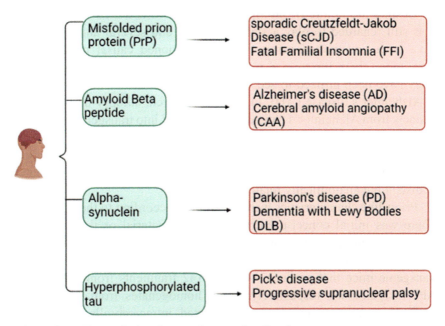

FIGURE 3.1 Types of prions in neurodegenerative disorders.

3.3.1 AMYLOID-B PRIONS

Plaques of A, the characteristic feature of Alzheimer's disease (AD), are formed when filamentous β-sheet aggregates of small fragments deposited in specific brain regions' extracellular spaces.

Cerebral amyloid angiopathy can be caused by deposits in blood vessel walls as well as plaques.

When taken together, these risk factors greatly enhance an individual's likelihood of getting Alzheimer's disease (AD).[58] Less than 5% of Alzheimer's disease cases are autosomal dominant. Early research established a connection between Alzheimer's disease and mutations in the amyloid precursor protein (APP) and presenilin (PSEN1 and PSEN2) genes in families. The -secretase complex, of which PS1 and PS2 are subunits, degrades APP into peptides of varying lengths.[59]

The A sequence of APP has been found to be responsible for a number of familial forms of Alzheimer's disease.

Alzheimer's disease is caused by alterations in genes responsible for increased concentrations or an increased propensity to assemble (AD).

Despite the failure of multiple treatment efforts aimed at An in AD, A is still regarded to play a significant role, and several animal models have been constructed using the aforementioned causal mutations to learn more about the myriad mechanisms at play in AD pathogenesis.[60] They have been utilized to see whether the prion theory may be applied to Alzheimer's disease (AD). In the first research, autopsy-derived brain extracts from Alzheimer's patients were injected into transgenic mice with an APP mutation and high amounts of A.

There was a heavy concentration of amyloid plaques at the injection sites in the hippocampus and neocortex, and further deposits were found in distant but anatomically related places.[61-63]

Prion-like characteristics were found in A, according to these findings. There was initial concern that the injection material or the transgenic animals' immune systems would make them susceptible to disease. In light of these findings, the second set of experiments was carried out using transgenic mice that produce A40 and A42 fragments from APP23 and APP-PS1 animals, respectively. Brain homogenates from APP23 and APPPS1 transgenic animals were injected intracerebrally into young APP23 and APP-PS1 mice.[64] Intracerebral infusions of brain homogenates again elevated the deposition of nascent amyloid. The seeding response of isolates was suppressed by anti-A antibodies or formic acid pretreatment. Donor brain tissue contains a protein called A, which Gajdusek et al. found to act like prions in that it can generate or exacerbate disease pathology in experimental animal models. The results presented here lend credence to those conclusions.[65] Importantly, it was not clear why these initial trials failed to promote amyloid formation by injecting synthetic or pure A seeds into the brains of transgenic or wild-type mice.

It was not a complete surprise, given that prions created in a laboratory setting likewise failed to infect animals when given to them in a pure form. Synthetic forms of prions have greater infectious potential when combined with endogenous cofactors such as lipids and RNA, which have been shown to change the assembly of prions into more infectious templates.[66]

Propagation of Neurodegenerative disorders   63

To prove that A was responsible for the accumulation and disease, pure synthetic peptides were delivered into the brains of transgenic mice. After further incubation at higher concentrations, it was discovered that pure fibrils have nucleating characteristics.[67] The injection location developed plaques due to the pure synthetic fibrils, and more plaques were discovered in nearby areas. These results support the hypothesis that A plaques propagate along neural circuits, resulting in a stereotypical anatomical pattern in their appearance. Most notably, research showing that injections of pure synthetic A fibrils could cause amyloid plaques to spread in mice demonstrated that additional tissue components, which had been present in the brain-derived material utilized in the prior investigations, are not necessary.[68] This seminal research provided unequivocal proof that A can behave like a prion.

3.3.2   TAU PRION PROTEINS

The soluble form of tau is a short peptide that is naturally unfolded.[69] Neuronal axons have a high concentration of this protein, which binds to microtubules and aids in their stability. Tau builds up in neurons as NFT in a variety of age-related disorders.[70]

There are numerous morphologies for the filamentous inclusions' hyperphosphorylated filaments. Tau deposits are common in a variety of neurodegenerative conditions. Thus, in addition to the conventional tauopathies mentioned below, tau deposits are also present in synucleinopathies such as Parkinson's disease (PD) and dementia with Lewy bodies (DLB). Frontotemporal dementia, Pick's disease, progressive supranuclear palsy, and corticobasal degeneration are all examples of classic tauopathies.[71] Neurons are not the only cells that have tau; glial cells like astrocytes and oligodendrocytes have been found to contain trace amounts, too. Tau deposits in glial cells (coiled bodies) are observed in a variety of tauopathies, including argyrophilic grains disease (AGD), white matter tauopathy with globular glial inclusion, and others (tangles). Mutations in the tau gene can lead to familial tauopathies including frontotemporal dementia with pica (FTDP) and other inherited types of frontotemporal dementia (MAPT).[72] Scientists have discovered that repeated brain concussions and other damage in sports and soldiers are linked to environmental factors that can lead to the development of chronic traumatic encephalopathy (CTE). Other tauopathies also exhibit A, FUS, and TDP-43/TDP-43 inclusions within cells, in addition to the ubiquitous Tau inclusions. The potential of MAPT mutations to produce disease and the prevalence of tau inclusions in sporadic tauopathies provide compelling evidence that the development of tau aggregation is a critical pathogenic mechanism.[73] Distinct cellular pathologies, preferred anatomical distributions of the aggregates, and symptom patterns characterize the several tauopathies that have been identified. There are six distinct tau isoforms in the human genome, all of which originate from alternative mRNA splicing and hence help account for this variation.[74-76]

In particular, the focus on the microtubule-binding domain (3R tau) is repeated four times in the other three isoforms, whereas three additional isoforms contain three repetitions (4R tau). It is interesting to note that the levels of these various isoforms vary widely among different tauopathies. Distinct tau isoforms may play different functions in disease pathology in a subsequent section on the subject of tau strains.[77-80] Researchers were curious about the potential for tau aggregates to spread and behave like prions in light of recent discoveries on the prion-like qualities of other protein aggregates and descriptions of the development of tau illness. In preliminary in vitro testing, recombinant tau seeds were found to accelerate inclusion formation in HEK293 cells. Both shortened and full-length tau variants (4R tau) were able to seed aggregation formation in separate cellular assays.

Furthermore, insoluble fractions from diseased human brains were used to seed in vitro-grown HEK293 cells containing tau inclusions. When the brain homogenate of transgenic mice expressing the mutant form of tau (P301S) was injected into the cortex or hippocampus of young transgenic mice expressing full-length human tau (ALZ17), the disease progressed more quickly and tau was deposited as NFT, neuropil threads, and glial globular inclusions.[81-85] Studies using homogenized brain material from individuals with various forms of tauopathies were also shown to produce deposits of tau opathy in animals expressing full-length human 4R tau or in wild-type mice. When sick brain material was injected into the brains of people with Parkinson's, Alzheimer's, or CBD disease, it replicated their respective clinical symptoms in vivo.[86-90] Wild-type animals injected with sonicated transgenic mouse brain material induced inclusion development, but only in the injection site. Synthetic tau, with the P301S or P301L mutation, was administered to predisposed transgenic mice's brains in similar trials, and these experiments led to early illness onset with a variety of

Propagation of Neurodegenerative disorders 65

pathologies, including dysfunctional or lost neurons, gliosis, and behavioral abnormalities.

Purified recombinant tau protein was able to induce disease without the assistance of any additional hosts or cofactors. Not just in AD, but also in other tauopathies, tau inclusions appear to include well-delineated anatomical regions that adhere to predefined temporal-spatial patterns. As noted above, tau pathology in Alzheimer's disease (AD) may be divided into six distinct phases, whereas in AGD, there are three distinct stages of disease development. Grain-rich tau is initially seen in the ambient gyrus, followed by the medial temporal lobe and the Cingulate Gyrus. AGD sufferers experience a steady decline in cognitive abilities as a result of these neuropathological changes.

Animal models have been used to investigate the pathological development of various tauopathies, including those proposed by Braak et al. and others. Synthetic tau fibrils injected intracerebrally led to inclusions that spread in a time-dependent manner between restricted anatomical regions.[91]

Synaptic connections may have a greater role in shaping this pattern of NFTs than the closeness of the related locations. Different genetic tau models of early AD, including those with region-specific promoters, have been demonstrated to display tau aggregates in nonexpressing regions; limited transgenic tau expression in the entorhinal cortex led to non-transgenic tau aggregates (NFTs) in the corresponding limbic regions. Research suggests that tau disease is not a cellular phenomenon but rather behaves like a prion.[92]

3.3.3 α-SYNUCLEIN PRIONS

Like the aggregation-prone proteins mentioned before, this one is a small protein with a poorly defined tertiary structure and a high propensity to be in a folded state. Syn, a membrane-binding protein, is abundant in presynaptic terminals.[93] When two membranes are joined, it causes them to curve and form a tube by inserting itself between the phospholipid head groups of the outer membrane. The function of Syn as a chaperone in controlling the kinetics of endo- and exocytosis is also being studied.[94]

By virtue of its dynamic structural properties, Syn is capable of displaying a wide range of different functions. This means that new aggregates may develop, for example, near the membrane where the

Syn is heavily concentrated. DLB, Parkinson's disease (PD), and other uncommon disorders with pure autonomic dysfunction all have high levels of aggregated Syn.[95] Lewy pathology must be confirmed postmortem in order to correctly diagnose Parkinson's disease or DLB.

Neurons in MSA sufferers have Syn inclusions, however this is only seen in the latter stages of the illness. This Syn accumulates in two different types of cells: Schwann cells (called glial cytoplasmic inclusions in the case of Schwann cells) and oligodendrocytes (known as glial cytoplasmic inclusions).[96]

An oligodendropathy, MSA is the predominant one, and its origins are yet unexplained. Spontaneous occurrences of PD, DLB, and MSA make up the great majority of cases. As a result, scientists are now aware of a number of genetic variants that might cause family forms of Parkinson's disease (PD).

The gene load is negatively correlated with the age of onset in instances of gene multiplications, indicating that disease progression is affected by the amount of wild-type Syn.[97]

Since syn aggregates can act as seeds, they can initiate the transformation of a soluble precursor into a potentially dangerous assembly, as in vitro research has shown already two decades ago. Only a decade ago were scientists alerted to the idea that misfolded protein complexes may spread disease throughout the brain. Two investigations identified Lewy bodies in neural transplants given to Parkinson's patients more than ten years before death.[98] Lewy bodies in grafts were hypothesized to be activated by host factors in a non-cell-autonomous manner, and when it was proposed that cell-to-cell transferred misfolded Syn may be the trigger, opinions were divided.

Prion-like proliferation in the absence of sick material was required to demonstrate that Syn may act as a causal agent for synucleinopathies, and this was accomplished by demonstrating that pure Syn assemblies could do so. In the first two trials, wild-type and transgenic mice were given brain injections of aggregated mouse Syn lacking the C-terminus.[99]

Time-dependent protein spreading and aggregation was triggered by these synthetic assemblies. Human recombinant protein-based syn aggregates also demonstrated the ability to cause synucleinopathy, although at a slower pace. Analysis of the seeding efficacy of different assemblies revealed that stable Syn fibrillar seeds had greater nucleating capacities than smaller but unstable synthetic oligomers that did not exhibit prion characteristics in vivo.[100]

Propagation of Neurodegenerative disorders 67

3.3.4 HUNTINGTON PRIONS

HD, in contrast to the majority of suspected prion-like illnesses, is passed on entirely via the family. Polyglutamine (polyQ) or trinucleotide disorder is characterized by a wide range of neurological symptoms, including gradual mental decline and motor dysfunction. When CAG repetitions grow too large, the protein becomes more likely to combine into abnormal assemblies, causing polyQ disorders. Exon 1 of the IT15 gene, which encodes the Htt protein, has glutamine repeats in people with hereditary HD.[101] The normal Htt protein contains between six and 35 glutamine residues, and no one has been reported to have HD if they have less than 36 glutamine residues. The disease is only partially penetrating at 35–41 repeats, and it is fully penetrating at 41 repeats or more. It has been found that a longer polyQ insert promotes protein assembly.[102] A correlation between the number of repetitions in an aggregating protein and its toxicity points to a connection between protein folding and toxicity. Despite the fact that HD is a degenerative disease, the relationship between aggregate formation and disease progression is not well understood. There is an association between neuronal Htt inclusions and striatal and frontoparietal cortex atrophy and progressive neuronal death.[103] There are inclusions in the perikaryon's cytosol and nucleus that are mostly made up of N-terminally truncated mutant Htt (mHTT).

It is not yet proven that nonscavenged assemblies, such as those found in inclusion bodies, are responsible for disease etiology and prion-like spread.

Scientists have observed the proliferation of misfolded versions of Htt in an in vitro experiment using mutant or aggregated Htt. Large amounts of membrane-bound mHtt can be transported to postsynaptic neurons or glial cells via a variety of ways.[104]

Non-cell-autonomous synaptic alterations and cell damage were demonstrated to be caused by the transferred spreading particles.

Using brain extracts from mutant mice or people with HD, researchers were able to determine that mHTT had a self-replicating nature in vitro. No studies have shown that Htt aggregates can successfully recruit the wild-type form. Transplantation of fibroblasts from people with mHTT-related disorders, like Parkinson's, into the striatum of wild-type mice, led to the transmission of the disease. Transmitted mHTT caused cell death and cognitive deficits in this experimental paradigm.[105] Neuronal tissue implanted into the striatum of HD patients has been shown to contain Htt aggregates. After just a few years, these brain transplants showed evidence of deterioration.

Tissue toxicity may be caused by factors other than defective genes, such as the host environment, even when no defective genes are expressed in a patient's transplanted tissue, according to the findings of this study.[106]

Although there is mounting evidence for a prion-like mechanism in HD sickness etiology, much more research is needed to definitively label HD as a prion disease.

3.4 PHYSICAL, FUNCTIONAL, AND PATHOGENIC CHARACTERISTICS OF PRIONS

Prion disorders are commonly associated with prions; however, they also play a natural function in bodies that does not lead to illness. In bacteria, yeast, fungus, and mammals, prion traits have been reported, but many more are likely to be found in the future.[107]

Yeast prions like Sup35p were among the first to be found. Translation is terminated by the Sup35p prion, which sequesters its functional form by binding and sequestering it.

Because the physiologically active and soluble form is no longer able to attach to DNA, it is suppressed. Thus, yeast cells will produce unique genetic products and different yeast phenotypes that may confer a survival advantage.[108]

An additional type of fungal prion is the heterokaryon incompatibility protein s (HET-s). There is a protein-based genetic factor called HET-s that controls programmed cell death in fungi. The prion domain is noninfectious due to its inherently disordered sequence, which is surrounded by a globular region.[109] This is reminiscent of the modular structure of polyQ prions like Htt and ataxins, whose infectiousness increases with the length of their polyQ tracts or after cleavage of their globular domain. Like other prion-like domains, polyQ sequences are often rich in polar or hydrophobic amino acids, which facilitate homotypic oligomerization. Since the HET-s protein acts as an inhibitor, prions with nucleating HET-s mutations can only be passed on from mother to daughter cells during mitosis (in cis).[110] This sequence mismatch will make the prion-like form of this cis-acting element less likely to seed and aggregate.

Propagation of Neurodegenerative disorders   69

Mammalian cells also contain nonpathogenic prion-like proteins. Examples that have been extensively studied include the cytoplasmic polyadenylation element-binding protein and the T-cell restricted intracellular antigen 1(TIA-1). Multiple RNA-binding domains as well as a glutamine-rich domain similar to the PrP domain are present in TIA-1. TDP-43-like stress granules or membraneless organelles are formed during reversible oligomerization and liquid–liquid phase separation, leading to membraneless organelles similar to TDP-43 and FUS. It is possible for the liquid TIA-1 complexes that form microaggregates to solidify in response to stress or situations that boost the production of TIA-1, leading to bigger cytoplasmic inclusions with an abundance of -sheets. A series of protein misfolding and amplification occurs when TIA-1 assembles into insoluble seeds under experimental circumstances, propagating its soluble precursor.

TIA-1, in contrast to TDP-43 and FUS, which have nearly comparable activities in mammalian cells, does not seem to be harmful. These examples demonstrate that proteins in diverse species may have amyloid or prion-like characteristics in both soluble and insoluble states. Each protein requires these features in order to perform its unique biological function.[111]

3.5 NEURODEGENERATIVE DISEASES AND PRIONS

Natural selection, or lack thereof, may have favored certain proteins to normally exist as amyloid or prion forms. Additional proteins have evolved to reside near to the limits of their own solubility due to evolutionary pressure.[112] As it turns out, a number of pathogenic and nonpathogenic proteins have inverse correlations with their aggregation rates, including the PrP, tau, A, and Syn. Rather than just being owing to their sequence, proteins' propensity for aggregation may be determined by factors such as hydrophobicity or polarity, not only by the sequence itself. Genetic mutations or unidentified environmental factors that influence protein production or folding could favor the thermodynamically stable amyloid form. Some glutamate-rich proteins, such A, tau, and aSyn, are known to be innately disordered and to contain a prion domain (PrP, TDP-43, or FUS) (Htt or ataxins).[113]

The hydrophobic or polar residues of amyloidogenic or prionlike proteins are often exposed and clustered between these residues during the earliest stages of misfolding and amyloid formation in order to shield them from the surrounding aqueous environment.[114]

A hydrophobic collapse will result in tiny, amorphous assemblies with a -sheet shape, which are hydrophobic. Stress granules, for example, undergo a functional and reversible conformational change (TDP-43, FUS, and TIA-1). These assemblies are not very damaging to cells because they are unstable and can be broken down by the cellular degradation machinery. Toxic, stable, and able to seed further aggregation stages, these assemblies can be generated when the configuration of small aggregations changes.[115] Aggregation occurs in vivo only after long periods of time due to the substantial kinetic barriers that these stages impose. Despite these kinetic limitations, proteins' propensity to generate nucleating molecules may be influenced in a number of ways. Syn are found in the brain in quantities that approach or even surpass their solubility, which is the case with Syn.[116]

In their natural physiological environment, these prion-like proteins are predisposed to amyloid production at all times. When proteins with prion-like features create spreading species is the question here, not why. Soluble precursor proteins may be seeded onto this stable template after they have passed the kinetic threshold in a shifting energy environment. The existence of soluble monomers in folding equilibrium with their seed is critical to the formation of fibrils.[117] To ensure homotypic seeding, not all monomers will be able to form complexes with the template. The sequences must be similar enough, and there must be a common intermediate assembly state, for this to be possible resembles the seed's shape in order for it to be able to accept the seed's monomer. It is impossible to directly seed heterotypic seeding between proteins like tau and Syn because of their lack of common sequence.[118] A rupturing protofibrillar particle that has the potential to hasten further aggregation processes may be made from the inclusion of misfolded assemblies even if there are none of the previously mentioned amplification barriers to do so.

3.6 TRANSPORT AND CELL-TO-CELL DIVERSION MECHANISMS

3.6.1 *TRANSMISSION OF PRIONS*

Studies are being conducted to learn more about the toxicity of proteopathic chemicals and how they cause disease. Researcher postulate that seeding-potent particles, which may replicate and spread from neuron to neuron, are responsible for the emergence and spread of toxic inclusions.

Propagation of Neurodegenerative disorders 71

Some researchers believe that illness initiation and progression may be the result of a cell-autonomous process that includes selective vulnerability.[119] A combination of genetic and environmental factors, this theory posits, leads to cellular damage and increases the susceptibility of already fragile neurons to further degeneration. It has been postulated, for instance, that a selective vulnerability could explain why protein aggregation gradually accumulates in connected brain areas, and that an inflammatory reaction in one location could spread and create sickness inside a neighboring brain area.[120]

The most well-known disease caused by the transformation of an endogenous protein into a toxic amyloid is prionsc.

After obtaining an alternate conformation (PrPsc), endogenous PrPc becomes toxic and self-perpetuates, caused by protein aggregation and subsequent spread. The transmission of infectious prion particles (PrPsc) in TSEs such as Kuru, CJD, and others is facilitated by neural connections.[121] It has been established that PrPsc prions propagate in the brain through neuronal connections rather than diffusion via axonal projections after they have entered the brain.[122]

When administered to the peripheral nervous system, PrPsc prions travel to the spinal cord and lower brainstem through peripheral organ neurons (prions replicate first in the lymphoreticular system).

Although it is commonly understood that cells pick up infectious particles and pass them on to their surrounding cells, the exact mechanism by which TSE prions spread from neurons to other cells remains unknown. The endoplasmic reticulum synthesizes PrPc, and exosomes deliver it to the cell's outer membrane.[123]

Endosomes, lysosomes, and multivesicular bodies may then become involved in the process of internalization and localization. Researchers have found that PrPsc replicates in lipid organelles and the plasma membrane in vitro studies.

3.6.2   DIAGNOSTIC STRATEGIES

Clinical experiments to reduce disease progression have mostly failed despite many attempts in recent years. It is possible that the medicine has not made it into the brain, or that means that either the therapeutic target has not been triggered or the therapeutic chemical is not performing as intended. The most serious shortcoming is that the majority of trials have only included patients who are already in the last stages of their illness, when it may be too late to save their lives. As a result, diagnostic techniques that can detect illness at an early stage are desired, allowing therapy to begin sooner. Before irrevocable harm is done, we need to begin therapy.[124]

For this, we need to create diagnostic instruments that are more sensitive and trustworthy. The discovery of prion strains offers a fresh perspective on how to approach this issue.

Knowing which prion strain a patient has could be useful in developing novel positron emission tomography (PET) tracers. PET ligands are delivered to the brain where they bind to their target with reversible kinetics. The -sheets of extracellular a plaques bind to many PET tracers with high affinity, which has led to their effective therapeutic application. PET tracers, however, still have some problems concerning their binding qualities.[125] Researchers do not know precisely how ligands attach to plaques because of the mystery surrounding an aggregation nature. However, in other brain areas where plaques have a unique architecture, some radiotracers show high affinity but have little affinity for deposits in the cortex or cerebellum.[126] The binding characteristics of PET ligands in patients' brains seem to be influenced by structural differences in PET ligands. Discovering the molecular structure of strains will hopefully lead to the development of imaging tools that can detect and diagnose specific forms of Alzheimer's disease and other prion-like illnesses. Tracers used in PET scans have been shown to bind to amyloid proteins like tau and Syn with high affinity in vitro.[127]

Other diagnostic methods may make advantage of seeding-potent particles found in peripheral tissues or fluids. Due to their widespread distribution beyond the brain, misfolded proteins can be detected in extremely low concentrations using methods such as the protein misfolding cyclic amplification (PMCA) assay (which will go into more depth about in the last section). To perform seeded amplification with biological material, the recombinant monomer utilized in PMCA is introduced to a reaction buffer.[128] In the presence of seeds, the soluble monomers incorporate themselves into the seed. Sonicating the amplified product yields seeding-competent assemblies. Multiple iterations of a seeded growth and amplification chain reaction are carried out. PMCA has been used for the diagnosis of CJD by detecting PrPsc, and it is also being used for the diagnosis of AD and PD at the present time.[128]

3.7 CONCLUSION

Prion-like processes that cause progressive protein misfolding illnesses are currently the subject of a wide range of studies. Further research is needed to confirm the prion theory, which now encompasses other neurodegenerative disorders. Proteins that misfold in a neurodegenerative illness may seed and increase damage, according to the developing picture. Protein inclusions and disease pathology are transmitted via specific anatomical channels as a consequence. Proteinaceous particles that form clusters may be hazardous to cells and non-cells alike. Seeding nucleation may be hindered by a variety of reasons. Understanding the pathology of the disease and the architecture of different prion strains may lead to the development of novel therapeutics and diagnostics. This study gives us hope that one day we will be able to develop disease-modifying treatments for neurodegenerative diseases by preventing the spread of seeding-potent assemblies.

KEYWORDS

- **prion viruses**
- **prion-like proteins**
- **Lewy bodies**
- **amyotrophic lateral sclerosis**
- **argyrophilic grains disease**
- **polyQ disorders**

REFERENCES

1. Prusiner, S. B. Novel Proteinaceous Infectious Particles Cause Scrapie. *Science* **1982,** *216,* 136–144.
2. Caughey, B.; Race, R. E.; Chesebro, B. Detection of Prion Protein mRNA in Normal and Scrapie-Infected Tissues and Cell Lines. *J. Gen. Virol.* **1988,** 69 (Pt 3), 711–716.
3. Pan, K. M. et al. Conversion of Alpha-Helices Into Beta-Sheets Features in the Formation of the Scrapie Prion Proteins. *Proc. Natl. Acad. Sci. USA* **1993,** *90,* 10962–10966.
4. Prusiner, S. B. Prions. *Proc. Natl. Acad. Sci. USA* **1998,** *95,* 13363–13383.

5. Williamson, J.; Goldman, J.; Marder, K. S. Genetic Aspects of Alzheimer Disease. *Neurologist* **2009**, *15*, 80–86.

6. Armstrong, R. A.; Nochlin, D.; Bird, T. D. Neuropathological Heterogeneity in Alzheimer's Disease: A Study of 80 Cases Using Principal Components Analysis. *Neuropathology* **2000**, *20*, 31–37.

7. Chui, H. C.; Teng, E. L.; Henderson, V. W.; Moy, A. C. Clinical Subtypes of Dementia of the Alzheimer Type. *Neurology* **1985**, *35*, 1544–1550.

8. Askanas, V.; Engel, W. K. Inclusion-Body Myositis: A Myodegenerative Conformational Disorder Associated with Abeta, Protein Misfolding, and Proteasome Inhibition. *Neurology* **2006**, *66*, S39–S48.

9. Glenner, G. G.; Wong, C. W. Alzheimer's Disease: Initial Report of the Purification and Characterization of a Novel Cerebrovascular Amyloid Protein. *Biochem. Biophys. Res. Commun.* **1984**, *120*, 885–890.

10. Goedert, M. et al. From Genetics to Pathology: Tau and Alpha-Synuclein Assemblies in Neurodegenerative Diseases. *Philos Trans R Soc Lond B Biol Sci.* **2001**, *356*, 213–227.

11. Polymeropoulos, M. H. et al. Mutation in the Alpha-Synuclein Gene Identified in Families with Parkinson's Disease. *Science* **1997**, *276*, 2045–2047.

12. Zarranz, J. J. et al. The New Mutation, E46K, of Alpha-Synuclein Causes Parkinson and Lewy Body Dementia. *Ann. Neurol.* **2004**, *55*, 164–173.

13. Ibanez, P. et al. Causal Relation Between Alpha-Synuclein Gene Duplication and Familial Parkinson's Disease. *Lancet* **2004**, *364*, 1169–1171.

14. Singleton, A. B. et al. alpha-Synuclein Locus Triplication Causes Parkinson's Disease. *Science* **2003**, *302*, 841.

15. Chartier-Harlin, M. C. et al. Alpha-Synuclein Locus Duplication as a Cause of Familial Parkinson's Disease. *Lancet* **2004**, *364*, 1167–1169.

16. Ironside, J. W.; Ritchie, D. L.; Head, M. W. Phenotypic Variability in Human Prion Diseases. *Neuropathol Appl Neurobiol.* **2005**, *31*, 565–579.

17. Wadsworth, J. D.; Collinge, J. Update on Human Prion Disease. *Biochim. Biophys. Acta* **2007**, *1772*, 598–609.

18. Hsiao, K. et al. Linkage of a Prion Protein Missense Variant to Gerstmann-Straussler Syndrome. *Nature* **1989**, *338*, 342–345.

19. Gajdusek, D. C. Unconventional Viruses and the Origin and Disappearance of Kuru. *Science* **1977**, *197*, 943–960.

20. Prusiner, S. B. Prion diseases and the BSE crisis. *Science.* **1997**, *278*, 245–251.

21. Bessen, R. A. et al. Non-Genetic Propagation of Strain-Specific Properties of Scrapie Prion Protein. *Nature* **1995**, *375*, 698–700.

22. Telling, G. C. et al. Evidence for the Conformation of the Pathologic Isoform of the Prion Protein Enciphering and Propagating Prion Diversity. *Science* **1996**, *274*, 2079–2082.

23. Safar, J. et al. Eight Prion Strains Have PrP(Sc) Molecules with Different Conformations. *Nat. Med.* **1998**, *4*, 1157–1165.

24. Legname, G. et al. Continuum of Prion Protein Structures Enciphers a Multitude of Prion Isolate-Specified Phenotypes. *Proc. Natl. Acad. Sci. USA* **2006**, *103*, 19105–19110.

25. Tanaka, M.; Collins, S. R.; Toyama, B. H.; Weissman, J. S. The Physical Basis of How Prion Conformations Determine Strain Phenotypes. *Nature* **2006**, *442*, 585–589.

26. Toyama, B. H.; Kelly, M. J.; Gross, J. D.; Weissman, J. S. The Structural Basis of Yeast Prion Strain Variants. *Nature* **2007**, *449*, 233–237.

Propagation of Neurodegenerative disorders

27. Frost, B.; Ollesch, J.; Wille, H.; Diamond, M. I. Conformational Diversity of Wild-Type Tau Fibrils Specified by Templated Conformation Change. *J. Biol. Chem.* **2009**, *284*, 3546–3551.
28. Petkova, A. T. et al. Self-Propagating, Molecular-Level Polymorphism in Alzheimer's Beta-Amyloid Fibrils. *Science* **2005**, *307*, 262–265.
29. Yonetani, M. et al. Conversion of Wild-Type Alpha-Synuclein into Mutant-Type Fibrils and Its Propagation in the Presence of A30P Mutant. *J. Biol. Chem.* **2009**, *284*, 7940–7950.
30. von Bergen, M. et al. Assembly of Tau Protein into Alzheimer Paired Helical Filaments Depends on a Local Sequence Motif ((306)VQIVYK(311)) Forming Beta Structure. *Proc. Natl. Acad. Sci. USA* **2000**, *97*, 5129–5134.
31. Fishman, S. L.; Murray, J. M.; Eng, F. J.; Walewski, J. L.; Morgello, S.; Branch, A. D. Molecular and Bioinformatic Evidence of Hepatitis C Virus Evolution in Brain. *J. Infect. Dis.* **2008**, *197* (4), 597–607. DOI: 10.1086/526519.
32. Fletcher, N. F.; McKeating, J. A. Hepatitis C Virus and the Brain. *J. Viral. Hepat.* **2012**, *19* (5), 301–306. DOI: 10.1111/j.1365-2893.2012.01591.x.
33. Frank, S. Treatment of Huntington's Disease. *Neurother. J. Am. Soc. Exp. NeuroTher.* **2014**, *11* (1), 153–160. DOI: 10.1007/s13311-013-0244-z.
34. Frontzek, K.; Lutz, M. I.; Aguzzi, A.; Kovacs, G. G.; Budka, H. Amyloid-Beta Pathology and Cerebral Amyloid Angiopathy Are Frequent in Iatrogenic Creutzfeldt–Jakob Disease After Dural Grafting. *Swiss Med. Wkly.* **2016**, *146*, w14287. DOI: 10.4414/smw.2016.14287.
35. Frost, B.; Diamond, M. I. Prion-Like Mechanisms in Neurodegenerative Diseases. *Nat. Rev. Neurosci.* **2010**, *11* (3):155–159. DOI: 10.1038/nrn2786.
36. Gaughwin, P. M.; Ciesla, M.; Lahiri, N.; Tabrizi, S. J.; Brundin, P.; Bjorkqvist, M. Hsa-miR-34b Is a Plasma-Stable microRNA That Is Elevated in Pre-Manifest Huntington's Disease. *Hum. Mol. Genet.* **2011**, *20* (11), 2225–2237. DOI: 10.1093/hmg/ddr111.
37. Geekiyanage, H.; Chan, C. MicroRNA-137/181c Regulates Serine Palmitoyltransferase and in Turn Amyloid Beta, Novel Targets in Sporadic Alzheimer's Disease. *J. Neurosci. Off. J. Soc. Neurosci.* **2011**, *31* (41), 14820–14830. DOI: 10.1523/JNEUROSCI.3883-11.2011.
38. Geekiyanage, H.; Jicha, G. A.; Nelson, P. T.; Chan, C. Blood serum miRNA: non-invasive biomarkers for Alzheimer's disease. *Exp Neurol.* **2012**, 235(2):491–496. DOI: 10.1016/j.expneurol.2011.11.026.
39. Goedert, M. Neurodegeneration. Alzheimer's and Parkinson's Diseases: The Prion Concept in Relation to Assembled Abeta, Tau, and Alpha-Synuclein. *Science* **2015**, *349* (6248), 1255555. DOI: 10.1126/science.1255555.
40. Goedert, M.; Falcon, B.; Clavaguera, F.; Tolnay, M. Prion-Like Mechanisms in the Pathogenesis of Tauopathies and Synucleinopathies. *Curr. Neurol. Neurosci. Rep.* **2014**, *14* (11), 495. DOI: 10.1007/s11910-014-0495-z.
41. Goedert, M.; Masuda-Suzukake, M.; Falcon, B. Like Prions: The Propagation of Aggregated Tau and Alpha-Synuclein in Neurodegeneration. *Brain J. Neurol.* 2016. DOI: 10.1093/brain/aww230.
42. González-Scarano, F.; Martín-García, J. The Neuropathogenesis of AIDS. *Nat. Rev. Immunol.* **2005**, *5* (1), 69–81. DOI: 10.1038/nri1527.

43. Grad, L. I.; Fernando, S. M.; Cashman, N. R. From Molecule to Molecule and Cell to Cell: Prion-Like Mechanisms in Amyotrophic Lateral Sclerosis. *Neurobiol. Dis.* **2015,** *77,* 257–265. DOI: 10.1016/j.nbd.2015.02.009.

44. Heaton, R. K.; Franklin, D. R.; Ellis, R. J.; McCutchan, J. A.; Letendre, S. L.; Leblanc, S. et al. HIV-Associated Neurocognitive Disorders Before and During the Era of Combination Antiretroviral Therapy: Differences in Rates, Nature, and Predictors. *J. Neurovirol.* **2011,** *17* (1), 3–16. DOI: 10.1007/s13365-010-0006-1.

45. Hebert, S. S.; Horre, K.; Nicolai, L.; Papadopoulou, A. S.; Mandemakers, W.; Silahtaroglu, A. N. et al. Loss of microRNA Cluster miR-29a/b-1 in Sporadic Alzheimer's Disease Correlates with Increased BACE1/Beta-Secretase Expression. *Proc. Natl. Acad. Sci. USA* **2008,** *105* (17), 6415–6420. DOI: 10.1073/pnas.0710263105.

46. Hernandez-Rapp, J.; Martin-Lanneree, S.; Hirsch, T. Z.; Launay, J. M.; Mouillet-Richard, S. Hijacking PrP(c)-Dependent Signal Transduction: When Prions Impair Abeta Clearance. *Front. Aging Neurosci.* **2014,** *6*, 25. DOI: 10.3389/fnagi.2014.00025.

47. Hill, J. M.; Lukiw, W. J. MicroRNA (miRNA)-Mediated Pathogenetic Signaling in Alzheimer's Disease (AD). *Neurochem. Res.* **2016,** *41* (1–2), 96–100. DOI: 10.1007/s11064-015-1734-7.

48. Hill, J. M.; Clement, C.; Pogue, A. I.; Bhattacharjee, S.; Zhao, Y.; Lukiw, W. J. Pathogenic Microbes, the Microbiome, and Alzheimer's Disease (AD) *Front. Aging Neurosci.* **2014,** *6*, 127. DOI: 10.3389/fnagi.2014.00127.

49. Hock, E. M.; Polymenidou, M. Prion-Like Propagation as a Pathogenic Principle in Frontotemporal Dementia. *J. Neurochem.* **2016,** *138* (Suppl 1), 163–183. DOI: 10.1111/jnc.13668.

50. Hong, Z.; Shi, M.; Chung, K. A.; Quinn, J. F.; Peskind, E. R.; Galasko, D. et al. DJ-1 and Alpha-Synuclein In Human Cerebrospinal Fluid as Biomarkers of Parkinson's Disease. *Brain J. Neurol.* **2010,** 133(Pt 3):713–726. DOI: 10.1093/brain/awq008.

51. Idda, M. L.; Munk, R.; Abdelmohsen, K.; Gorospe, M. Noncoding RNAs in Alzheimer's disease. *Wiley Interdiscip Rev RNA.* 2018 DOI: 10.1002/wrna.1463.

52. Itzhaki, R. F. Herpes simplex virus type 1 and Alzheimer's Disease: Increasing Evidence for a Major Role of the Virus. *Front. Aging Neurosci.* **2014,** *6*, 202. DOI: 10.3389/fnagi.2014.00202.

53. Jarosz-Griffiths, H. H.; Noble, E.; Rushworth, J. V.; Hooper, N. M. Amyloid-Beta Receptors: The Good, the Bad, and the Prion Protein. *J. Biol. Chem.* **2016,** *291* (7), 3174–3183. DOI: 10.1074/jbc.R115.702704.

54. Jucker, M.; Walker, L. C. Pathogenic Protein Seeding in Alzheimer Disease and Other Neurodegenerative Disorders. *Ann. Neurol.* **2011,** *70* (4), 532–540. DOI: 10.1002/ana.22615.

55. Karim, S.; Mirza, Z.; Kamal, M. A.; Abuzenadah, A. M.; Azhar, E. I.; Al-Qahtani, M. H. et al. The Role of Viruses in Neurodegenerative and Neurobehavioral Diseases. *CNS Neurol. Disord. Drug. Targets.* **2014,** *13* (7), 1213–1223. DOI: 10.2174/18715 2731307141015122638.

56. Katsarou, K.; Rao, A. L.; Tsagris, M.; Kalantidis, K. Infectious Long Non-Coding RNAs. *Biochimie.* **2015,** *117*, 37–47. DOI: 10.1016/j.biochi.2015.05.005.

57. Khan, M. B.; Lang, M. J.; Huang M-B, Raymond, A.; Bond, V. C.; Shiramizu, B. et al. Nef Exosomes Isolated from the Plasma of Individuals with HIV-Associated

Dementia (HAD) Can Induce Aβ(1-42) Secretion in SH-SY5Y Neural Cells. *J. Neurovirol.* **2016,** *22* (2), 179–190. DOI: 10.1007/s13365-015-0383-6.

58. Khodr, C. E.; Becerra, A.; Han, Y.; Bohn, M. C. Targeting Alpha-Synuclein with a microRNA-Embedded Silencing Vector in the Rat Substantia Nigra: Positive and Negative Effects. *Brain Res.* **2014,** *1550,* 47–60. DOI: 10.1016/j.brainres.2014.01.010.

59. Khoo, S. K.; Petillo, D.; Kang, U. J.; Resau, J. H.; Berryhill, B.; Linder, J. et al. Plasma-Based Circulating MicroRNA Biomarkers for Parkinson's Disease. *J. Parkinson's Dis.* **2012,** *2* (4), 321–331. DOI: 10.3233/JPD-012144.

60. Kumar, P.; Dezso, Z.; MacKenzie, C.; Oestreicher, J.; Agoulnik, S.; Byrne, M. et al. Circulating miRNA Biomarkers for Alzheimer's Disease. *PLoS ONE.* **2013,** *8* (7). e69807. DOI: 10.1371/journal.pone.0069807.

61. Braak, H.; Braak, E. Neuropathological Staging of Alzheimer-Related Changes. *Acta Neuropathol.* **1991,** *82,* 239–259.

62. Seeley, W. W.; Crawford, R. K.; Zhou, J.; Miller, B. L.; Greicius, M. D. Neurodegenerative Diseases Target Large-Scale Human Brain Networks. *Neuron* **2009,** *62,* 42–52.

63. Hobson, P.; Meara, J. The Detection of Dementia and Cognitive Impairment in a Community Population of Elderly People with Parkinson's Disease by Use of the CAMCOG Neuropsychological Test. *Age Ageing* **1999,** *28,* 39–43.

64. Cudkowicz, M.; Qureshi, M.; Shefner, J. Measures and Markers in Amyotrophic Lateral Sclerosis. *NeuroRx* **2004,** *1,* 273–283.

65. Glatzel, M.; Aguzzi, A. PrP(C) Expression in the Peripheral Nervous System Is a Determinant of Prion Neuroinvasion. *J. Gen. Virol.* **2000,** *81,* 2813–2821.

66. Brown, P.; Preece, M. A.; Will, R. G. "Friendly Fire" in Medicine: Hormones, Homografts, and Creutzfeldt-Jakob Disease. *Lancet* **1992,** *340,* 24–27.

67. Beekes, M.; McBride, P. A.; Baldauf, E. Cerebral Targeting Indicates Vagal Spread of Infection in Hamsters Fed with Scrapie. *J. Gen. Virol.* **1998,** *79* (Pt 3):601–607.

68. Fraser, H. Neuronal Spread of Scrapie Agent and Targeting of Lesions Within the Retino-Tectal Pathway. *Nature* **1982,** *295,* 149–150.

69. Brandner, S. et al. Normal Host Prion Protein (PrPC) Is Required for Scrapie Spread Within the Central Nervous System. *Proc. Natl. Acad. Sci. USA* **1996,** *93,* 13148–13151.

70. Magalhaes, A. C. et al. Uptake and Neuritic Transport of Scrapie Prion Protein Coincident with Infection of Neuronal Cells. J Neurosci. **2005,** *25,* 5207–5216.

71. Fevrier, B. et al. Cells Release Prions in Association with Exosomes. *Proc. Natl. Acad. Sci. USA* **2004,** *101,* 9683–9688.

72. Gousset, K. et al. Prions Hijack Tunnelling Nanotubes for Intercellular Spread. *Nat. Cell Biol.* **2009,** *11,* 328–336.

73. Gerdes, H. H.; Carvalho, R. N. Intercellular Transfer Mediated by Tunneling Nanotubes. *Curr. Opin. Cell Biol.* **2008,** *20,* 470–475.

74. Li, J. Y. et al. Lewy Bodies in Grafted Neurons in Subjects with Parkinson's Disease Suggest Host-to-Graft Disease Propagation. *Nat. Med.* **2008,** *14,* 501–503.

75. Kordower, J. H.; Chu, Y.; Hauser, R. A.; Olanow, C. W.; Freeman, T. B. Transplanted Dopaminergic Neurons Develop PD Pathologic Changes: A Second Case Report. *Mov. Disord.* **2008,** *23,* 2303–2306.

76. Kordower, J. H.; Chu, Y.; Hauser, R. A.; Freeman, T. B.; Olanow, C. W. Lewy Body-Like Pathology in Long-Term Embryonic Nigral Transplants in Parkinson's Disease. *Nat. Med.* **2008,** *14,* 504–506.

77. Desplats, P. et al. Inclusion Formation and Neuronal Cell Death Through Neuron-to-Neuron Transmission of Alpha-Synuclein. *Proc. Natl. Acad. Sci. USA* **2009,** *106,* 13010–13015.
78. Yang, W.; Dunlap, J. R.; Andrews, R. B.; Wetzel, R. Aggregated Polyglutamine Peptides Delivered to Nuclei Are Toxic to Mammalian Cells. *Hum. Mol. Genet.* **2002,** *11,* 2905–2917.
79. Lee, H. J. et al. Assembly-Dependent Endocytosis and Clearance of Extracellular Alphasynuclein. *Int. J. Biochem. Cell Biol.* **2008,** *40,* 1835–1849.
80. Frost, B.; Jacks, R. L.; Diamond, M. I. Propagation of Tau Misfolding from the Outside to the Inside of a Cell. *J. Biol. Chem.* **2009,** *284,* 12845–12852.
81. Ren, P. H. et al. Cytoplasmic Penetration and Persistent Infection of Mammalian Cells by Polyglutamine Aggregates. *Nat. Cell Biol.* **2009,** *11,* 219–225.
82. Krammer, C. et al. The Yeast Sup35NM Domain Propagates as a Prion in Mammalian Cells. *Proc. Natl. Acad. Sci. USA* **2009,** *106,* 462–467.
83. Meyer-Luehmann, M. et al. Exogenous Induction of Cerebral Beta-Amyloidogenesis Is Governed by Agent and Host. *Science* **2006,** *313,* 1781–1784.
84. Clavaguera, F. et al. Transmission and Spreading of Tauopathy in Transgenic Mouse Brain. *Nat Cell Biol.* **2009,** *11,* 909–913.
85. Werdelin, O.; Ranlov, P. Amyloidosis in Mice Produced by Transplantation of Spleen Cells from Casein-Treated Mice. *Acta Pathol. Microbiol. Scand.* **1966,** *68,* 1–18. [PubMed] [Google Scholar].
86. Westermark, G. T.; Westermark, P. Serum Amyloid A and Protein AA: Molecular Mechanisms of a Transmissible Amyloidosis. *FEBS Lett.* **2009,** *583,* 2685–2690.
87. Lundmark, K. et al. Transmissibility of Systemic Amyloidosis by a Prion-Like Mechanism. *Proc. Natl. Acad. Sci. USA* **2002,** *99,* 6979–6984.
88. Mendez, O. E.; Shang, J.; Jungreis, C. A.; Kaufer, D. I. Diffusion-weighted MRI in Creutzfeldt-Jakob Disease: A Better Diagnostic Marker Than CSF Protein 14-3-3? J Neuroimaging. **2003,** *13,* 147–151.
89. Asuni, A. A.; Boutajangout, A.; Quartermain, D.; Sigurdsson, E. M. Immunotherapy Targeting Pathological Tau Conformers in a Tangle Mouse Model Reduces Brain Pathology with Associated Functional Improvements. *J. Neurosci.* **2007,** *27,* 9115–9129.
90. Masliah, E. et al. Effects of Alpha-Synuclein Immunization in a Mouse Model of Parkinson's Disease. *Neuron.* **2005,** *46,* 857–868.
91. Nekooki-Machida, Y. et al. Distinct Conformations of In Vitro and In Vivo Amyloids of Huntingtin-Exon1 Show Different Cytotoxicity. *Proc. Natl. Acad. Sci. USA* **2009,** *106,* 9679–9684.
92. Ren, P. H.; Lauckner, J. E.; Kachirskaia, I.; Heuser, J. E.; Melki, R.; Kopito, R. R. Cytoplasmic Penetration and Persistent Infection of Mammalian Cells by Polyglutamine Aggregates. *Nat. Cell Biol.* **2009,** *11* (2), 219–225. DOI: 10.1038/ncb1830.
93. Roth, W.; Hecker, D.; Fava, E. Systems Biology Approaches to the Study of Biological Networks Underlying Alzheimer's Disease: Role of miRNAs. *Methods Mol. Biol.* **2016,** *1303,* 349–377. DOI: 10.1007/978-1-4939-2627-5_21.
94. Rudge, P.; Jaunmuktane, Z.; Adlard, P.; Bjurstrom, N.; Caine, D.; Lowe, J. et al. Iatrogenic CJD due to pituitary-Derived Growth Hormone with Genetically Determined Incubation Times of up to 40 Years. *Brain J. Neurol.* **2015,** *138* (Pt 11), 3386–3399. DOI: 10.1093/brain/awv235.

Propagation of Neurodegenerative disorders 79

95. Sala Frigerio, C.; Lau, P.; Salta, E.; Tournoy, J.; Bossers, K.; Vandenberghe, R. et al. Reduced Expression of hsa-miR-27a-3p in CSF of Patients with Alzheimer Disease. *Neurology* **2013**, 81(24):2103–2106. DOI: 10.1212/01.wnl.0000437306.37850.22.

96. Sarkies, P.; Miska, E. A. Molecular Biology: Is There Social RNA? *Science* **2013**, 341(6145):467–468. DOI: 10.1126/science.1243175.

97. Saylor, D.; Dickens, A. M.; Sacktor, N.; Haughey, N.; Slusher, B.; Pletnikov, M. et al. HIV-Associated Neurocognitive Disorder-Pathogenesis and Prospects for Treatment. *Nat. Rev. Neurol.* **2016**, *12* (5):309. DOI: 10.1038/nrneurol.2016.53.

98. Schipper, H. M.; Maes, O. C.; Chertkow, H. M.; Wang, E. MicroRNA Expression in Alzheimer Blood Mononuclear Cells. *Gene Regul. Syst. Biol.* **2007**, *1*, 263–274.

99. Schmitz, M.; Wulf, K.; Signore, S. C.; Schulz-Schaeffer, W. J.; Kermer, P.; Bahr, M. et al. Impact of the cellular prion protein on amyloid-beta and 3PO-tau processing. *J Alzheimers Dis JAD*. **2014**, 38(3):551–565. DOI: 10.3233/JAD-130566.

100. Sheinerman, K. S.; Tsivinsky, V. G.; Crawford, F.; Mullan, M. J.; Abdullah, L.; Umansky, S. R. Plasma microRNA Biomarkers for Detection of Mild Cognitive Impairment. *Aging* **2012**, 4(9):590–605. DOI: 10.18632/aging.100486.

101. Sobue, G. MicroRNA in Neurodegenerative Disorders. *Rinsho Shinkeigaku* **2013**, *53* (11):942–944. DOI: 10.5692/clinicalneurol.53.942.

102. Soreq, L.; Salomonis, N.; Bronstein, M.; Greenberg, D. S.; Israel, Z.; Bergman, H. et al. Small RNA Sequencing-Microarray Analyses in Parkinson Leukocytes Reveal Deep Brain Stimulation-Induced Splicing Changes That Classify Brain Region Transcriptomes. *Front. Mol. Neurosci.* **2013**, *6*, 10. DOI: 10.3389/fnmol.2013.00010.

103. Stohr, J.; Watts, J. C.; Mensinger, Z. L.; Oehler, A.; Grillo, S. K.; DeArmond, S. J. et al. Purified and Synthetic Alzheimer's Amyloid Beta (Abeta) Prions. *Proc. Natl. Acad. Sci. USA.* **2012**, *109* (27), 11025–11030. DOI: 10.1073/pnas.1206555109.

104. Torniainen-Holm, M.; Suvisaari, J.; Lindgren, M.; Härkänen, T.; Dickerson, F.; Yolken, R. H. Association of Cytomegalovirus and Epstein–Barr Virus with Cognitive Functioning and Risk of Dementia in the General Population: 11-Year Follow-Up Study. *Brain Behav. Immun.* **2018**, *69*, 480–485. DOI: 10.1016/j.bbi.2018.01.006.

105. Turner, M. R.; Kiernan, M. C.; Leigh, P. N.; Talbot, K. Biomarkers in Amyotrophic Lateral Sclerosis. *Lancet Neurol.* **2009**, *8* (1):94–109. DOI: 10.1016/S1474-4422(08)70293-X.

106. Turner, R. S.; Chadwick, M.; Horton, W. A.; Simon, G. L.; Jiang, X.; Esposito, G. An Individual with Human Immunodeficiency Virus, Dementia, and Central Nervous System Amyloid Deposition. *Alzheimers Dement* **2016**, *4*, 1–5. DOI: 10.1016/j.dadm. 2016.03.009.

107. Valentine, J. S.; Doucette, P. A.; Zittin Potter, S. Copper–Zinc Superoxide Dismutase and Amyotrophic Lateral Sclerosis. *Annu. Rev. Biochem.* **2005**, *74*, 563–593. DOI: 10.1146/annurev.biochem.72.121801.161647.

108. Walker, L. C.; Jucker, M. Neurodegenerative Diseases: Expanding the Prion Concept. *Annu. Rev. Neurosci.* **2015**, *38*, 87–103. DOI: 10.1146/annurev-neuro-071714-033828.

109. Walker, L. C.; Schelle, J.; Jucker, M. The Prion-Like Properties of Amyloid-Beta Assemblies: Implications for Alzheimer's Disease. *Cold Spring Harb. Perspect. Med.* 2016. DOI: 10.1101/cshperspect.a024398.

110. Wang, W. X.; Rajeev, B. W.; Stromberg, A. J.; Ren, N.; Tang, G.; Huang, Q. et al. The Expression of microRNA miR-107 Decreases Early in Alzheimer's Disease

and May Accelerate Disease Progression Through Regulation of Beta-Site Amyloid Precursor Protein-Cleaving Enzyme 1. *J. Neurosci. Off. J. Soc. Neurosci.* **2008,** *28* (5), 1213–1223. DOI: 10.1523/JNEUROSCI.5065-07.2008.

111. Watts, J. C.; Condello, C.; Stohr, J.; Oehler, A.; Lee, J.; DeArmond, S. J. et al. Serial Propagation of Distinct Strains of Abeta Prions from Alzheimer's Disease Patients. *Proc. Natl. Acad. Sci. USA.* **2014,** *111* (28), 10323–10328. DOI: 10.1073/pnas. 1408900111.

112. Whitehouse, I. J.; Miners, J. S.; Glennon, E. B.; Kehoe, P. G.; Love, S.; Kellett, K. A. et al. Prion Protein Is Decreased in Alzheimer's Brain and Inversely Correlates with BACE1 Activity, Amyloid-Beta Levels and Braak Stage. *PLoS ONE.* **2013,** *8* (4), e59554. DOI: 10.1371/journal.pone.0059554.

113. Xue, Y. C.; Feuer, R.; Cashman, N.; Luo, H. Enteroviral Infection: The Forgotten Link to Amyotrophic Lateral Sclerosis? *Front. Mol. Neurosci.* **2018,** *11*, 63. DOI: 10.3389/fnmol.2018.00063.

114. Yelamanchili, S. V.; Chaudhuri, A. D.; Chen, L. N.; Xiong, H.; Fox, H. S. MicroRNA-21 Dysregulates the Expression of MEF2C in Neurons in Monkey and Human SIV/HIV Neurological Disease. *Cell Death Dis.* **2010,** *1*, e77. DOI: 10.1038/cddis.2010.56.

115. Zhao, Y.; Bhattacharjee, S.; Dua, P.; Alexandrov, P. N.; Lukiw, W. J. microRNA-Based Biomarkers and the Diagnosis of Alzheimer's Disease. *Front. Neurol.* **2015,** *6*, 162. DOI: 10.3389/fneur.2015.00162.

116. Luk, K. C.; Kehm, V.; Carroll, J.; Zhang, B.; O'Brien, P.; Trojanowski, J. Q. et al. Pathological Alpha-Synuclein Transmission Initiates Parkinson-Like Neurodegeneration in Nontransgenic Mice. *Science* **2012,** *338*, 949–953.

117. Watts, J. C.; Giles, K.; Oehler, A.; Middleton, L.; Dexter, D. T.; Gentleman, S. M. et al. Transmission of Multiple System Atrophy Prions to Transgenic Mice. *Proc. Natl. Acad Sci. USA* **2013,** *110*, 19555–19560.

118. Eisele, Y. S.; Obermuller, U.; Heilbronner, G.; Baumann, F.; Kaeser, S. A.; Wolburg, H. et al. Peripherally Applied Abeta-Containing Inoculates Induce Cerebral Beta-Amyloidosis. *Science* **2010,** *330*, 980–982.

119. Clavaguera, F.; Hench, J.; Lavenir, I.; Schweighauser, G.; Frank, S.; Goedert, M. et al. Peripheral Administration of Tau Aggregates Triggers Intracerebral Tauopathy in Transgenic Mice. *Acta Neuropathol.* **2014,** *127*, 299–301.

120. Sacino, A. N.; Brooks, M.; Thomas, M. A.; McKinney, A. B.; Lee, S.; Regenhardt, R. W. et al. Intramuscular Injection of Alpha-Synuclein Induces CNS Alpha-Synuclein Pathology and a Rapid-Onset Motor Phenotype in Transgenic Mice. *Proc. Natl. Acad. Sci. USA* **2014,** *111*, 10732–10737.

121. Lohmann, S.; Bernis, M. E.; Tachu, B. J.; Ziemski, A.; Grigoletto, J.; Tamguney, G. Oral and Intravenous Transmission of Alpha-Synuclein Fibrils to Mice. *Acta Neuropathol.* **2019,** *138*, 515–533.

122. Pattison, I. H.; Gordon, W. S.; Millson, G. C. Experimental Production of Scrapie in Goats. *J. Comp. Pathol.* **1959,** *69*, 300–312.

123. Chandler, R. L. Encephalopathy in Mice Produced by Inoculation with Scrapie Brain Material. *Lancet* **1961,** *1*, 1378–1379.

124. Brandner, S.; Jaunmuktane, Z. Prion Disease: Experimental Models and Reality. *Acta Neuropathol.* **2017,** *133*, 197–222.

Propagation of Neurodegenerative disorders

125. Comoy, E. E.; Mikol, J.; Luccantoni-Freire, S.; Correia, E.; Lescoutra-Etchegaray, N.; Durand, V. et al. Transmission of Scrapie Prions to Primate After an Extended Silent Incubation Period. *Sci. Rep.* **2015,** *5,* 11573.
126. Recasens, A.; Dehay, B.; Bove, J.; Carballo-Carbajal, I.; Dovero, S.; Perez-Villalba, A. et al. Lewy Body Extracts from Parkinson Disease Brains Trigger Alpha-Synuclein Pathology and Neurodegeneration in Mice and Monkeys. *Ann. Neurol.* **2014,** *75,* 351–362.
127. Beck, E.; Daniel, P. M.; Alpers, M.; Gajdusek, D. C.; Gibbs, C. J. Jr. Experimental "Kuru" in Chimpanzees a Pathological Report. *Lancet* **1966,** *2,* 1056–1059.
128. Gajdusek, D. C.; Gibbs, C. J.; Alpers, M. Experimental Transmission of a Kuru-Like Syndrome to Chimpanzees. *Nature* **1966,** *209,* 794–796.

CHAPTER 4

Gene Therapy: A Promising Strategy for the Treatment of Brain Disease

ABSTRACT

In order to cure sickness, nucleic acids are being used according to a method called "gene therapy," which also includes substitution for faulty genes with healthy ones. Treatment options for illnesses of the nervous system are generally inadequate, making gene therapy methods vital. Human clinical studies using gene treatments are already underway, and they promise to be both a useful research tool and a potentially life-changing treatment option. Researchers need a thorough familiarity with the many existing gene therapy approaches in order to complete gene therapy projects successfully and develop novel strategies for treating diseases with genes. In this chapter, talk about the benefits and drawbacks of using viral and nonviral vectors to transport genes to the CNS, as well as their potential future uses. There has been talk of controlling transgene expression using optogenetics and designer receptors that can only be triggered by designer drugs. Topics include gene editing, gene silencing, and gene overexpression. Finally, we detail the success of these strategies in treating include neurodegenerative diseases, lysosomal storage diseases, and Duchenne muscular dystrophy in animal models and human therapeutic trials. To aid neuroscientists in selecting the most suitable tools for their investigations and the creation of novel gene treatments, aim to provide a synopsis of gene therapy methods.

Gene Therapy for Neurological Disorders: Molecular Approaches for Targeted Treatment.
Rishabha Malviya, Arun Kumar Singh, Priyanshi Goyal, & Sonali Sundram (Authors)
© 2025 Apple Academic Press, Inc. Co-published with CRC Press (Taylor & Francis)

4.1 INTRODUCTION

Several neurological diseases have achieved significant strides in therapy, and the list of those diseases is expanding as a result of these advancements.[1,2] Yet, there are many illnesses and ailments for which effective treatments have not yet been discovered. Some neurological diseases are resistant to typical small-molecule therapies because of the nervous system and the difficulty of delivering drugs to particular targets in the CNS without causing undesirable side effects, research into drug transport to the CNS has proven to be a frustrating and fruitless endeavor. Because it permits the stable or titratable expression of a gene product in very specific target cells, intracerebral delivery of genetic materials encoding therapeutic agents (protein, RNA, etc.) shows promise in treating a wide range of neurological disorders, including those caused by genetic mutations and acquired or sporadic diseases.[3-5] Gene therapy involves the construction of therapeutic DNA or RNA structures, the development of gene transfer vectors, and the introduction of therapeutic genes into the cells of interest, and gene expression is regulated as part of gene therapy. In this article, take a look at the most widely used methods for delivering DNA to the brain, including both viral and nonviral vectors. Each vector's salient features are described, and their advantages and disadvantages are weighed. Here, talk about Exclusively Activated by Designer Drugs, Cre/loxP Recombination, and Optogenetic Methods in Designer Receptors for regulating gene expression in space and time.[6,7]

In addition, evaluate strategies for vector-based transport and expression of several transgenes. Examples of classic gene therapy include gene overexpression, gene silencing (through RNAi or other techniques), and the modification of genetic material using tools like CRISPR/Cas9. In this article, describe a number of case reports from both clinical practice and laboratory investigations to illustrate the success of a wide range of gene therapy techniques for neurological illnesses.[8-11] Figure 4.1 diagrammatically represents *in-vivo* gene therapy with AAVs.

4.2 VIRAL VECTORS

The idea that introducing a new gene into an organism may cure or prevent illness is important to the field of medicine known as gene therapy. First,

Gene Therapy: A Promising Strategy 85

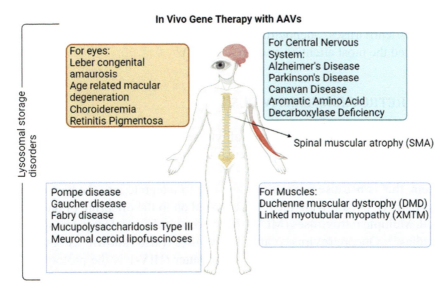

FIGURE 4.1 In vivo gene therapy with AAVs.

the desired genetic material (often a gene) must be delivered to the desired cells.[12] This is challenging regardless of the cell type; nevertheless, it is especially challenging in neurons, which constitute the brain's circuits and are commonly disturbed in neurological illnesses.[13] One of the best ways to get genes into the brain, where they can be produced consistently and for a long time, is to utilize a virus as a delivery vehicle. To effectively carry genetic material into target cells without generating disease or other undesirable side effects in the host, scientists have manipulated naturally occurring viruses to serve as viral vectors.[14] There are several different viruses that have been utilized to develop viral vectors; some of these viruses are quite harmful and can cause fatal diseases like AIDS and rabies. The possibility of producing a "wild-type" or infectious virus is minimal because the vectors have been created so that genes crucial for infection are either absent or delivered in various packaging structures.[15] Whether the vectors of an RNA virus or a DNA virus are able to integrate into the host cell's genome is determined by the kind of virus or even if the vectors are lentiviruses or eukaryotic (episomal).[16]. Using an integrated vector, therapeutic genes can be expressed in the correct cells for an extended length of time. Neuronal cells, which do not divide on their own, respond well to transduction utilizing viral vectors maintained as episomes. There are many different types of viral vectors, but those generated from retro-viruses/lentiviruses, adenoviruses, AAVs, and herpes simplex virus have attracted the most attention and study (HSV).[17]

4.3 RETROVIRUS/LENTIVIRUS

There are more different types of viruses in the RNA virus family, retroviruses, than in any other genus. Viral RNA may be transformed into proviral DNA with the use of reverse transcriptase. Incredible as it may seem, this is because retroviruses are able to integrate into the host cell's genomic DNA, allowing them to be passed on to the offspring of the host cell. Multiple retroviruses (MLVs) have been used as vectors in transgenic studies.[18] Oncoretroviruses and lentiviruses (also known as gamma retroviruses) are prime examples of the latter (HIV-1 is the prototypical lentivirus). Transduction of cultivated cells ex vivo with MLV vectors is followed by transplantation and it has been proven that transferring genes to hematopoietic cells works. The central nervous system (CNS) is an attractive target for gene therapy, but viral vectors are unable to deliver DNA to nondividing cells like neurons. Lentiviral vectors have the ability to transduce both quiescent and actively dividing cells, which means that they can potentially transport, integrate, and sustain the expression of transgenes in vivo.[19] Lentiviral vectors are commonly utilized for CNS gene transfer because of their ability to transduce multiple brain cell subtypes and induce extremely steady transgene expression (CNS). From then on, lentiviral vectors will be the primary area of interest.[20] Terminal repeats enclose the three most essential genes gag, pol, and env in the RNA genomes of retroviruses, including lentiviruses (LTRs). Viral structural proteins are encoded by the gag gene, while the pol gene encodes enzymes involved in reverse transcriptase and integration. For viruses to infect a host cell, they need to use envelope glycoproteins, which are encoded by the env gene. When a virus binds to a host cell, its membrane, and the host cell's membrane fuse, allowing the virus' nucleic acid core to leak into the cytoplasm. Because of a process called reverse transcription, the RNA genome of a virus may be converted into DNA.[21] The viral preintegration complex, which consists of viral DNA and proteins, must next enter the nucleus and integrate into the host genome. In order for HIV-1, the most studied lentivirus, to replicate, four genes (vif, vpr, vpu, and nef) encoding virulence components are added (gag, pol, and env). In vivo transduction of neurons with an HIV-derived lentiviral vector is described for the first time in this study. It has been shown that the early lentiviral vectors were capable of packaging the whole HIV-1 protein complement apart from the envelope protein. Recent developments in lentiviral vector technology have made the method more reliable and reduced the possibility of producing a Viable Strain of a Virus.[22] All four genes responsible for making auxiliary proteins are missing from current lentiviral vectors. In the third generation of lentiviral vectors, the HIV U3 in the 50 LTR has been replaced with a constitutive promoter, rendering the Tat protein superfluous for vector genome transcription.[23] Therefore, the tat gene was not included in the final product since it was removed during production.

Gene rev was previously located on the packaging plasmid, but in more advanced systems, it is given in trans from a different plasmid. Four distinct plasmids were used to produce transducing particles, and the resulting gene delivery technique offers substantial biosafety benefits. Moreover, in self-inactivated (SIN) lentiviral vectors, the U3 region of 30 LTR is often eliminated from the transfer construct.[24] Virus promoters and enhancers are located in the U3 region. Both LTRs become transcriptionally inactive when a vector lacking the 30 U3 is transduced into a cell. This is because the 50 LTR experiences a replicative inversion. A third-generation packaging method was used to create most lentiviral vectors that are produced by cotransfecting vector packing into 293T cells which requires a transfer plasmid with many assistance plasmids encoding structural and functional proteins, as depicted in Figure 4.1. There are now viable cell lines for packing that express these crucial aids.[25] Animal studies and a human clinical trial using gamma retrovirus-based vectors incorporation of the insertion of lentiviral or other retroviral vectors into the host genome cause insertional mutagenesis, as was observed in a study for X-linked severe combined immunodeficiency. Nonintegrating vectors were developed to eliminate the potential for insertional mutagenesis.[26] Episomal DNA, which makes up the great majority of viral genomes, is extremely stable, making nonintegrating lentiviral vectors ideal for gene expression in nondividing cells. Integrase coding area mutations produce faulty lentiviral vectors.[27] Successful transcription may occur even if a genome lacks the integrase required for efficient transcription, albeit protein output would be much lower than with traditional vectors. Eye administration of viral vectors protects against retinal degeneration by using a mouse as a model. Using a lentiviral genome of the host cell's nucleus, we were able to generate long-lasting transgenic expression in the mouse cerebral cortex.[28]

Different envelope glycoproteins from the original virus can be used to make lentiviral vectors (pseudotyping). Among viral envelope glycoproteins, vesicular stomatitis virus is by far the most common (VSV-G).[29] VSV-G receptors, also known as low-density lipoprotein receptors, are membrane proteins expressed by virtually all cell types. This includes neurons and glia. VSV-G is more trophotropic and structurally stable, allowing for ultracentrifugation to concentrate the virus to extraordinarily high concentrations. A number of different glycoproteins, such as VSV-G and rabies virus glycoprotein, are used by pseudotyped lentiviral vectors for transporting genetic material to the brain (RV-G).[30] These glycoproteins are helpful for both long-range neuronal communication and axonal reversal. Motor neurons in the spinal cord may produce transgenic DNA if RV-G is injected into them. Transgenic expression in the substantia nigra's projection neurons is induced by injecting a vector derived from the equine infectious anemia virus into a thigh muscle.[31] RV-G improves retrograde axonal transmission when used in conjunction with HIV-based lentiviral vectors in the brains of mice and monkeys. Antibodies against glycoproteins from some of the lentiviral vectors used for the transduction of CNS cells in culture and animals are Mokola virus, LCMV, Ross River virus, and MLV.[32]

Lentiviral vectors are gaining popularity for their ability to transduce signals selectively in the brain. Specifically, the promoters utilized by these vectors permit the production of desired genes in only the intended cell types.[33] The transgenic expression can be maximized with a ubiquitous promoter if cell-type specificity is not an issue. Combining the cytomegalovirus (CMV) enhancer with the chicken-actin (CAG), phosphoglycerate kinase (PGK), or elongation factor-1 alpha (EF-1) promoters increases gene expression in the brain. Despite its potency, the CMV promoter is vulnerable to transcriptional inhibition due to DNA methylation, which has led to a steady decline in transgenic production.[34] Select CpG sites are messed with so that CMV does not silence genes. When possible, it is desirable to use a promoter sequence that is highly efficient in the target cell type. If, for example, transgenes were solely expressed in astrocytes, then the released trophic factor would be disseminated locally, preventing the risk of detrimental anterograde transfer. There are both ubiquitous promoters and various cell-type-specific promoters.[35] Highly specialized for neuronal expression are the promoters for synapsin 1 and NSE (neuron-specific enolase). It has been shown, via in vivo and in vitro investigations, that the GFAP promoter is only used for expression by astrocytes (encodes an acidic protein found in glial cells). The oligodendrocyte myelin basic protein (MBP) gene is regulated by promoters.[36] Extreme difficulties arise when using viral vectors to deliver a large number of promoters that are particular to individual types of endogenous neurons. Because of their decreased potency or loss of cell-type selectivity, the vectors' shorter forms may be unusable. Additional promoter screening or the development of synthetic promoters will be required for future work.[37]

4.4 ADENOVIRUS

The icosahedral protein capsid of adenovirus (Ad) contains its genome of roughly 36 kilobase pairs (kb) of DNA that has two strands.[38] The danger of insertional mutagenesis is low since it is uncommon for viral DNA to become permanently incorporated into a host genome. Adenovirus is a promising vector candidate due to its high packing capacity, ease of propagating high-titer viral stock, and infectivity across different kinds of cells (including nondividing cells). Adenovirus serotype 5 is the most often utilized adenoviral vector; however, other serotypes and nonhuman adenoviruses have also been employed successfully.[39] Taking off the viral sequence responsible for replication and replacing it with a transgenic expression cassette creates a recombinant adeno-associated virus vector. When it comes to foreign DNA, wild-type adenoviruses have a very limited storage capacity of just 2 kilobase pairs. When the E1 region is cut off, around 5 kb of space is made available for cloning. In order to multiply vectors, E1-expressing cell lines are required. These include HEK293.[40] The E1 region is crucial for the security of gene therapy treatments to be removed because doing so improves cloning efficiency and renders the vector replication defective.[41] It is not necessary to enter the E3 area to create vectors. Recombinant vectors with insert sizes up to 8 kb can be made by removing the first E1 and third E3 regions of Ad in a noncontiguous fashion (e.g., the AdEasy method). Adenovirus genomes are eliminated in helper-dependent adenoviral vectors, which remove the viral genome (thus the names "gutless" or "gutted") noncoding inverted terminal repeats and packing signal.[42] There will be more room for transgenes if the host cell's immune response is lowered in this way. The largest transgene that can be accommodated by these vectors is around 36 kbp in length. Even if their adaptive immunity is weakened, they may still be able to trigger the innate immune response in vivo. Neurons and glial cells can be transduced in vivo using helper-dependent vectors.[43] Most expressed genes are found in glial cells rather than neurons because the Ad5 vector is poorly adapted for brain delivery. Vectors derived from canine adenovirus 2 (CAdV2 or CAV-2) efficiently engage in retrograde axonal transport and transduce neurons selectively.[44] Immune responses to CAV-2 vectors are weaker than those to vectors derived from human adenovirus serotype 5. Ad5 adenoviruses have had the fiber knob domain of canine adenovirus serotype 2 inserted into them to improve their tropism. After injecting the Ad5-CGW-CK2 vector into the mouse brain, only certain types of neurons are affected.[45] Adenoviral vectors share many of the same advantages as perfect vectors, but they are not commonly used on account of issues, including the potential for irreparable brain injury, in the cerebral cortex and spinal cord host immunological response and the unavailability of helper-free manufacturing procedures. However, oncolytic adenoviruses or possibly an earlier generation of adenoviruses might be effective against malignant brain tumors.[46]

4.5 VIRUS LINKED TO ADENOVIRUSES

Among the Dependovirus family is the Parvoviridae genus, which houses AAV. It poses no danger to humans and is completely safe to be around. The genome of an adeno-associated virus (AAV) virion is around 4.7 kilobase pairs in size, and it is encased in an icosahedral protein capsid. T-shaped inverted terminal repeats (ITRs) separate the rep and cap genes that make up the AAV genome (ITRs).[47] Many different proteins are encoded by the rep gene. Each copy of the cap gene in an AAV produces one of the three structural proteins (VP1, VP2, and VP3) that make up the virus's capsid.[48] However, rAAV vectors only include the ITRs, which are required for genome replication, integration, and packaging into the capsid. Each structural protein (VP1, VP2, and VP3) in the capsid of an adeno-associated virus (AAV) is encoded by its own copy of the cap gene.[48] In rAAV vectors, just the ITRs exist, yet they are required for genomic replication, integration, and capsid packaging.

Gene Therapy: A Promising Strategy

To replicate, AAV requires the presence of other viruses like adenoviruses and herpes viruses. Despite the rarity of chromosome 19 integration, in some cases, wild-type AAV can result in a dormant infection without the aid of a helper virus. To put it simply, targeting integration is impossible with rAAV vectors since they lack Rep, a requirement for doing so. Due to its low toxicity, high transduction effectiveness, and strong, long-lasting expression of transgenes, there has been a lot of success using AAV human illness models in animals and vectors for human gene therapy. The first vectors for CNS gene transfer were created using AAV serotype 2[49] (AAV2). AAV2's therapeutic potential is limited by the little brain region it can transduce after being injected. Multiple novel serotypes of AAV have been isolated. Different serotypes of AAV viruses are defined based on their capsid sequences.[50] Researcher argue that a virus is of a novel serotype when neutralizing sera against all previously described serotypes fails to produce a strong cross-reaction. To enter and spread within cells, different AAV serotypes use a wide variety of strategies, including receptor recognition and other entry/trafficking pathways. Therefore, the serotype and level of production of the transgenic influence its tropism toward nerve cells. When making vectors not based on AAV2, the ITRs and rep genes are often substituted with the cap gene of the desired serotype.[51] Cross-packing, also called pseudo-typing, is a name for this strategy. In this way, an AAV8 capsid might be used to transport a transgene containing AAV2 ITRs. Both AAV2/8 and AAV8 can be used to refer to the across-packingtant adeno-associated virus (AAV) vector. Taymans et al. found that all but AAV2 could transduce comparable quantities of brain tissue in their particular areas of interest and that they selectively target neurons for DNA synthesis in the mouse brain.[52]

Many different AAV vectors were tested by Broekman et al. to determine which would be the most effective in delivering genes to targeted parts of the mouse brain. The striatum, hippocampus, and thalamus all have neurons that can be transduced with cDNA for -glucuronidase encoded by AAV7, AAV8, AAV9, and rh.10 vectors, but astrocytes and oligodendrocytes cannot. While certain serotypes are only capable of transducing cells within the normal diffusion range, others may be able to transduce cells over extremely long distances in either the forward (anterograde) or backward (retrograde) motion of axons. To be injected into the ventral tegmental region (VTA), all three vectors propagated; however, the AAV9 vector spread the farthest, followed by the AAVrh[53] 10 vectors, and then by the AAV1. After injecting AAV8 and AAV9 into the adult mouse brain, researchers observed both transport in both directions (antegrade and retrograde) in a single, one-way circuit. Transduction of spinal cord neurons by AAV1 is possible following intracortical injection and subsequent propagation along axons in an anterograde orientation.[54]

Since BBB-permeable vectors may transport therapeutic genes to the brain without intracranial injections, they have attracted many researchers' work done in the realm of gene therapy. Foust et al. were the first to show that AAV9 could transduce CNS cells in both neonatal and adult mice. Evidence for motor neuron transduction in adult rats was discovered by Duque et al. in 2009 when self-complementary AAV9 vectors were injected intravenously.[55] Extensive research has shown that several different AAV serotypes can successfully cross the brain's blood–brain barrier. Researchers have discovered that AAVrh.10 is as successful as AAV9, and often more so, in a wide range of these settings. To improve targeting specificity and transduction efficiency, many synthetic AAV vectors have been produced in addition to the many naturally occurring AAV serotypes. AAV2 capsid tyrosine phosphorylation suppresses transgene expression and nuclear import.[56]

Mutating surface-exposed tyrosine residues improves the transduction capability of working effectively in living organisms (in vivo) and laboratory settings (in vitro). All AAV serotypes can be treated with this technique.[57] Transgene expression differs from that of wild-type AAV when it is both higher and more extensive after injection of AAV serotype 8 or 9 mutant vectors subretinally or intravitreally. A hybrid capsid library may be made by combining the capsids of several wild-type viruses. DNA recombination and directed evolution were employed by Gray et al. (2010) to target tissue damage induced by seizures with gene therapy by creating novel adeno-associated virus (AAV) vectors. Three libraries of capsids were produced using in vivo directed evolution (mutation, shuffling, and random insertion), Dalkara et al. (2013) were able to successfully isolate an AAV variant that efficiently traveled to reach every layer of the retina in mice and apes (7m8).[58]

The Cre-expressing target cell was precisely transduced using AAV libraries by Deverman et al. (2016), and new capsids were constructed using Cre-expressing mice. Extensive research showed that AAV-PHP.B is at least 40-fold more effective in transducing astrocytes and neurons than the gold standard, AAV9.[59]

Gene Therapy: A Promising Strategy

AAV vectors provide some advantages over other gene transfer methods, including the possibility of effective gene transfer, lasting transgenic expression, low toxicity, and lack of immunogenicity. Because of these benefits, AAV vectors have replaced all previous strategies to transport genetic material to the brain. However, because of AAV's little storage capacity, it is difficult, if not impossible, to deliver large transgenes or cell-specific transcription regulatory elements. Some possible methods for the concatemerization of AAV vectors include trans-splicing, homologous recombination, and hybridization.[60] The expression of a gene of interest can be stimulated using vectors like dural and tri-AAV. After co-transduction with three separate adeno-associated virals (AAV) vectors, Mdx4cv mice expressed full-length human dystrophin in their tibialis anterior muscles.[61]

4.6 NONVIRAL VECTORS

Naked plasmid DNA has been proposed as the most secure, least expensive, and most readily available method of gene transfer. Plasmids can only boost gene expression to a certain extent, although this might be useful if transgene expression needs to be repeatedly turned on and off. Instead of using viral vectors, which can trigger unwanted immunological responses and frequent insertional mutagenesis, plasmid DNA can be used instead.[62] Naked DNA has a limited efficacy of entering cells, and transfection reagents can be dangerous. There is an atypical case in neurons. There is a chance that the nucleic acids will be broken down by some nucleases. DNA is a very large molecule with a negative charge that makes it tough for cells to take up and transport to the nucleus. DNA is often joined with compounds to ease transport and expression in nonviral gene delivery techniques.[63]

4.7 NANOPARTICLES

Plasmid DNA can be better protected from degradation during transport to the target cells if it is encapsulated in lipids or synthetic polymers.[64] PEGylated liposomes have a longer half-life in circulation and are taken up less readily by the mononuclear phagocytic system. Several different types of nanoparticles, including lipid and polymer ones, have been employed for gene transfer.

Multiple ligands may be combined into one molecule to form a hybrid nanoparticle with improved targeting efficacy and accuracy. Since most therapeutic drugs are unable because they cannot cross the blood–brain barrier (BBB) and cannot effectively treat neurological disorders (CNS), and introducing new genes into the brain through the circulatory system is a challenging task as shown in Figure 4.2.[65] Using transvascular administration of short interfering RNA (siRNA) and a synthetic peptide derived from the glycoprotein of the rabies virus, gene silencing in specific brain neuronal cells was accomplished (RVG).[66] Combining this shRNA, which zeroes in on the beta-site APP cleaving enzyme 1 antisense (BACE1-AS) transcript, with a second shRNA, with another shRNA was found to be effective by Liu et al, with an amino acid that decreases tau fibrils, significantly improved the efficacy of the treatment (D-peptide). To formulate nanoparticles containing the therapeutic plasmid and two brain-specific peptides (D-peptide and RVG29 peptides), investigators bonded the peptides to dendrigraft poly-L-lysines.[67] These nanoparticles dramatically decreased BACE1 enzyme and neurofibrillary tangle levels in a rodent model of Alzheimer's illness (AD). Two mouse models of spinocerebellar ataxia type 3 showed improvement in neuropathology and motor behavior difficulties when treated with stable nucleic acid-lipid particles encasing siRNAs against the mutant ataxin-3 gene product.[68] Using monoclonal antibodies that bind to receptors on the blood–brain barrier (BBB) and brain cellular membranes, the modified liposomes can be transported intracerebrally, allowing for nonviral gene delivery to the central nervous system (such as the transferrin receptor).[69] Such "Trojan horse" liposomes have been used in animal models of Parkinson's disease and lysosomal storage diseases.

It was discovered that ultrasound imaging microbubbles (MB) can cause reversible BBB rupture when combined with focused ultrasound (FUS) bursts, all without causing any damage to brain tissue.[70] Cationic microspheres can be used to transport plasmid DNA and other gene therapy materials from the bloodstream to the brain, where they can be exposed to FUS. Cationic MB platforms loaded with glial cell-derived neurotrophic factor (GDNF) were shown to have neuroprotective effects in a mouse model of Parkinson's disease.[71] For example, Mead et al. DNA "brain penetrating" nanoparticles (DNA-BPNs) were coinjected with MB into the tail veins of rats, and then transgenic expression was induced within 24 hours and maintained for at least 28 days using magnetic resonance

Gene Therapy: A Promising Strategy

imaging-guided FUS. Nearly half of the cells were transfected in the FUS-treated area.[72] Both neurons and astrocytes were considered. Even with precautions, there is still a chance that these nonviral vectors may have unintended consequences. Viral vectors are widely employed for gene transfer because their transfer efficiency is higher than that of nonviral vectors. Therefore, repeated injections into the brain parenchyma are out of the question since plasmid-based vectors only provide temporary gene expression. Because of this, they cannot be used to treat conditions that call for constant expression of the transgene.[73]

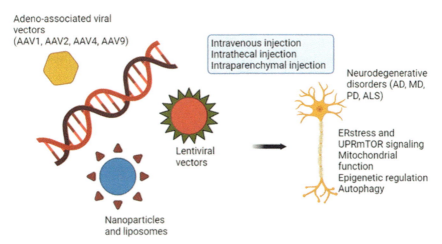

FIGURE 4.2 Nanoparticles and liposomes used in neurons.[63]

4.8 TRANSPOSONS IN DNA

DNA transposons are snippets of genetic material that can move around the genome via transposing. DNA transposons are therefore a valuable tool for gene transfer. Transposon gene delivery systems include two plasmids: one with the transgene and another with the transposase.[74] Both the transposon and the transposase gene could be put into the same plasmid. Transposases are injected into cells and bind to terminal repeat sequences on the plasmid, allowing the gene of interest (GOI) to be cut out of the host cell's DNA using a plasmid that was provided by a donor.[75] The Sleeping Beauty (SB) transposon has been used well as a nonviral gene delivery strategy in a variety of animal models and is the most studied transposon in vertebrates.

Originally discovered in insect cells, the PiggyBac (PB) transposon has since been shown to transpose in mammalian and human cells, suggesting that it could be used as a vector in gene therapy as shown in Figure 4.3.[76] Transgenic expression was maintained in mouse lungs following direct intravenous infusion of transposon vector/polyethyleneimine complexes. In mice with human glioblastoma xenografts, tumor development was suppressed and survival was increased when SB transposons encoding antiangiogenic genes were administered.[77]

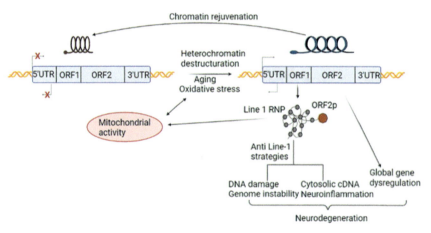

FIGURE 4.3 Transposons in DNA.

Maintaining transgenic expression for long periods of time using viral vectors is made possible by transposons, which combine the benefits of nonviral delivery strategies (improved safety profile and decreased manufacturing cost) with such systems.[78] In theory, transgenes can be deleted from cells by making transposase, suggesting that gene transfer is reversible. Therefore, transposons are of interest for their potential application in producing pluripotent stem cells (iPSCs) for the goal of treating disorders, particularly neurological ailments. DNA transposons, like viral vectors, carry the potential for insertional mutagenesis.[79] Studies have been conducted lately on the insertion rates of SB and PB transposons, HIV lentivirus, and MLV retrovirus in human CD41 T cells. When compared to the PB, MLV, and HIV transposons, it has been shown that the SB transposon randomly inserts into expressed genes. These results suggest that the SB transposon is more suitable for human usage.[80]

Gene Therapy: A Promising Strategy 97

4.9   TRANSGENE EXPRESSION CONTROL

Using cell-type-specific promoters like those described for lentiviral vectors allows researchers employing both viral and nonviral vectors to control gene expression. There are promoters out there who are rather sizable; thus, it is important to monitor the overall vector construct size to ensure it does not exceed the constraints of the vector packing.[81] A variety of techniques for altering gene expression will be discussed here.

4.10   REGULATABLE PROMOTERS

Several different regulatory mechanisms can be utilized to manipulate transgene expression. For instance, the tetracycline (tet) regulatory mechanism has been studied extensively and is widely employed. This method relies on the cluster of genes in *Escherichia coli* that determines whether or not the bacteria will respond negatively to the antibiotic tetracycline.[82] Transactivator (tTA; Tet repressor and herpes simplex virus VP16 hybrid) is used in the Tet-Off system to initiate transcription from tetracycline-operated minimal promoters (tetO). Doxycycline (Dox; a tetracycline analogue) inhibits the interaction between tetracycline response element-activating factor (tetA) and tetracycline response element-binding protein (tetO). In Hela cells, reporter gene expression could be enhanced by a factor of 105 using these methods.[83] Researchers Manfredsson et al. successfully transferred an AAV vector encoding the Tet-Off system to maintain dynamic expression of nigrostriatal GDNF in an animal model. When rapid induction of gene expression is needed, or when prolonged periods of silence gene expression are desired, the Tet-On technique may be the method of choice. The Tet-On strategy flips the script by employing a reverse tTA (rtTA), which exhibits the opposite behaviors of a regular tTA. Doxycycline binds to the tetO region, where rtTA is found, and it may increase promoters and gene expression.[84] Researchers found that GDNF gene transfer improvement in motor skills in a rat model of Parkinson's illness utilizing Tet-On lentiviral vectors was shown to preserve nigral dopaminergic neurons. Assessing the applicability of tet-regulated gene expression requires considering "leaky" expression in the absence of tet in the Tet-On system and residual expression in the Tet-Off system.[85]

4.11 OPTOGENETICS

Genetic techniques allow for the spatiotemporal modulation of neuronal depolarization and hyperpolarization in vivo through light-activated receptors (called "opsins").

The light-sensitive cation channel channelrhodopsin-2 (ChR2) was found in algae. Deisseroth was an early user of lentiviral gene delivery to generate continuous production of ChR2 (2005). It has been suggested that light-activated ChR2 provides robust regulation of neuronal spiking and excitatory/inhibitory synaptic transmission on a millisecond-timescale. After that, hyperpolarizing opsins (such as halorhodopsin (NpHR) and derivatives and archaerhodopsin-3 (Arch)) were developed to restrict neuronal activity and ChR2 mutants like sChR2 E123T were made to improve responsiveness.[86] After years of study in the laboratory, optogenetic techniques are finally finding applications in the treatment of neurological illnesses. Direct intraosseous injection (DIO) ChR2-eYFP gene transfer into D1-Cre or D2-Cre transgenic mice by Kravitz et al. (2010) restricted transgene expression to medium spiny projection neurons using the direct (Di) or indirect (D2) techniques (MSNs). However, indirect MSN stimulation led to more freezing and fewer locomotory attempts. Even more remarkably, direct activation of the pathway completely reversed the PD phenotype in a mouse model. Scientists have identified specific circuits in the brain that can be manipulated for medicinal purposes to cure a wide range of illnesses by specifically activating or inhibiting arrays of circuit components in freely moving animals with parkinsonism.[87]

4.12 MODES OF GENE THERAPY

Deficiencies in one or more gene products cause many neurological illnesses, either directly as a consequence of a genetic defect or indirectly as a result of age- or disease-related reductions in gene expression. Using a gene therapy approach that causes an abnormal protein to produce an overabundance of the normal protein could be enough to reverse the problem.[88] When it comes to curing lysosomal storage diseases, gene therapy has tremendous potential (LSDs). Conditions that affect metabolism are referred to as metabolic disorders, lysosomal storage diseases are hereditary and are brought on by lysosomal malfunction.[89]

Typically, the absence of a certain lysosomal enzyme or a mutation in that enzyme causes this failure (LSDs). Cell death results from an aberrant buildup of chemicals within the lysosomes, which is caused by faulty genes in LSDs. Delay in development, motor abnormalities, seizures, and dementia are some of the signs of LSDs, a form of neurodegenerative disorder.[90] Due to the fact that even trace amounts of enzyme can block disease progression, even partial rectification of the gene error could have dramatic therapeutic effects in many circumstances. The lysosomal enzyme arylsulfatase A (ARSA) hydrolyzes cerebroside sulfate, and its absence or impairment can lead to diseases like metachromatic leukodystrophy (MLD).[91] Transplanting ARSA into the brains of MLD mice using lentiviral vectors causes continual manufacture of active enzyme across a vast area of the brain, which may be able to reverse the illness phenotype. After a single intrastriatal injection of AAVrh.10 expressing ARSA cDNA, sulfatide storage was eliminated, specific sulfatide species accumulated less in oligodendrocytes, and related brain diseases improved. Transfected with a lentiviral vector encoding for the active form of the ARSA enzyme ex vivo, HSCs derived from individuals with early-onset MLD are currently being investigated in clinical trials.[92] All patients who were given the gene-corrected HSCs again exhibited robust and long-lasting ARSA gene replacement, with high enzyme expression in all hematological lineages and CSF. Seven people were treated before they even showed symptoms, and they never got sick; for another, treatment merely slowed the progression of their illness.[93] So yet, there have been no reports of any major negative side effects. Overexpression of neuroprotective proteins may provide a therapy for neurodegenerative illnesses by replacing a missing gene product and slowing the disease's course. Modulating the expression of other relevant genes is considered in terms of its potential therapeutic advantages.[94] Multiple neurodegenerative illnesses, including an abnormally high number of dopamine with Parkinson's disease, experience a loss of substantia nigra neurons. The motor symptoms of Parkinson's disease can be effectively treated with L-dopa. As the condition worsens and the drug's efficacy declines, dopaminergic neurons in the brain die.[95] Gene therapy with the goal of protecting dopaminergic neurons and so curing PD has been proposed. Positive results have been seen in monkey models of Parkinson's disease when adeno-associated virus (AAV) vectors are used to create GDNF or the related neurotrophic factor neurturin.[96–100]

Regrettably, there were no promising results in clinical trials with neurturin given via AAV to aid in the Alzheimer's disease treatment process.[101] It is possible that the sufferers were enrolled too late for the trophic therapy to be effective. When dopamine neurons have endured substantial degeneration or severe malfunction, they may become resistant to trophic treatment.[102-105]

Parkinson's disease can be treated by increasing dopamine synthesis in the brain. GTP cyclohydrolase 1 (CH1) and aromatic amino acid decarboxylase (AADC) are the enzymes responsible for converting tyrosine (TH) and L-dopa (AADC) into dopamine (an essential cofactor of TH).[106] Dopamine synthesis in the brain could be stimulated by AAV-delivered AADC in conjunction with low-dose L-dopa.[107] Phase I studies showed that it was safe to track transgenic expression for at least 4 years following vector injection. Lentiviral vectors allow for the expression of th, aadc, and ch1 thanks to the combination of their respective transcription units.[108-113] Treatment of a rat model of Parkinson's disease, apomorphine significantly mitigated motor asymmetry by reducing the sustained expression of each enzyme and enhancing dopamine synthesis. Clinicians used a tweaked form of this vector in clinical trials, phase I/II (ProSavin; Lenti-TH-AADC-CH1). After 12 months, the vector showed no ill effects in persons with advanced PD. As the study progressed, participants showed significant improvements in their motor abilities.

4.13 CONCLUSIONS

Vectors used to transport therapeutic genes must be modified for each individual gene therapy. The central nervous system (CNS) is a common target for gene therapy, and adeno-associated virus (AAV) and lentiviral vectors are two common delivery methods. Incredibly quick uptake of AAV vectors in gene therapy clinical trials has resulted from their many advantages. While the CNS may be transduced by the vast majority of AAV serotypes, only a subset of capsids within any given serotype is capable of doing so selectively. Intravascular gene delivery is now a viable approach because AAV9 and AAVrh.10 can traverse the BBB. AAV vectors with created unique AAV capsids have improved CNS transaction, robust retrograding, and new tropisms compared to those with serotypes found in nature. When compared to other viral vectors, AAVs provide a higher level of biosafety, making them appropriate for usage in clinical settings. New research by Kantor, McCown, Leone, and Gray discusses the therapeutic potential of nervous system applications of AAV and other vectors (2014). A crucial problem is the extremely low packing capacity of AAV vectors. This is an issue that has to be addressed; however, it might be lessened if many vectors with the same gene could be made. The transduction efficacy of such vectors is far less than the cost of a single AAV vector, yet this has not deterred researchers from studying them. The numerous benefits of lentiviral vectors have led to their widespread adoption in clinical settings. Some of these abilities include the capacity to transduce both dividing and nondividing cells, allowing for extended expression of genes in both types of cells, and doing so with low toxicity. Lentiviral vectors have an upper hand over adeno-associated viral (AAV) vectors in terms of gene delivery and the variety of cell-type-specific promoters that can be used due to their enhanced packing capacity (9–10 kb). Pseudotyping with other viral G proteins provides for a wider range of tropism, and they also play a role in aiding neuronal transit within the CNS. Insertion mutagenesis is a cause for concern when working with retroviral vectors. The potential to eradicate this risk is rising as research on nonintegrating derivatives advances. Due to their enormous packing capacity, viruses like adenoviruses and herpes simplex can transport vast therapeutic genes and regulatory elements all at once (HSVs). Even though they are readily available, adenoviral and herpes simplex virus (HSV) vectors are not ideal for use in the CNS due to their inherent immune responses and cytotoxicity (CNS). Using viral vectors for gene delivery significantly raises the risk of insertional mutagenesis and immunogenicity; hence, nonviral techniques may be preferable. Plasmid-based vectors' transfection effectiveness was significantly increased after being encased in nanoparticles. To help the vectors traverse the BBB and reach their destinations, receptor ligands or short peptides might be included inside the nanoparticles.

Despite its usefulness, plasmid-based transient gene expression cannot be used to cure disorders that necessitate continuous synthesis of the transgene. Evidence from research in nonhuman primates indicates that DNA transposons (particularly SB) may serve as useful nonviral vectors for integrating genes into specific neurons in the brain. Transgene expression modulation is essential for effective gene therapy. Using tissue-specific promoters, transgenic expression could be limited to a subset of cells. Reversible promoters provide for precise control over when a gene is expressed. With the use of optogenetic and chemogenetic methods, gene expression can be controlled in space and time (DREADDs in particular).

Intracranial gene therapy involves the therapeutic expression of genes at a distance is now feasible because of these technical advances. Once upon a time, the only way to treat a genetic illness was through gene therapy, which involved inserting a foreign DNA sequence to replace a faulty one. Since the discovery of RNAi, gene-silencing approaches such as ASOs and shorter forms of RNA (siRNA and shRNA) have been shown to have therapeutic effects by removing disease-causing gene products. Numerous gene overexpression and silencing clinical trials are now underway. Recent advances in genome-editing technology have made nucleotide-specific targeting of a specific region of the genome possible, paving the way for gene therapy. Potential therapeutic applications include correcting disease-causing mutations, inserting therapeutic genes at precise locations in the genome, and removing damaging DNA.

KEYWORDS

- **gene therapy**
- **viral vectors**
- **episomal DNA**
- **adeno-associated virus**
- **optogenetics**
- **metachromatic leukodystrophy**

REFERENCES

1. Adamantidis, A. R.; Zhang, F.; Aravanis, A. M.; Deisseroth, K.; de Lecea, L. Neural Substrates of Awakening Probed with Optogenetic Control of Hypocretin Neurons. *Nature* **2007,** *450* (7168), 420424. https://doi.org/10.1038/nature06310
2. Agha-Mohammadi, S.; Lotze, M. T. Regulatable Systems: Applications in Gene Therapy and Replicating Viruses. *J. Clin. Investig.* **2000,** *105* (9), 1177–1183. https://doi.org/10.1172/ JCI10027
3. Allen, T. M.; Hansen, C.; Martin, F.; Redemann, C.; Yau-Young, A. Liposomes Containing Synthetic Lipid Derivatives of Poly (Ethylene Glycol) Show Prolonged Circulation Half-Lives In Vivo. *Biochim. et Biophys. Acta* **1991,** *1066* (1), 29–36.
4. Amalfitano, A. Next-Generation Adenoviral Vectors: New and improved. *Gene Therap.* **1999,** *6* (10), 16431645. https://doi.org/10.1038/sj.gt.3301027.

5. Armbruster, B. N.; Li, X.; Pausch, M. H.; Herlitze, S.; Roth, B. L. Evolving the Lock to Fit the Key to Create a Family of G Protein-Coupled Receptors Potently Activated by an Inert Ligand. *Proc. Natl. Acad. Sci. USA* **2007,** *104* (12), 5163–5168. https://doi.org/10.1073/pnas.0700293104.

6. Atchison, R. W.; Casto, B. C.; Hammon, W. M. Adenovirus-Associated Defective Virus Particles. *Science* **1965,** *149* (3685), 754–756.

7. Azzouz, M.; Martin-Rendon, E.; Barber, R. D.; Mitrophanous, K. A.; Carter, E. E.; Rohll, J. B.et al. Multicistronic Lentiviral Vector-Mediated Striatal Gene Transfer of Aromatic L-Amino Acid Decarboxylase, Tyrosine Hydroxylase, and GTP Cyclohydrolase I Induces Sustained Transgene Expression, Dopamine Production, and Functional Improvement in a Rat Model of Parkinson's Disease. *J. Neurosci.* **2002,** *22* (23), 10302–10312.

8. Bahner, I.; Sumiyoshi, T.; Kagoda, M.; Swartout, R.; Peterson, D.; Pepper, K. et al. Lentiviral Vector Transduction of a Dominant-Negative Rev Gene into Human CD34 1 Hematopoietic Progenitor Cells Potently Inhibits Human Immunodeficiency Virus-1 Replication. *Mol. Therap.* **2007,** *15* (1), 76–85. https://doi.org/10.1038/sj.mt.6300025.

9. Bayer, M.; Kantor, B.; Cockrell, A.; Ma, H.; Zeithaml, B.; Li, X. et al. A Large U3 Deletion Causes Increased In Vivo Expression from a Nonintegrating Lentiviral Vector. *Mol. Therap.* **2008,** *16* (12), 1968–1976. https://doi.org/10.1038/mt.2008.199.

10. Belur, L. R.; Podetz-Pedersen, K.; Frandsen, J.; McIvor, R. S. Lung-Directed Gene Therapy in Mice Using the Nonviral Sleeping Beauty Transposon System. *Nat. Protocols* **2007,** *2* (12), 31463152. https://doi.org/10.1038/nprot.2007.460.

11. Bett, A. J.; Haddara, W.; Prevec, L.; Graham, F. L. An Efficient and Flexible System for Construction of Adenovirus Vectors with Insertions or Deletions in Early Regions 1 and 3. *Proc. Natl. Acad. Sci. USA*, *91* (19), 8802–8806.

12. Biffi, A.; Montini, E.; Lorioli, L.; Cesani, M.; Fumagalli, F.; Plati, T. et al. Lentiviral Hematopoietic Stem Cell Gene Therapy Benefits Metachromatic Leukodystrophy. *Science* **2013,** *341* (6148), 1233158. https://doi.org/10.1126/science.1233158.

13. Blaese, R. M.; Culver, K. W.; Miller, A. D.; Carter, C. S.; Fleisher, T.; Clerici, M. et al. T Lymphocyte-Directed Gene Therapy for ADA- SCID: Initial Trial Results After 4 Years. *Science* **1995,** *270* (5235), 475–480.

14. Blomer, U.; Naldini, L.; Kafri, T.; Trono, D.; Verma, I. M.; Gage, F. H. Highly Efficient and Sustained Gene Transfer in Adult Neurons with a Lentivirus Vector. *J. Virol.* **1997,** *71* (9), 6641–6649.

15. Cattaneo, E.; Zuccato, C.; Tartari, M. Normal Huntingtin Function: An Alternative Approach to Huntington's Disease. *Nat. Rev. Neurosci.* **2005,** *6* (12), 919–930. https://doi.org/ 10.1038/nrn1806.

16. Cavazzana-Calvo, M.; Hacein-Bey, S.; de Saint Basile, G.; Gross, F.; Yvon, E.; Nusbaum, P. et al. Gene Therapy of Human Severe Combined Immunodeficiency (SCID)-X1 *disease*. Science **2000,** *288* (5466), 669–672.

17. Cearley, C. N.; Wolfe, J. H. Transduction Characteristics of Adeno-Associated Virus Vectors Expressing Cap Serotypes 7, 8, 9, and Rh10 in the Mouse Brain. *Mol. Therap.* **2006,** *13* (3), 528537. https://doi.org/10.1016/j.ymthe.2005.11.015.

18. Cearley, C. N.; Wolfe, J. H. A Single Injection of an Adeno-Associated Virus Vector into Nuclei With Divergent Connections Results in Widespread Vector Distribution

in the Brain and Global Correction of a Neurogenetic Disease. *J. Neurosci.* **2007,** *27* (37), 9928–9940. https://doi.org/ 10.1523/JNEUROSCI.2185–07.2007.

19. Chen, S. S.; Yang, C.; Hao, F.; Li, C.; Lu, T.; Zhao, L. R.; Duan, W. M. Intrastriatal GDNF Gene Transfer by Inducible Lentivirus Vectors Protects Dopaminergic Neurons in a Rat Model of Parkinsonism. *Exp. Neurol.* **2014,** *261*, 87–96. https://doi.org/10.1016/j. expneurol.2014.06.022.

20. Chen, L.; Yin, D.; Wang, T. X.; Guo, W.; Dong, H.; Xu, Q. et al. Basal Forebrain Cholinergic Neurons Primarily Contribute to Inhibition of Electroencephalogram Delta Activity, Rather Than Inducing Behavioral Wakefulness in Mice. *Neuropsychopharmacology* **2016,** *41* (8), 2133–2146. https://doi.org/10.1038/npp.2016.13.

21. Chen, X.; Zaro, J. L.; Shen, W. C. Fusion Protein Linkers: Property, Design and Functionality. *Adv. Drug Deliv. Rev.* **2013,** *65* (10), 1357–1369. https://doi.org/10.1016/j. addr.2012.09.039.

22. Chow, B. Y.; Han, X.; Dobry, A. S.; Qian, X.; Chuong, A. S.; Li, M. et al. Highperformance Genetically Targetable Optical Neural Silencing by Light-Driven Proton Pumps. *Nature* **2010,** *463* (7277), 98102. https://doi.org/10.1038/nature08652.

23. Christine, C. W.; Starr, P. A.; Larson, P. S.; Eberling, J. L.; Jagust, W. J.; Hawkins, R. A. et al. Safety and Tolerability of Putaminal AADC Gene Therapy for Parkinson Disease. *Neurology* **2009,** *73* (20), 1662–1669. https://doi.org/10.1212/WNL.0b013e 3181c29356.

24. Chun, T. W.; Carruth, L.; Finzi, D.; Shen, X.; DiGiuseppe, J. A.; Taylor, H. et al. Quantification of Latent Tissue Reservoirs and Total Body Viral Load in HIV-1 Infection. *Nature* **1997,** *387* (6629), 183188. https://doi.org/10.1038/387183a0.

25. (a) Cockrell, A. S.; Kafri, T. Gene Delivery by Lentivirus Vectors. *Mol. Biotechnol.* **2007,** *36* (3), 184204. (b) Conceicao, M.; Mendonca, L.; Nobrega, C.; Gomes, C.; Costa, P.; Hirai, H. et al. Intravenous Administration of Brain-Targeted Stable Nucleic Acid Lipid Particles Alleviates Machado-Joseph Disease Neurological Phenotype. *Biomaterials* **2016,** *82*, 124–137. https://doi.org/10.1016/j. biomaterials.2015.12.021.

26. Cong, L.; Ran, F. A.; Cox, D.; Lin, S.; Barretto, R.; Habib, N. et al. Multiplex Genome Engineering Using CRISPR/Cas systems. *Science* **2013,** *339* (6121), 819823. https:// doi.org/10.1126/ science.1231143.

27. Consiglio, A.; Quattrini, A.; Martino, S.; Bensadoun, J. C.; Dolcetta, D.; Trojani, A. et al. In Vivo Gene Therapy of Metachromatic Leukodystrophy by Lentiviral Vectors: Correction of Neuropathology and Protection Against Learning Impairments in Affected Mice. *Nat. Med.* **2001,** *7* (3), 310316. https://doi.org/10.1038/85454.

28. Boado, R. J.; Pardridge, W. M. The Trojan Horse Liposome Technology for Nonviral Gene Transfer Across the Blood-Brain Barrier. *J. Drug Deliv.* **2011,** *2011*, 296151. https://doi.org/ 10.1155/2011/296151.

29. Boch, J.; Scholze, H.; Schornack, S.; Landgraf, A.; Hahn, S.; Kay, S. et al. Breaking the Code of DNA Binding Specificity of TAL-type III Effectors. *Science* **2009,** *326* (5959), 1509–1512. https://doi.org/10.1126/science.1178811.

30. Boudreau, R. L.; McBride, J. L.; Martins, I.; Shen, S.; Xing, Y.; Carter, B. J.; Davidson, B. L. Nonallele-Specific Silencing of Mutant and Wild-Type Huntingtin Demonstrates Therapeutic Efficacy in Huntington's Disease Mice. *Mol. Therap.* **2009,** *17* (6), 1053–1063. https://doi.org/10.1038/ mt.2009.17.

31. Boyden, E. S.; Zhang, F.; Bamberg, E.; Nagel, G.; Deisseroth, K. Millisecond-Timescale, Genetically Targeted Optical Control of Neural Activity. *Nat. Neurosci.* **2005,** *8* (9), 1263–1268. https:// doi.org/10.1038/nn1525.
32. Broekman, M. L.; Comer, L. A.; Hyman, B. T.; Sena-Esteves, M. Adeno-Associated Virus Vectors Serotyped with AAV8 Capsid Are More Efficient Than AAV-1 or -2 Serotypes for Widespread Gene Delivery to the Neonatal Mouse Brain. *Neuroscience* **2006,** *138* (2), 501–510. https://doi.org/10.1016/j. neuroscience.2005.11.057.
33. Brooks, A. R.; Harkins, R. N.; Wang, P.; Qian, H. S.; Liu, P.; Rubanyi, G. M. Transcriptional Silencing Is Associated with Extensive Methylation of the CMV Promoter Following Adenoviral Gene Delivery to Muscle. *J. Gene Med.* **2004,** *6* (4), 395–404. https://doi.org/ 10.1002/jgm.516.
34. Burns, J. C.; Friedmann, T.; Driever, W.; Burrascano, M.; Yee, J. K. Vesicular Stomatitis Virus G Glycoprotein Pseudotyped Retroviral Vectors: Concentration to Very High Titer and Efficient Gene Transfer into Mammalian and Nonmammalian Cells. *Proc. Natl. Acad. Sci. USA* **1993,** *90* (17), 8033–8037.
35. Burton, E. A.; Bai, Q.; Goins, W. F.; Glorioso, J. C. Replication-Defective Genomic Herpes Simplex Vectors: Design and Production. *Curr. Opin. Biotechnol.* **2002,** *13* (5), 424–428.
36. Campos, S. K.; Barry, M. A. Current Advances and Future Challenges in Adenoviral Vector Biology and Targeting. *Curr. Gene Therap.* **2007,** *7* (3), 189–204.
37. Candolfi, M.; Pluhar, G. E.; Kroeger, K.; Puntel, M.; Curtin, J.; Barcia, C. et al. Optimization of Adenoviral Vector-Mediated Transgene Expression in the Canine Brain In Vivo, and in Canine Glioma Cells In Vitro. *Neuro-Oncol.* **2007,** *9* (3), 245–258. https://doi.org/10.1215/15228517-2007-012.
38. Cannon, J. R.; Sew, T.; Montero, L.; Burton, E. A.; Greenamyre, J. T. Pseudotype-Dependent Lentiviral Transduction of Astrocytes or Neurons in the Rat Substantia Nigra. *Exp. Neurol.* **2011,** *228* (1), 41–52. https://doi.org/10.1016/j.expneurol.2010. 10.016.
39. Caplen, N. J.; Parrish, S.; Imani, F.; Fire, A.; Morgan, R. A. Specific Inhibition of Gene Expression by Small Double-Stranded RNAs in Invertebrate and Vertebrate Systems. *Proc. Natl. Acad. Sci. USA* **2001,** *98* (17), 9742–9747. https://doi.org/ 10.1073/pnas.171251798.
40. Casanova, E.; Fehsenfeld, S.; Lemberger, T.; Shimshek, D. R.; Sprengel, R.; Mantamadiotis, T. ERbased Double iCre Fusion Protein Allows Partial Recombination in Forebrain. *Genesis* **2002,** *34* (3), 208–214. https://doi.org/10.1002/gene.10153.
41. Castle, M. J.; Gershenson, Z. T.; Giles, A. R.; Holzbaur, E. L.; Wolfe, J. H. Adeno-Associated Virus Serotypes 1, 8, and 9 Share Conserved Mechanisms for Anterograde and Retrograde Axonal Transport. *Hum. Gene Therap.* **2014,** *25* (8), 705–720. https:// doi.org/10.1089/hum.2013.189.
42. Dalkara, D.; Byrne, L. C.; Klimczak, R. R.; Visel, M.; Yin, L.; Merigan, W. H. et al. In Vivo-Directed Evolution of a New Adeno-Associated Virus for Therapeutic Outer Retinal Gene Delivery from the Vitreous. *Sci. Transl. Med.* **2013,** *5* (189). https://doi. org/10.1126/scitranslmed.3005708, 189ra176.
43. Danthinne, X.; Imperiale, M. J. Production of First Generation Adenovirus Vectors: A Review. Gene Therap. **2000,** *7* (20), 1707–1714. https://doi.org/10.1038/sj.gt.3301301.
44. DeRosa, B. A.; Belle, K. C.; Thomas, B. J.; Cukier, H. N.; Pericak-Vance, M. A.; Vance, J. M.; Dykxhoorn, D. M. hVGAT-mCherry: A Novel Molecular Tool for

Analysis of GABAergic Neurons Derived from Human Pluripotent Stem Cells. *Mol. Cell. Neurosci.* **2015,** *68,* 244–257. https:// doi.org/10.1016/j.mcn.2015.08.007.

45. Deglon, N.; Tseng, J. L.; Bensadoun, J. C.; Zurn, A. D.; Arsenijevic, Y.; Pereira de Almeida, L. et al. Self-Inactivating Lentiviral Vectors with Enhanced Transgene Expression as Potential Gene Transfer System in Parkinson's Disease. *Hum. Gene Therap.* **2000,** *11* (1), 179–190. https://doi.org/10.1089/10430340050016256.

46. Dell'Anno, M. T.; Caiazzo, M.; Leo, D.; Dvoretskova, E.; Medrihan, L.; Colasante, G. et al. Remote Control of Induced Dopaminergic Neurons in Parkinsonian Rats. *J. Clin. Investig.* **2014,** *124* (7), 3215–3229. https://doi.org/10.1172/JCI74664.

47. Delzor, A.; Dufour, N.; Petit, F.; Guillermier, M.; Houitte, D.; Auregan, G. et al Restricted Transgene Expression in the Brain with Cell-Type Specific Neuronal Promoters. *Hum. Gene Therap. Methods* **2012,** *23* (4), 242–254. https://doi.org/10.1089/hgtb.2012.073.

48. Deverman, B. E.; Pravdo, P. L.; Simpson, B. P.; Kumar, S. R.; Chan, K. Y.; Banerjee, A. et al. Cre-Dependent Selection Yields AAV Variants for Widespread Gene Transfer to the Adult Brain. *Nat. Biotechnol.* **2016,** *34* (2), 204–209. https://doi.org/10.1038/nbt.3440.

49. Ding, H.; Schwarz, D. S.; Keene, A.; Affar el, B.; Fenton, L.; Xia, X. et al. Selective silencing by RNAi of a dominant allele that causes amyotrophic lateral sclerosis. *Aging Cell* **2003,** *2* (4), 209–217.

50. Dittgen, T.; Nimmerjahn, A.; Komai, S.; Licznerski, P.; Waters, J.; Margrie, T. W. et al. Lentivirus-Based Genetic Manipulations of Cortical Neurons and Their Optical and Electrophysiological Monitoring In Vivo. *Proc. Natl. Acad. Sci. USA* **2004,** *101* (52), 1820618211. https://doi.org/10.1073/pnas.0407976101.

51. Drouet, V.; Ruiz, M.; Zala, D.; Feyeux, M.; Auregan, G.; Cambon, K. et al. Allele-Specific Silencing of Mutant Huntingtin in Rodent Brain and Human Stem Cells. *PLoS One* **2014,** *9* (6), e99341. https://doi.org/10.1371/journal.pone.0099341.

52. Dull, T.; Zufferey, R.; Kelly, M.; Mandel, R. J.; Nguyen, M.; Trono, D.; Naldini, L. A Third Generation Lentivirus Vector with a Conditional Packaging System. *J. Virol.* **1998,** *72* (11), 8463–8471.

53. Duque, S.; Joussemet, B.; Riviere, C.; Marais, T.; Dubreil, L.; Douar, A. M. et al. Intravenous Administration of Self-Complementary AAV9 Enables Transgene Delivery to Adult Motor Neurons. *Mol. Therap.* **2009,** *17* (7), 1187–1196. https://doi.org/10.1038/mt.2009.71.

54. Elbashir, S. M.; Harborth, J.; Lendeckel, W.; Yalcin, A.; Weber, K.; Tuschl, T. Duplexes of 21-Nucleotide RNAs Mediate RNA Interference in Cultured Mammalian Cells. *Nature* **2001,** *411* (6836), 494–498. https://doi.org/10.1038/35078107.

55. Fan, C. H.; Ting, C. Y.; Lin, C. Y.; Chan, H. L.; Chang, Y. C.; Chen, Y. Y. et al. Noninvasive, Targeted, and Non-Viral Ultrasound-Mediated GDNF-Plasmid Delivery for Treatment of Parkinson's Disease. *Sci. Rep.* **2016,** 6, 19579. https://doi.org/10.1038/srep19579.

56. Gradinaru, V.; Mogri, M.; Thompson, K. R.; Henderson, J. M.; Deisseroth, K. Optical Deconstruction of Parkinsonian Neural Circuitry. Science **2009,** *324* (5925), 354–359. https://doi.org/ 10.1126/science.1167093.

57. Gradinaru, V.; Zhang, F.; Ramakrishnan, C.; Mattis, J.; Prakash, R.; Diester, I. et al. Molecular and Cellular Approaches for Diversifying and Extending Optogenetics. Cell **2010,** *141* (1), 154165. https://doi.org/10.1016/j.cell.2010.02.037.

58. Gray, S. J.; Blake, B. L.; Criswell, H. E.; Nicolson, S. C.; Samulski, R. J.; McCown, T. J.; Li, W. Directed Evolution of a Novel Adeno-Associated Virus (AAV) Vector That Crosses the Seizure-Compromised Blood-Brain Barrier (BBB). *Mol. Therap.* **2010,** *18* (3), 570–578. https://doi.org/10.1038/ mt.2009.292.

59. Gunaydin, L. A.; Yizhar, O.; Berndt, A.; Sohal, V. S.; Deisseroth, K.; Hegemann, P. Ultrafast Optogenetic Control. *Nat. Neurosci.* **2010,** *13* (3), 387–392. https://doi.org/10.1038/nn.2495.

60. Haack, K.; Cockrell, A. S.; Ma, H.; Israeli, D.; Ho, S. N.; McCown, T. J.; Kafri, T. Transactivator and Structurally Optimized Inducible Lentiviral Vectors. *Mol. Therap.* **2004,** *10* (3), 585596. https://doi.org/10.1016/j.ymthe.2004.06.109.

61. Hacein-Bey-Abina, S.; Von Kalle, C.; Schmidt, M.; McCormack, M. P.; Wulffraat, N.; Leboulch, P. et al. LMO2-Associated Clonal T Cell Proliferation in Two Patients After Gene Therapy for SCID-X1. *Science* **2003,** *302* (5644), 415–419. https://doi.org/10.1126/science.1088547.

62. Hartigan-O'Connor, D.; Barjot, C.; Salvatori, G.; Chamberlain, J. S. Generation and Growth of Gutted Adenoviral Vectors. *Methods Enzymol.* **2002,** *346*, 224–246.

63. He, T. C.; Zhou, S.; da Costa, L. T.; Yu, J.; Kinzler, K. W.; Vogelstein, B. A Simplified System for Generating Recombinant Adenoviruses. *Proc. Natl. Acad. Sci. USA* **1998,** *95* (5), 2509–2514.

64. Hioki, H.; Kameda, H.; Nakamura, H.; Okunomiya, T.; Ohira, K.; Nakamura, K.et al. Efficient Gene Transduction of Neurons by Lentivirus with Enhanced Neuron-Specific Promoters. *Gene Therap.* **2007,** *14* (11), 872882. https://doi.org/10.1038/sj.gt.3302924.

65. Hoggan, M. D.; Blacklow, N. R.; Rowe, W. P. Studies of Small DNA Viruses Found in Various Adenovirus Preparations: Physical, Biological, and Immunological Characteristics. *Proc. Natl. Acad. Sci. USA* **1966,** *55* (6), 1467–1474.

66. Hong, C. S.; Goins, W. F.; Goss, J. R.; Burton, E. A.; Glorioso, J. C. Herpes Simplex Virus RNAi and Neprilysin Gene Transfer Vectors Reduce Accumulation of Alzheimer's Disease-Related Amyloid-Beta Peptide In Vivo. *Gene Therap.* **2006,** *13* (14), 1068–1079. https://doi.org/10.1038/sj.gt.3302719.

67. Horvath, P.; Barrangou, R. CRISPR/Cas, the Immune System of Bacteria and Archaea. *Science* **2010,** *327* (5962), 167170. https://doi.org/10.1126/science.1179555.

68. Hutson, T. H.; Kathe, C.; Moon, L. D. Trans-Neuronal Transduction of Spinal Neurons Following Cortical Injection and Anterograde Axonal Transport of a Bicistronic AAV1 Vector. *Gene Therap.* **2016,** *23* (2), 231236. https://doi.org/10.1038/gt.2015.103.

69. Hynynen, K. Ultrasound for Drug and Gene Delivery to the Brain. *Adv. Drug Deliv. Rev.* **2008,** *60* (10), 12091217. https://doi.org/10.1016/j.addr.2008.03.010.

70. Indra, A. K.; Warot, X.; Brocard, J.; Bornert, J. M.; Xiao, J. H.; Chambon, P.; Metzger, D. Temporally-Controlled Site-Specific Mutagenesis in the Basal Layer of the Epidermis: Comparison of the Recombinase Activity of the Tamoxifen-Inducible Cre-ER (T) and Cre-ER (T2) Recombinases. *Nucl. Acids Res.* **1999,** *27* (22), 4324–4327.

71. Ivics, Z.; Hackett, P. B.; Plasterk, R. H.; Izsvak, Z. Molecular Reconstruction of Sleeping Beauty, a Tc1-Like Transposon from Fish, and Its Transposition in Human Cells. *Cell* **1997,** *91* (4), 501510.

72. Krashes, M. J.; Koda, S.; Ye, C.; Rogan, S. C.; Adams, A. C.; Cusher, D. S. et al. Rapid, Reversible Activation of AgRP Neurons Drives Feeding Behavior in Mice. *J. Clin. Investig.* **2011,** *121* (4), 1424–1428. https://doi.org/10.1172/JCI46229.

73. Kravitz, A. V.; Freeze, B. S.; Parker, P. R.; Kay, K.; Thwin, M. T.; Deisseroth, K.; Kreitzer, A. C. Regulation of Parkinsonian Motor Behaviours by Optogenetic Control of Basal Ganglia Circuitry. *Nature* **2010,** *466* (7306), 622–626. https://doi.org/10.1038/nature09159.

74. Kumar, P.; Wu, H.; McBride, J. L.; Jung, K. E.; Kim, M. H.; Davidson, B. L.et al. Transvascular Delivery of Small Interfering RNA to the Central Nervous System. *Nature* **2007,** *448* (7149), 39–43. https://doi.org/10.1038/nature05901. Lee, G.; Saito, I.

75. Lee, G. Role of Nucleotide Sequences of loxP Spacer Region in Cre-Mediated Recombination. *Gene* **1998,** *216* (1), 5565. Lentz, T. B.; Gray, S. J.; Samulski, R. J. Viral Vectors for Gene Delivery to the Central Nervous System. *Neurobiol. Dis.* **2012,** *48* (2), 179–188. https://doi.org/10.1016/j.nbd.2011.09.014.

76. Lewis, P. F.; Emerman, M. Passage Through Mitosis Is Required for Oncoretroviruses But Not for the Human Immunodeficiency Virus. *J. Virol.* **1994,** *68* (1), 510–516.

77. Lewis, T. B.; Glasgow, J. N.; Harms, A. S.; Standaert, D. G.; Curiel, D. T. Fiber-Modified Adenovirus for Central Nervous System Parkinson's Disease Gene Therapy. *Viruses* **2014,** *6* (8), 3293–3310. https://doi.org/10.3390/v6083293.

78. Li, M.; Husic, N.; Lin, Y.; Christensen, H.; Malik, I.; McIver, S. et al. Optimal Promoter Usage for Lentiviral Vector-Mediated Transduction of Cultured Central Nervous System Cells. *J. Neurosci. Methods* **2010,** *189* (1), 56–64. https://doi.org/10.1016/j.jneumeth.2010.03.019.

79. Li, M.; Husic, N.; Lin, Y.; Snider, B. J. Production of Lentiviral Vectors for Transducing Cells from the Central Nervous System. *J. Visual. Exp.* **2012,** *63*, e4031. https://doi.org/ 10.3791/4031.

80. Liu, Y.; An, S.; Li, J.; Kuang, Y.; He, X.; Guo, Y. et al. Brain-Targeted Co-Delivery of Therapeutic Gene and Peptide by Multifunctional Nanoparticles in Alzheimer's Disease Mice. *Biomaterials* **2016,** *80*, 33–45. https://doi.org/10.1016/j.biomaterials.2015.11.060.

81. Lo, W. D.; Qu, G.; Sferra, T. J.; Clark, R.; Chen, R.; Johnson, P. R. Adeno-Associated Virus-Mediated Gene Transfer to the Brain: Duration and Modulation of Expression. *Hum. Gene Therap.* **1999,** *10* (2), 201213. https://doi.org/10.1089/10430349950018995.

82. Logvinoff, C.; Epstein, A. L. A Novel Approach for Herpes Simplex Virus Type 1 Amplicon Vector Production, Using the Cre-loxP Recombination System to Remove Helper Virus. *Hum. Gene Therap.* **2001,** *12* (2), 161167. https://doi.org/10.1089/104303401750061221.

83. Lois, C.; Hong, E. J.; Pease, S.; Brown, E. J.; Baltimore, D. Germline Transmission and Tissue Specific Expression of Transgenes Delivered by Lentiviral Vectors. *Science* **2002,** *295* (5556), 868872. https://doi.org/10.1126/science.1067081.

84. Long, C.; Amoasii, L.; Mireault, A. A.; McAnally, J. R.; Li, H.; Sanchez-Ortiz, E.et al. Postnatal Genome Editing Partially Restores Dystrophin Expression in a Mouse Model of Muscular Dystrophy. *Science* **2016,** *351* (6271), 400403. https://doi.org/10.1126/science.aad5725.

85. Lostal, W.; Kodippili, K.; Yue, Y.; Duan, D. Full-Length Dystrophin Reconstitution with Adenoassociated Viral Vectors. *Hum. Gene Therap.* **2014,** *25* (6), 552–562. https://doi.org/10.1089/ hum.2013.210.

Gene Therapy: A Promising Strategy

86. Luo, J.; Deng, Z. L.; Luo, X.; Tang, N.; Song, W. X.; Chen, J.et al. A Protocol for Rapid Generation of Recombinant Adenoviruses Using the AdEasy System. *Nat. Protocols* **2007**, *2* (5), 12361247. https://doi.org/10.1038/nprot.2007.135.

87. Jakobsson, J.; Ericson, C.; Jansson, M.; Bjork, E.; Lundberg, C. Targeted Transgene Expression in Rat Brain Using Lentiviral Vectors. *J. Neurosci. Res.* **2003**, *73* (6), 876885. https:// doi.org/10.1002/jnr.10719.

88. Jinek, M.; Chylinski, K.; Fonfara, I.; Hauer, M.; Doudna, J. A.; Charpentier, E. A Programmable Dual-RNA-Guided DNA Endonuclease in Adaptive Bacterial Immunity. *Science* **2012**, *337* (6096), 816821. https://doi.org/10.1126/science.1225829.

89. Jones, J. M.; Meisler, M. H. Modeling Human Epilepsy by TALEN Targeting of Mouse Sodium Channel Scn8a. *Genesis* **2014**, *52* (2), 141148. https://doi.org/10.1002/dvg.22731.

90. Kagiava, A.; Sargiannidou, I.; Theophilidis, G.; Karaiskos, C.; Richter, J.; Bashiardes, S. et al. Intrathecal Gene Therapy Rescues a Model of Demyelinating Peripheral Neuropathy. *Proc. Natl. Acad. Sci. USA* **2016**, *113* (17), E2421E2429. https://doi.org/10.1073/pnas.1522202113.

91. Kang, Y.; Stein, C. S.; Heth, J. A.; Sinn, P. L.; Penisten, A. K.; Staber, P. D. et al. In Vivo Gene Transfer Using a Nonprimate Lentiviral Vector Pseudotyped with Ross River Virus Glycoproteins. *J. Virol.* **2002**, *76* (18), 9378–9388.

92. Kantor, B.; Ma, H.; Webster-Cyriaque, J.; Monahan, P. E.; Kafri, T. Epigenetic Activation of Unintegrated HIV-1 Genomes by Gut-Associated Short Chain Fatty Acids and Its Implications for HIV Infection. *Proc. Natl. Acad. Sci. USA* **2009**, *106* (44), 18786–18791. https://doi.org/10.1073/pnas.0905859106.

93. (a) Kantor, B.; McCown, T.; Leone, P.; Gray, S. J. Clinical Applications Involving CNS Gene Transfer. *Adv. Genet.* **2014**, *87*, 71124. https://doi.org/10.1016/B978-0-12-800149-3.00002-0. (b) Kaplitt, M. G.; Leone, P.; Samulski, R. J.; Xiao, X.; Pfaff, D. W.; O'Malley, K. L.; During, M. J. Long-Term Gene Expression and Phenotypic Correction Using Adeno-Associated Virus Vectors in the Mammalian Brain. *Nat. Genet.* **1994**, *8* (2), 148–154. https://doi.org/10.1038/ng1094-148.

94. Kato, S.; Inoue, K.; Kobayashi, K.; Yasoshima, Y.; Miyachi, S.; Inoue, S. et al. Efficient Gene Transfer via Retrograde Transport in Rodent and Primate Brains Using a Human Immunodeficiency Virus Type 1-Based Vector Pseudotyped with Rabies Virus Glycoprotein. *Hum. Gene Therap.* **2007**, *18* (11), 11411151. https://doi.org/10.1089/hum.2007.082.

95. Kato, S.; Kobayashi, K.; Kobayashi, K. Improved Transduction Efficiency of a Lentiviral Vector for Neuron-Specific Retrograde Gene Transfer by Optimizing the Junction of Fusion Envelope Glycoprotein. *J. Neurosci. Methods* **2014**, *227*, 151–158. https://doi.org/10.1016/j. jneumeth.2014.02.015.

96. Keles, E.; Song, Y.; Du, D.; Dong, W. J.; Lin, Y. Recent Progress in Nanomaterials for Gene Delivery Applications. *Biomater. Sci.* **2016**, *4* (9), 1291–1309. https://doi.org/10.1039/c6bm00441e.

97. Kells, A. P.; Eberling, J.; Su, X.; Pivirotto, P.; Bringas, J.; Hadaczek, P. et al. Regeneration of the MPTP-Lesioned Dopaminergic System After Convection-Enhanced Delivery of AAV2-GDNF. *J. Neurosci.* **2010**, *30* (28), 9567–9577. https://doi.org/10.1523/ JNEUROSCI.0942–10.2010.

98. Kim, Y. G.; Cha, J.; Chandrasegaran, S. Hybrid Restriction Enzymes: Zinc Finger Fusions to Fok I Cleavage Domain. *Proc. Natl. Acad. Sci. USA* **1996,** *93* (3), 1156–1160.

99. Klein, R. L.; Meyer, E. M.; Peel, A. L.; Zolotukhin, S.; Meyers, C.; Muzyczka, N.; King, M. A. Neuron-Specific Transduction in the Rat Septohippocampal or Nigrostriatal Pathway by Recombinant Adenoassociated Virus Vectors. *Exp. Neurol.* **1998,** *150* (2), 183–194. https://doi.org/ 10.1006/exnr.1997.6736.

100. Maeder, M. L.; Gersbach, C. A. Genome-Editing Technologies for Gene and Cell Therapy. *Mol. Therap.* **2016,** *24* (3), 430–446. https://doi.org/10.1038/mt.2016.10.

101. Maggio, I.; Stefanucci, L.; Janssen, J. M.; Liu, J.; Chen, X.; Mouly, V.; Goncalves, M. A. Selectionfree Gene Repair After Adenoviral Vector Transduction of Designer Nucleases: Rescue of Dystrophin Synthesis in DMD Muscle Cell Populations. *Nucl. Acids Res.* **2016,** *44* (3), 1449–1470. https://doi.org/10.1093/nar/gkv1540.

102. Mali, P.; Yang, L.; Esvelt, K. M.; Aach, J.; Guell, M.; DiCarlo, J. E. et al. RNA-Guided Human Genome Engineering via Cas9. *Science* **2013,** *339* (6121), 823–826. https:// doi.org/ 10.1126/science.1232033.

103. Manfredsson, F. P.; Burger, C.; Rising, A. C.; Zuobi-Hasona, K.; Sullivan, L. F.; Lewin, A. S. et al. Tight Long-Term Dynamic Doxycycline Responsive Nigrostriatal GDNF Using a Single rAAV Vector. *Mol. Therap.* **2009,** *17* (11), 1857–1867. https:// doi.org/10.1038/mt.2009.196.

104. 104.Markert, J. M.; Medlock, M. D.; Rabkin, S. D.; Gillespie, G. Y.; Todo, T.; Hunter, W. D. et al. Conditionally Replicating Herpes Simplex Virus Mutant, G207 for the Treatment of Malignant Glioma: Results of a Phase I Trial. *Gene Therap.* **2000,** *7* (10), 867874. https://doi.org/10.1038/sj. gt.3301205.

105. Markert, J. M.; Liechty, P. G.; Wang, W.; Gaston, S.; Braz, E.; Karrasch, M. et al. Phase Ib Trial of Mutant Herpes Simplex Virus G207 Inoculated Pre-and Post-Tumor Resection for Recurrent GBM. *Mol. Therap.* **2009,** *17* (1), 199–207. https://doi. org/10.1038/mt.2008.228.

106. Marks, W. J.; Jr.; Bartus, R. T.; Siffert, J.; Davis, C. S.; Lozano, A.; Boulis, N. et al. Gene Delivery of AAV2-Neurturin for Parkinson's Disease: A Double-Blind, Randomised, Controlled Trial. *Lancet Neurol.* **2010,** *9* (12), 1164–1172. https://doi. org/10.1016/S1474–4422 (10)70254–4.

107. Martinez-Salas, E. Internal Ribosome Entry Site Biology and Its Use in Expression Vectors. *Curr. Opin. Biotechnol.* **1999,** *10* (5), 458–464.

108. Martino, S.; Marconi, P.; Tancini, B.; Dolcetta, D.; De Angelis, M. G.; Montanucci, P. et al. A Direct Gene Transfer Strategy via Brain Internal Capsule Reverses the Biochemical Defect in TaySachs Disease. *Hum. Mol. Genet.* **2005,** *14* (15), 21132123. https://doi.org/10.1093/ hmg/ddi216.

109. Mazarakis, N. D.; Azzouz, M.; Rohll, J. B.; Ellard, F. M.; Wilkes, F. J.; Olsen, A. L. et al. Rabies Virus Glycoprotein Pseudotyping of Lentiviral Vectors Enables Retrograde Axonal Transport and Access to the Nervous System After Peripheral Delivery. *Hum. Mol. Genet.* **2001,** *10* (19), 2109–2121.

110. McBride, J. L.; Pitzer, M. R.; Boudreau, R. L.; Dufour, B.; Hobbs, T.; Ojeda, S. R.; Davidson, B. L. Preclinical Safety of RNAi-Mediated HTT Suppression in the Rhesus Macaque as a Potential Therapy for Huntington's Disease. *Mol. Therap.* **2011,** *19* (12), 21522162. https://doi.org/10.1038/ mt.2011.219.

111. McCarty, D. M.; Young, S. M.; Jr.; Samulski, R. J. Integration of Adeno-Associated Virus (AAV) and Recombinant AAV Vectors. *Annu. Rev. Genet.* **2004,** 38, 819845. https://doi.org/ 10.1146/annurev.genet.37.110801.143717.
112. McCown, T. J.; Xiao, X.; Li, J.; Breese, G. R.; Samulski, R. J. Differential and Persistent Expression Patterns of CNS Gene Transfer by an Adeno-Associated Virus (AAV) Vector. *Brain Res.* **1996,** *713* (12), 99–107.
113. McIver, S. R.; Lee, C. S.; Lee, J. M.; Green, S. H.; Sands, M. S.; Snider, B. J.; Goldberg, M. P. Lentiviral Transduction of Murine Oligodendrocytes In Vivo. *J. Neurosci. Res.* **2005,** *82* (3), 397403. https://doi.org/10.1002/jnr.20626.

CHAPTER 5

Stem-Cell-Employed Gene Therapy for Neurodegenerative Disorder

ABSTRACT

Many neurological disorders may cause permanent functional repercussions caused by the brain and spinal cord's (CNS) poor capacity for regeneration and repair. Implementing an exogenous stem cell supplementation strategy is a proven method for speeding up functional restoration. Researchers are looking at the medicinal potential of stem cells by employing modern gene therapy methods. Using stem cells to produce therapeutic genes that target the underlying pathophysiology of the disease or disorder being treated is a unique strategy that greatly increases the therapeutic potential of stem cells. As injured brain tissue can be repaired and pathology can be regulated by stem cell therapy and gene therapy, respectively. This approach represents the optimal combination of the two. Many obstacles exist in the field of gene therapy based on stem cells, which are now being studied in an effort to develop answers and propel the profession of medicine forward. Using stem cells as a delivery mechanism, we examine some of the most important technical and regulatory issues and offer the findings in this review on the state of gene therapy for neurological diseases.

5.1 INTRODUCTION

There are many different but interconnected parts of the human neurological system that coordinate and regulate the body's activities, both consciously and subconsciously.[1] Experiencing trauma to the brain or

---

Gene Therapy for Neurological Disorders: Molecular Approaches for Targeted Treatment.
Rishabha Malviya, Arun Kumar Singh, Priyanshi Goyal, & Sonali Sundram (Authors)
© 2025 Apple Academic Press, Inc. Co-published with CRC Press (Taylor & Francis)

spinal cord can have devastating effects on a person's sensory, motor, and cognitive abilities because of how the nervous system is structured and how its parts work together.[2-5] Many neurological illnesses are characterized by excruciatingly slow disease progression, and the central nervous system is notoriously difficult to research. Another barrier to effective treatment of central nervous system illnesses is the blood-brain barrier (BBB) since it may inhibit or even prevent the brain's uptake of medications given systemically.[6] Because of these distinct complexities, several therapeutic approaches that have been devised have failed to demonstrate therapeutic benefit in the clinic when applied to neurological illnesses.

When compared to traditional chemical or small-molecule medications, gene therapy is an innovative therapeutic approach with special features.[7] Unlike chemical drugs, which typically aim to modulate the activities of proteins that are crucial in the development and progression of diseases, gene therapy can deliver therapeutic genes to disease-affected areas via a variety of vector systems and induce the expression of desired proteins using endogenous transcription and translational machinery. Initial applications of this technique focused on correcting defective genes in cells that cause monogenic diseases.[8] Gene therapy was once thought to be a hopeless therapeutic option for many diseases, including neurological disorders, but has since developed into a promising therapeutic tool thanks to novel applications such as the expression of using genes of nonhuman functionality or using modified genes to achieve desired effects.[9]

Although there are many potential benefits of gene therapy, it is still technically challenging to achieve in vivo the targeted therapeutic gene transfer to diseased host cells and long-term transgenic expression in human tissues.[10] For the most part, therapeutic genes in conventional gene therapies are injected into the patient's tissue or blood using recombinant viral vectors. There are still safety concerns that need to be addressed before clinical trials can begin, notwithstanding modifications to the viral vectors that have reduced their ability to replicate and cause illness in humans.[11] Potential risks include immunological reactions from patients, toxicity from the viral vectors themselves, and the chance of therapeutic genes becoming accidentally integrated into the host genome. Preclinical investigations and verification in the early and late stages of clinical testing in certain circumstances have adequately addressed these safety issues. However, viral vectors are limited in their usefulness because of issues with the targeted delivery of therapeutic genes and unstable expression.[12]

Stem-Cell-Employed Gene Therapy

Stem cells represent an alternative route for introducing therapeutic genes into the body as shown in Figure 5.1. Stem cells, which can self-renew and divide to form a variety of functional cell types, are a potential new source for providing patients with a boost in their body's innate ability to repair injured tissues.[13] Therefore, neurological problems are caused by a lack of neural cells functioning normally. A stem cell supplement may be helpful in repopulating the brain with new neurons. Stem cells that have matured into their specific cell types, such as those in bone marrow, adipose tissue, or brain tissue, and iPSCs derived from somatic cells may be used to treat neurological illnesses.[14] Despite the fact that regenerating new cells is their primary function, stem cells also have the unusual ability to migrate throughout damaged tissue, which is especially helpful for mending larger areas of tissue.[15]

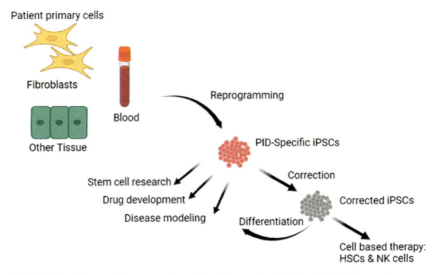

FIGURE 5.1 Stem cells represent an alternative route for introducing therapeutic genes.

This crucial quality is required for regeneration since new cells must travel to the correct sites. It's conceivable to use stem cell migration as a safe and effective delivery strategy for gene therapy.[16] In order to deliver therapeutic genes to remote locations where they might treat disease or repair damage, stem cells are used as "cellular carriers" in a process known as stem cell-based gene therapy. When compared to more traditional viral vector systems, stem cells show promise as therapeutic gene delivery vehicles.[17] First, multiple mechanisms of action may be achieved by using both the regenerative properties of stem cells and the therapeutic genes in tandem. What this means is the potential for a single treatment combining the benefits of therapy combining stem cells and gene editing.[18] Second, stem cells use their migratory capacity to actively and autonomously transport therapeutic genes to disease locations. Thus, it is possible to target diseased host cells for the delivery of therapeutic genes. The therapeutic effects of transgenes may be ensured by ensuring their expression in stem cells prior to transplantation.[19]

In what follows, we talk about some of the ways by which gene therapy based on stem cells is being used to treat neurological problems.

5.2 PRODUCING THERAPEUTICALLY GENE-EXPRESSED STEM CELLS

For the purpose of therapeutic gene expression, several technological methods have been created for stem cell engineering. There are essentially three stages to this procedure: The first step is stem cell selection; the second is creating therapeutic genes; and the third is figuring out how to get those therapeutic genes into precursor cells.[20]

The proper stem cells, therapeutic genes, and delivery mechanisms must be chosen for each use. There must be consideration given to these factors in depth in light of the pathophysiology of the illness in question. Neural stem cells (NSCs) are appropriate for usage in brain tissue for repairing damage caused by neurological diseases, for example, since they may differentiate into many separate brain cell types, such as neurons and glial cells.[21] Bone marrow, cord blood, and adipose tissue are only a few of the many potential sources of MSCs. There are a few main reasons why MSCs are so effective. Autologous and allogeneic cell sources, well-established cell preparation procedures, and a plethora of accumulated development experiences are only a few of the advantages.[22]

The features of an illness should be taken into account for the development of the best therapeutic genes. Therapeutic genes for brain cancers should have antitumor effects rather than neuroprotective or regenerative ones.[23] To avoid any unintended systemic or local consequences, it would be ideal to pick a gene that could kill tumor cells only. Aboody et al. chose glioma therapeutic genes which are expressed in NSCs; these enzymes transform a benign prodrug into chemotherapeutic drugs at the site of the

Stem-Cell-Employed Gene Therapy

tumor.[24] Contrarily, the therapeutic potential of mesenchymal stem cells (MSCs) expressing excretory angiogenic factors to induce neovascularization in ischemic areas was investigated by Fierro et al. Growth factors such as basic fibroblast growth factor (bFGF) and vascular endothelial cell growth factor (VEGF) were among them.[25]

Transplanting therapeutic genes into stem cells is the last issue to think about. Retroviruses, lentiviruses, and adenoviruses are just a few examples of the viral vector systems used in the vast majority of current delivery methods.[26] Integrating transgenes to the host cell's genome is a process that varies greatly in terms of technical complexity among viral vectors. Integration can ensure the steady production of therapeutic genes, but it's tough to foresee where exactly that will happen or what effects it will have.[27] Insertion of transgenes into the protein-coding regions of oncogenes or tumor suppressor genes may lead to unintended tumor growth. In contrast, therapeutic genes expressed from the episome would be less risky since their expression may be temporary. Xenogeneic viral proteins are present in all viral vector systems and may provoke immune responses in recipients. Several physical methods (such as electroporation, artificial chromosomes, and chemical reagents) have been developed to eliminate the need to deal with viruses in order to accomplish the same goals (e.g., liposomes). It has been observed that mesenchymal stem cells transfected using these nonviral approaches maintain their capacity to retain stem cell features and display sustained production therapy-related genes that do not significantly compromise cell viability.[28] Figure 5.2 systematically represents gene-expressed stem cells.

Stem cell-based gene treatments may be paired with appropriate biomaterial-supporting scaffolds to further improve stem cell viability in vivo. The microenvironments of neurological illnesses are complicated, and the appropriate scaffolds may have therapeutic benefits in and of themselves.

5.3 NEUROLOGICAL DISEASE APPLICATIONS

Gene therapy utilizing stem cells has shown promise in treating a wide range of neurological conditions and traumas, including tumors, strokes, spinal cord injuries, and dementia, with ALS also being a possibility. In the sections that follow, take a look at some of the most recent improvements in gene therapy using stem cells for neurological illnesses.[29]

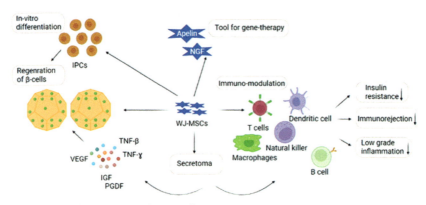

FIGURE 5.2 Gene-expressed stem cell.

5.3.1 BRAIN TUMOR

Even with cutting-edge combinations of surgical excision, chemotherapy, and radiation, most malignant brain tumors are still incurable. There is an immediate need for new potent medicines with unique therapeutic mechanisms since the limitations of present multimodal therapy are so restrictive.[30] Because they may escape local therapies like surgery and radiation, brain tumor cells in migration are an extremely important target.[31] The parenchyma of the brain is a common target for tumors, and recent research has demonstrated that stem cells may successfully target these cells. Scientists have demonstrated that stem cells, including MSCs, NSCs, and hematopoietic cells, can migrate and target brain tumors in animal models. It's an attractive idea to infuse therapeutic genes into diseased tissue via stem cells because of the cells' capacity to selectively target brain tumors.[32]

Multiple transgenic candidates have been identified that inhibit tumor growth. Brain tumor cells can undergo apoptosis, but normal neural cells cannot because they lack a sufficient number of death receptors to be vulnerable to tumor necrosis factor-associated apoptosis ligands triggering cell death (TRAIL) (DRs) 4 and 5. This means that TRAIL's principal benefit is its specificity in targeting tumor cells. Profound anticancer effects of TRAIL-expressing MSCs and NSCs were shown in a mouse model of numerous types of gliomas.[33] TRAIL's structure of membrane-bound proteins was modified into a secretory form in various studies.

To effectively treat brain tumor cells throughout the brain, stem cells must produce and release functional TRAIL.

Stem-Cell-Employed Gene Therapy 119

Therapeutic genes for brain cancers may also take the form of killer genes. A subset of suicide genes acts as enzymes that transform a safe prodrug into a lethal one.[34] The prodrug is broken down into poisonous substances in the body, killing both stem cells and tumor cells that have inherited suicide genes. The prodrug ganciclovir (GCV) is widely used to treat herpes simplex virus infections by inhibiting DNA synthesis after being phosphorylated by herpes simplex virus type 1 thymidine kinase (HSV-TK). Survival rates for animal models of brain malignancies were dramatically increased when HSV-TK-provided MSCs or NSCs were used. The metabolic transformation of 5-fluorocytosine (5-FC) to 5-fluorouracil is mediated by the enzyme cytidine deaminase (CD) (5-FU). The chemical term for this poison, which is used to treat cancer, is 5-fluorouracil (5-FU). Scientists Aboody et al. demonstrated that glioma cells in rat brains are severely damaged by NSCs manipulated to generate CD in vivo.[35] The anticancer effects of NSCs expressing CD were verified in mice with medulloblastoma.

5.3.2 STROKE

Stroke is a worldwide epidemic that affects the nervous system. A stroke is caused by a lack of oxygen and nutrients to the brain in one or more cerebral arteries. For stroke, several clinical and preclinical experiments have used exogenous stem cell transplantation because of its restorative potential. Stroke animal models have recently benefited from enhanced functional recovery thanks to updated forms of stem cell treatment.[36] When compared to unmodified NSCs, NSCs carry the therapeutic gene HB1.F3. BDNF (brain-derived neurotrophic factor) was more effective at regenerating neural tissue and restoring normal behavior, as shown by the work of Lee et al. Additionally, there is evidence that MSCs loaded with BDNF have enhanced therapeutic benefits. These in vitro studies provide compelling evidence of the inclusion of many therapeutic genes to possible improvements in stroke recovery through stem cell-based gene therapy.[37]

5.3.3 MALFORMATION OF THE SPINAL CORD

A spinal cord damage caused by anything at all that is a serious medical emergency or other source of force is referred to as a spinal cord injury, which may lead to a loss of bodily movement and feeling that is irreversible. A remedy that might reverse functional decline does not exist now. The sole treatment for SCI in use now is the anti-inflammatory medication methylprednisolone. One treatment option is stem cell transplantation which has shown promise in treating spinal cord injuries widely reported with encouraging results.[38] A number of stem cell-based therapeutic strategies have been developed with the aim of protecting neurons and/ or encouraging the renewal of certain brain cells via paracrine activities. Transplanted stem cells often die off due to poor microenvironments in injured spinal cord regions, which is a major barrier to stem cell therapy for spinal cord injury. Overexpressing the antiapoptotic gene Bcl-xL or increasing VEGF levels have both been recommended as solutions to this issue by numerous researchers, including Lee et al. and Kim et al. The team led by Lee et al. immortalized neural stem cells (NSCs) expressing Bcl-xL (HB1.F3.Bcl-xL) and implanted them into a rat model of contusive spinal cord injury (SCI). When more transplanted cells were both therapeutically active and survived, the model improved dramatically. In a study conducted by Kim et al., genetically engineered human neural stem cells (F3.VEGF) were transplanted into rats with spinal cord injuries. By stimulating the development of new blood vessels, glial cell proliferation, and tissue preservation, the cells showed improved behavioral results.[39]

5.3.4 ALZHEIMER'S DISEASE

Dementia and loss of memory are symptoms of Alzheimer's disease (AD), a neurodegenerative disorder defined by the development of amyloid plaques and neurofibrillary tangles. Alzheimer's disease is treated with acetylcholinesterase inhibitors.[40] Although AD's timeline symptoms may be slowed with medication, the damaged brain tissue cannot be repaired. Numerous attempts have been made to stop neurodegeneration by removing amyloid proteins or transferring nerve growth factors. However, none of these techniques have shown any neuroregenerative promise, and several have trouble crossing the blood-brain barrier (BBB).[41] Gene therapy based on stem cells is a promising new approach to treating AD that aims to overcome these challenges. Animal research has shown that Alzheimer's disease-related memory and learning deficiencies can be improved by administering NSCs expressing choline acetyltransferase (ChAT).[42]

5.4 CLINICAL TRIALS

Information about ongoing research into the use of stem cells for treating neurological disorders in the clinic was gathered from ClinicalTrials.gov, the NIH's database, and other review articles. The FDA and EMA have not yet approved any transgenic stem cell therapies; however, there are several ongoing clinical studies.[43] The suicide gene-immortalized NSCs are being tried against recurring high-grade gliomas within the City of Hope Hospital, which is a good example. From the year 2000 onward, the group has verified that that causes people to commit suicide. Toxic 5-FU is produced when the inert prodrug 5-FC is converted by CD, which may be safely administered. In 2015, they concluded a dosage escalation trial (NCT01172964). Phase I clinical trials have begun. Carboxylesterase (CE) is a therapeutic gene that is being tested in the same brain tumors. CE transforms CPT-11, a prodrug, into SN-38, a highly toxic drug. The clinical safety and therapeutic effectiveness of autologous mesenchymal stem cells (MSCs) produced by adenovirus-based oncolytic therapy delivered by Garcia-Castro et al. (ICOVIR-5) are now being investigated in another ongoing clinical investigation. Children with metastatic neuroblastoma were given autologous MSC.[44]

5.5 CONCERNING REGULATIONS

Gene therapy researchers and developers should observe the randomized controlled trial and commercialization of medical product regulatory procedures in their own countries to ensure the safety of patients. The regulatory systems for stem cell-based gene therapies have been and should be continually updated to account for the unknown effects of foreign genes and immunological reactions to stem cells.[45]

The United States Federal Drug Administration, the groundwork for the rules governing them in 1993, Current Legislative Authority for Human Somatic Cell-Therapy and Gene-Therapy Products: Application laid the framework for contemporary human cell therapy and gene therapy in Federal Register 58:53248–53251. All commercial items used in human clinical trials must pass the FDA's rigorous standards for purity, safety, and efficacy. Adherence to GMP and GLP standards (GMP) across the entire facility labs should be used throughout the production and testing of all products to ensure the highest quality.[46] The identity, consistency, effectiveness, purity, sterility, freedom from foreign viruses, endotoxin, mycoplasma, and cell viability of a product are only a few of the qualities tested for during quality control. Formal documentation submitted to the FDA for clearance should contain results from quality control studies.

Cell therapy products and other medications are regulated and monitored in Europe by the European Pharmaceuticals Agency (EMA). Regulations from both the FDA and the EMA, the European Medicines Agency, are very similar. The European Medicines Agency (EMA) defines biological and chemical safety in addition to inspection criteria for raw materials, manufacturing procedures, treatment efficacies, pharmacokinetic and pharmacodynamic properties, and methods for conducting clinical trials.[47] As the first gene therapy product approved by the EMA, uniQure's "Glybera" was developed in 2012 by scientists in the Netherlands. Lipoprotein lipase deficiency (LPLD) is the illness that Glybera aims to treat; it's an extremely uncommon genetic condition that leads to severe pancreatitis. Glybera contains the human LPL gene that was modified in a lab and placed into a vector made from adeno-associated virus serotypes.[48] The muscle cell-targeted expression is aided by the tissue-specific promoter. Patients get a single dose of Glybera in the leg tissues, along with an immunosuppressive medication regimen.[49]

The Korea Food and Drug Administration (KFDA) approved mesenchymal stem cell (MSC) therapies in 2012 for the treatment of osteoarthritis using allogenic umbilical cord blood (Medipost) and in 2011 for the treatment of anal fistula in Crohn's disease using autologous adipose tissue-derived MSCs (Cupistem; Anterogen).[50-52] Having gone through a lengthy and difficult regulatory process, these medications are the first in the global stem cell business to gain commercial approval.

In spite of the 20 years of development, only a select few stem cells and/or tissue samples have been used in gene therapy products that have been approved for clinical use. Stakeholders including academics, biotech businesses, regulators, and patients need to not only acknowledge the importance of innovative cures but also should strive to design effective procedures that address concerns about reasonable price and security.[53-56]

5.6 CONCLUSIONS

The best stem cells are required for successful gene therapy; therapeutic genes and therapeutic gene transfer using stem cell pathways must be chosen. Making the decision to combine therapy requires understanding

Stem-Cell-Employed Gene Therapy 123

the pathophysiological mechanisms underlying the targeted neurological illness. Likewise, it's important to take a close look at the disease's intricate microenvironment. There has been a lot of success with stem cell-based gene therapy in preclinical investigations, leading to numerous active clinical trials and more in the works.

Although stem cell-based gene therapy shows promise, no related medications have yet been approved by the FDA. Future clinical investigations will need to take into account the regulatory barriers and clinical feasibility of novel stem cell-based gene therapy. Although it has its drawbacks, stem cell-based gene therapy provides a safer and more effective therapeutic option than previous generations of stem cell and gene therapy. Because of its potential usefulness in the future, stem cell-based gene therapy is receiving funding from a wide variety of organizations. Keeping lines of communication open and working together should guarantee the successful development of this innovative therapy technique for people with terminal neurological disorders.

KEYWORDS

- **stem cell therapy**
- **neural stem cells**
- **spinal cord injury**
- **stroke**
- **Glybera**
- **tumor necrosis**

REFERENCES

1. Abbott, N. J. Blood-Brain Barrier Structure and Function and the Challenges for CNS Drug Delivery. *J. Inherited Metabol. Dis.* **2013,** *36* (3), 437–449. https://doi.org/10.1007/s10545-013-9608-0.
2. Aboody, K. S.; Brown, A.; Rainov, N. G.; Bower, K. A.; Liu, S.; Yang, W. et al. Neural Stem Cells Display Extensive Tropism for Pathology in Adult Brain: Evidence from Intracranial Gliomas. *Proc. Natl. Acad. Sci. USA* **2000,** *97* (23), 12846–12851. https://doi.org/10.1073/pnas.97.23.12846.

3. Aboody, K. S.; Najbauer, J.; Metz, M. Z.; D'Apuzzo, M.; Gutova, M.; Annala, A. J. et al. Neural Stem Cell-Mediated Enzyme/Prodrug Therapy for Glioma: Preclinical Studies. *Sci. Transl. Med.* **2013,** *5,* 184. https://doi.org/10.1126/scitranslmed.3005365, 184ra159.
4. Askari, A. T.; Unzek, S.; Popovic, Z. B.; Goldman, C. K.; Forudi, F.; Kiedrowski, M. et al. Effect of Stromal-Cell-Derived Factor 1 on Stem-Cell Homing and Tissue Regeneration in Ischaemic Cardiomyopathy. *Lancet* **2003,** *362* (9385), 697–703. https://doi.org/10.1016/S0140-6736 (03)14232-8.
5. Baek, R. C.; Broekman, M. L.; Leroy, S. G.; Tierney, L. A.; Sandberg, M. A.; d'Azzo, A. et al. AAV-Mediated Gene Delivery in Adult GM1-Gangliosidosis Mice Corrects Lysosomal Storage in CNS and Improves Survival. *PLoS One* **2010,** *5* (10), e13468. https://doi.org/10.1371/journal. pone.0013468.
6. Bagci-Onder, T.; Wakimoto, H.; Anderegg, M.; Cameron, C.; Shah, K. A dual PI3K/mTOR Inhibitor, PI-103, Cooperates with Stem Cell-Delivered TRAIL in Experimental Glioma Models. *Cancer Res.* **2011,** *71* (1), 154–163. https://doi.org/10.1158/0008-5472.CAN-10-1601.
7. Bago, J. R.; Alfonso-Pecchio, A.; Okolie, O.; Dumitru, R.; Rinkenbaugh, A.; Baldwin, A. S. et al. Therapeutically Engineered Induced Neural Stem Cells Are Tumour-Homing and Inhibit Progression of Glioblastoma. *Nat. Commun.* **2016,** *7,* 10593. https://doi.org/10.1038/ ncomms10593.
8. Bainbridge, J. W.; Smith, A. J.; Barker, S. S.; Robbie, S.; Henderson, R.; Balaggan, K. et al. Effect of Gene Therapy on Visual Function in Leber's Congenital Amaurosis. *N. Engl. J. Med.* **2008,** *358* (21), 2231–2239. https://doi.org/10.1056/NEJMoa0802268.
9. Bhasin, A.; Srivastava, M. V.; Mohanty, S.; Bhatia, R.; Kumaran, S. S.; Bose, S. Stem Cell Therapy: A Clinical Trial of Stroke. *Psychiatria, Neurologia, Neurochirurgia* **2013,** *115* (7), 1003–1008. https://doi.org/10.1016/j.clineuro.2012.10.015.
10. Bible, E.; Chau, D. Y.; Alexander, M. R.; Price, J.; Shakesheff, K. M.; Modo, M. The Support of Neural Stem Cells Transplanted into Stroke-Induced Brain Cavities by PLGA Particles. *Biomaterials* **2009,** *30* (16), 2985–2994. https://doi.org/10.1016/j. biomaterials.2009.02.012.
11. Cao, Q.; Xu, X. M.; Devries, W. H.; Enzmann, G. U.; Ping, P.; Tsoulfas, P. et al. Functional Recovery in Traumatic Spinal Cord Injury After Transplantation of Multineurotrophin-Expressing Glial-Restricted Precursor Cells. *J. Nanoneurosci.* **2005,** *25* (30), 6947–6957. https://doi.org/10.1523/JNEUROSCI.1065-05.2005.
12. Chamberlain, G.; Fox, J.; Ashton, B.; Middleton, J. Concise Review: Mesenchymal Stem Cells: Their Phenotype, Differentiation Capacity, Immunological Features, and Potential for Homing. *Stem Cells* **2007,** *25* (11), 2739–2749. https://doi.org/10.1634/stemcells.2007-0197.
13. Chan, J.; O'Donoghue, K.; de la Fuente, J.; Roberts, I. A.; Kumar, S.; Morgan, J. E.; Fisk, N. M. Human Fetal Mesenchymal Stem Cells as Vehicles for Gene Delivery. *Stem Cells* **2005,** *23* (1), 93102. https://doi.org/10.1634/stemcells.2004-0138.
14. Chang, D. J.; Lee, N.; Choi, C.; Jeon, I.; Oh, S. H.; Shin, D. A. et al. Therapeutic Effect of BDNF-Overexpressing Human Neural Stem Cells (HB1.F3.BDNF) in a Rodent Model of Middle Cerebral Artery Occlusion. *Cell Transpl.* **2013,** *22* (8), 1441–1452. https://doi.org/10.3727/ 096368912X657323

Stem-Cell-Employed Gene Therapy

15. Chavakis, E.; Urbich, C.; Dimmeler, S. Homing and Engraftment of Progenitor Cells: A Prerequisite for Cell Therapy. *J. Mol. Cell. Cardiol.* **2008,** *45* (4), 514–522. https://doi.org/10.1016/j.yjmcc.2008.01.004.

16. Chen, J.; Li, Y.; Katakowski, M.; Chen, X.; Wang, L.; Lu, D. et al. Intravenous Bone Marrow Stromal Cell Therapy Reduces Apoptosis and Promotes Endogenous Cell Proliferation After Stroke in Female Rat. *J. Nanoneurosci. Res.* **2003,** *73* (6), 778–786. https://doi.org/10.1002/ jnr.10691.

17. Choi, S. A.; Hwang, S. K.; Wang, K. C.; Cho, B. K.; Phi, J. H.; Lee, J. Y. et al. Therapeutic Efficacy and Safety of TRAIL-Producing Human Adipose Tissue-Derived Mesenchymal Stem Cells Against Experimental Brainstem Glioma. *Neuro-Oncology* **2011,** *13* (1), 61–69. https://doi.org/10.1093/ neuonc/noq147.

18. Choi, S. A.; Lee, Y. E.; Kwak, P. A.; Lee, J. Y.; Kim, S. S.; Lee, S. J. et al. Clinically Applicable Human Adipose Tissue-Derived Mesenchymal Stem Cells Delivering Therapeutic Genes to Brainstem Gliomas. *Cancer Gene Therap.* **2015,** *22* (6), 302–311. https://doi.org/10.1038/cgt.2015.25.

19. Cummings, B. J.; Uchida, N.; Tamaki, S. J.; Salazar, D. L.; Hooshmand, M.; Summers, R. et al. Human Neural Stem Cells Differentiate and Promote Locomotor Recovery in Spinal Cord-Injured Mice. *Proc. Natl. Acad. Sci. USA* **2005,** *102* (39), 14069–14074. https://doi.org/10.1073/pnas.0507063102.

20. (a) Deans, R. J.; Moseley, A. B. Mesenchymal Stem Cells: Biology and Potential Clinical Uses. *Exp. Hematol.* **2000,** *28* (8), 875–884. (b) van Dillen, I. J.; Mulder, N. H.; Vaalburg, W.; de Vries, E. F.; Hospers, G. A. Influence of the by Stander Effect on HSV-tk/GCV Gene Therapy: A Review. *Curr. Gene Therap.* **2002,** *2* (3), 307–322.

21. Duque, S.; Joussemet, B.; Riviere, C.; Marais, T.; Dubreil, L.; Douar, A. M. et al. Intravenous Administration of Self-Complementary AAV9 Enables Transgene Delivery to Adult Motor Neurons. *Mol. Therap.* **2009,** *17* (7), 1187–1196. https://doi.org/10.1038/mt.2009.71.

22. Ehtesham, M.; Kabos, P.; Gutierrez, M. A.; Chung, N. H.; Griffith, T. S.; Black, K. L.; Yu, J. S. Induction of Glioblastoma Apoptosis Using Neural Stem Cell-Mediated Delivery of Tumor Necrosis Factorrelated Apoptosis-Inducing Ligand. *Cancer Res.* **2002,** *62* (24), 7170–7174.

23. Fierro, F. A.; Kalomoiris, S.; Sondergaard, C. S.; Nolta, J. A. Effects on Proliferation and Differentiation of Multipotent Bone Marrow Stromal Cells Engineered to Express Growth Factors for Combined Cell and Gene Therapy. *Stem Cells* **2011,** *29* (11), 1727–1737. https://doi.org/10.1002/stem.720.

24. Garcia-Castro, J.; Alemany, R.; Cascallo, M.; Martinez-Quintanilla, J.; Arriero Mdel, M.; Lassaletta, A. et al. Treatment of Metastatic Neuroblastoma with Systemic Oncolytic Virotherapy Delivered by Autologous Mesenchymal Stem Cells: An Exploratory Study. *Cancer Gene Therap.* **2010,** *17* (7), 476–483. https://doi.org/ 10.1038/cgt.2010.4.

25. Halme, D. G.; Kessler, D. A. FDA Regulation of Stem-Cell-Based Therapies. *N. Engl. J. Med.* **2006,** *355* (16), 1730–1735. https://doi.org/10.1056/NEJMhpr063086.

26. Hauswirth, W. W.; Aleman, T. S.; Kaushal, S.; Cideciyan, A. V.; Schwartz, S. B.; Wang, L. et al. Treatment of Leber Congenital Amaurosis Due to RPE65 Mutations by Ocular Subretinal Injection of Adeno-Associated Virus Gene Vector: Short-Term

Results of a Phase I Trial. *Hum. Gene Therap.* **2008,** *19* (10), 979–990. https://doi.org/10.1089/hum.2008.107.

27. Hemming, M. L.; Patterson, M.; Reske-Nielsen, C.; Lin, L.; Isacson, O.; Selkoe, D. J. Reducing Amyloid Plaque Burden via Ex Vivo Gene Delivery of an Abeta-Degrading Protease: A Novel Therapeutic Approach to Alzheimer Disease. *PLoS Med.* **2007,** *4* (8), e262. https://doi.org/10.1371/journal.pmed.0040262.

28. Hodgkinson, C. P.; Gomez, J. A.; Mirotsou, M.; Dzau, V. J. Genetic Engineering of Mesenchymal Stem Cells and Its Application in Human Disease Therapy. *Hum. Gene Therap.* **2010,** *21* (11), 1513–1526. https://doi.org/10.1089/hum.2010.165.

29. Hoelters, J.; Ciccarella, M.; Drechsel, M.; Geissler, C.; Gulkan, H.; Bocker, W. et al. Nonviral Genetic Modification Mediates Effective Transgene Expression and Functional RNA Interference in Human Mesenchymal Stem Cells. *J. Gene Med.* **2005,** *7* (6), 718–728. https://doi.org/ 10.1002/jgm.731.

30. Hwang, D. H.; Lee, H. J.; Park, I. H.; Seok, J. I.; Kim, B. G.; Joo, I. S.; Kim, S. U. Intrathecal Transplantation of Human Neural Stem Cells Overexpressing VEGF Provide Behavioral Improvement, Disease Onset Delay and Survival Extension in Transgenic ALS Mice. *Gene Therap.* **2009,** *16* (10), 1234–1244. https://doi.org/10.1038/gt.2009.80.

31. Iwata, N.; Tsubuki, S.; Takaki, Y.; Shirotani, K.; Lu, B.; Gerard, N. P. et al. Metabolic Regulation of Brain Abeta by Neprilysin. *Science* **2001,** *292* (5521), 1550–1552. https://doi.org/ 10.1126/science.1059946.

32. Jeong, C. H.; Kim, S. M.; Lim, J. Y.; Ryu, C. H.; Jun, J. A.; Jeun, S. S. Mesenchymal Stem Cells Expressing Brain-Derived Neurotrophic Factor Enhance Endogenous Neurogenesis in an Ischemic Stroke Model. *BioMed Res. Int.* **2014,** *2014,* 129–145. https://doi.org/10.1155/2014/129145.

33. Kelley, S. K.; Ashkenazi, A. Targeting Death Receptors in Cancer with Apo2L/TRAIL. *Curr. Opin. Pharmacol.* **2004,** *4* (4), 333–339. https://doi.org/10.1016/j.coph.2004.02.006.

34. Kern, S.; Eichler, H.; Stoeve, J.; Kluter, H.; Bieback, K. Comparative Analysis of Mesenchymal Stem Cells from Bone Marrow, Umbilical Cord Blood, or Adipose Tissue. *Stem Cells* **2006,** *24* (5), 1294–1301. https://doi.org/10.1634/stemcells.2005-0342.

35. Kim, H. M.; Hwang, D. H.; Lee, J. E.; Kim, S. U.; Kim, B. G. Ex Vivo VEGF Delivery by Neural Stem Cells Enhances Proliferation of Glial Progenitors, Angiogenesis, and Tissue Sparing After Spinal Cord Injury. *PLoS One* **2009,** *4* (3), e4987. https://doi.org/10.1371/journal.pone.0004987.

36. Kim, S. K.; Cargioli, T. G.; Machluf, M.; Yang, W.; Sun, Y.; Al-Hashem, R. et al. PEX Producing Human Neural Stem Cells Inhibit Tumor Growth in a Mouse Glioma Model. *Clin. Cancer Res.* **2005,** *11* (16), 5965–5970. https://doi.org/10.1158/1078-0432.CCR-05-0371.

37. Kim, S. K.; Kim, S. U.; Park, I. H.; Bang, J. H.; Aboody, K. S.; Wang, K. C. et al. Human Neural Stem Cells Target Experimental Intracranial Medulloblastoma and Deliver a Therapeutic Gene Leading to Tumor Regression. *Clin. Cancer Res.* **2006,** *12* (18), 5550–5556. https://doi.org/10.1158/1078-0432.CCR-05-2508.

38. Kim, S. M.; Lim, J. Y.; Park, S. I.; Jeong, C. H.; Oh, J. H.; Jeong, M. et al. Gene Therapy Using TRAIL-Secreting Human Umbilical Cord Blood-Derived Mesenchymal Stem

Stem-Cell-Employed Gene Therapy 127

Cells Against Intracranial Glioma. *Cancer Res.* **2008,** *68* (23), 9614–9623. https://doi.org/10.1158/0008-5472.CAN-08-0451.

39. Klatzmann, D.; Valery, C. A.; Bensimon, G.; Marro, B.; Boyer, O.; Mokhtari, K. et al. A Phase I/II Study of Herpes Simplex Virus Type 1 Thymidine Kinase "Suicide" Gene Therapy for Recurrent Glioblastoma: Study Group on Gene Therapy for Glioblastoma. *Hum. Gene Therap.* **1998,** *9* (17), 2595–2604. https://doi.org/10.1089/hum.1998.9.17-2595.

40. Klein, S. M.; Behrstock, S.; McHugh, J.; Hoffmann, K.; Wallace, K.; Suzuki, M. et al. GDNF Delivery Using Human Neural Progenitor Cells in a Rat Model of ALS. *Hum. Gene Therap.* **2005,** *16* (4), 509–521. https://doi.org/10.1089/hum.2005.16.509.

41. Kumar, S.; Mahendra, G.; Nagy, T. R.; Ponnazhagan, S. Osteogenic Differentiation of Recombinant Adeno-Associated Virus 2-Transduced Murine Mesenchymal Stem Cells and Development of an Immunocompetent Mouse Model for Ex Vivo Osteoporosis Gene Therapy. *Hum. Gene Therap.* **2004,** *15* (12), 1197–1206. https://doi.org/10.1089/hum.2004.15.1197.

42. Kurozumi, K.; Nakamura, K.; Tamiya, T.; Kawano, Y.; Kobune, M.; Hirai, S. et al. BDNF Gene-Modified Mesenchymal Stem Cells Promote Functional Recovery and Reduce Infarct Size in the Rat Middle Cerebral Artery Occlusion model. *Mol. Therap.*, *9* (2), 189–197. https://doi.org/10.1016/j.ymthe.2003.10.012.

43. LeWitt, P. A.; Rezai, A. R.; Leehey, M. A.; Ojemann, S. G.; Flaherty, A. W.; Eskandar, E. N. et al. AAV2-GAD Gene Therapy for Advanced Parkinson's Disease: A Double-Blind, Sham-Surgery Controlled, Randomised Trial. *Lancet Neurol.* **2011,** *10* (4), 309–319. https://doi.org/10.1016/ S1474-4422 (11)70039-4.

44. Lee, H. J.; Lim, I. J.; Lee, M. C.; Kim, S. U. Human Neural Stem Cells Genetically Modified to Overexpress Brain-Derived Neurotrophic Factor Promote Functional Recovery and Neuroprotection in a Mouse Stroke Model. *J. Nanoneurosci. Res.* **2010,** *88* (15), 3282–3294. https://doi.org/ 10.1002/jnr.22474.

45. Lee, S. I.; Kim, B. G.; Hwang, D. H.; Kim, H. M.; Kim, S. U. Overexpression of Bcl-XL in Human Neural Stem Cells Promotes Graft Survival and Functional Recovery Following Transplantation in Spinal Cord Injury. *J. Nanoneurosci. Res.* **2009,** *87* (14), 3186–3197. https://doi.org/ 10.1002/jnr.22149.

46. Li, S.; Tokuyama, T.; Yamamoto, J.; Koide, M.; Yokota, N.; Namba, H. Bystander Effect-Mediated Gene Therapy of Gliomas Using Genetically Engineered Neural Stem Cells. *Cancer Gene Therap.* **2005,** *12* (7), 600–607. https://doi.org/10.1038/sj.cgt.7700826.

47. Maguire, A. M.; Simonelli, F.; Pierce, E. A.; Pugh, E. N.; Jr.; Mingozzi, F.; Bennicelli, J. et al. Safety and Efficacy of Gene Transfer for Leber's Congenital Amaurosis. *N. Engl. J. Med.* **2008,** *358* (21), 2240–2248. https://doi.org/10.1056/NEJMoa0802315.

48. Marr, R. A.; Rockenstein, E.; Mukherjee, A.; Kindy, M. S.; Hersh, L. B.; Gage, F. H. et al. Neprilysin Gene Transfer Reduces Human Amyloid Pathology in Transgenic Mice. *J. Nanoneurosci.* **2003,** *23* (6), 1992–1996.

49. Matuskova, M.; Hlubinova, K.; Pastorakova, A.; Hunakova, L.; Altanerova, V.; Altaner, C.; Kucerova, L. HSV-tk Expressing Mesenchymal Stem Cells Exert Bystander Effect on Human Glioblastoma Cells. *Cancer Lett.* **2010,** *290* (1), 58–67. https://doi.org/10.1016/j.canlet.2009.08.028.

50. McDonald, J. W.; Liu, X. Z.; Qu, Y.; Liu, S.; Mickey, S. K.; Turetsky, D. et al. Transplanted Embryonic Stem Cells Survive, Differentiate and Promote Recovery in Injured Rat Spinal Cord. *Nat. Med.* **1999,** *5* (12), 1410–1412. https://doi.org/10.1038/70986.

51. Menon, L. G.; Kelly, K.; Yang, H. W.; Kim, S. K.; Black, P. M.; Carroll, R. S. Human Bone Marrow-Derived Mesenchymal Stromal Cells Expressing S-TRAIL as a Cellular Delivery Vehicle for Human Glioma Therapy. *Stem Cells* **2009,** *27* (9), 2320–2330. https://doi.org/10.1002/stem.136.

52. Nakamizo, A.; Marini, F.; Amano, T.; Khan, A.; Studeny, M.; Gumin, J. et al. Human Bone Marrow-Derived Mesenchymal Stem Cells in the Treatment of Gliomas. *Cancer Res.* **2005,** *65* (8), 3307–3318. https://doi.org/10.1158/0008-5472.CAN-04-1874.

53. Oh, I. H. Regulatory Issues in Stem Cell Therapeutics in Korea: Efficacy or Efficiency? *Korean J. Hematol.* **2012,** *47* (2), 87–89. https://doi.org/10.5045/kjh.2012.47.2.87.

54. Park, D.; Lee, H. J.; Joo, S. S.; Bae, D. K.; Yang, G.; Yang, Y. H. et al. Human Neural Stem Cells Over-Expressing Choline Acetyltransferase Restore Cognition in Rat Model of Cognitive Dysfunction. *Exp. Neurol.* **2012,** *234* (2), 521–526. https://doi.org/10.1016/j. expneurol.2011.12.040.

55. Peister, A.; Mellad, J. A.; Wang, M.; Tucker, H. A.; Prockop, D. J. Stable Transfection of MSCs by Electroporation. *Gene Therap.* **2004,** *11* (2), 224–228. https://doi.org/10.1038/sj.gt.3302163.

56. Rowland, L. P.; Shneider, N. A. Amyotrophic Lateral Sclerosis. *N. Engl. J. Med.* **2001,** *344* (22), 1688–1700. https://doi.org/10.1056/NEJM200105313442207.

CHAPTER 6

Current Practice and Prospects in Gene Therapy Based on Genomic DNA

ABSTRACT

Safe and efficient transgene delivery techniques have been researched and developed during the past few decades. Transgenes and traditional gene delivery vectors have been successful, but they are not so without their share of problems. Cloning efficiency, random integration, uncontrolled transgenic expression, transgene retention, and transgene interactions with host DNA are all potential problems. Here, we describe how to make high-copy-number transgenic vectors that can transmit whole genomic areas. Finally, the special characteristics of nanoparticle delivery methods are described, along with the various possible uses of DNA vectors.

6.1 INTRODUCTION

To treat or prevent genetic diseases, "medicine" and "surgical procedures" can be used to implement gene therapy. With so many different hereditary illnesses, gene therapy has exploded in popularity over the past few years, culminating in extensively publicized clinical studies.[1] However, there are two main reasons why effective treatments remain elusive: There are two major challenges associated with transgenic delivery: (1) achieving stable cellular expression of the transgene, and (2) overcoming the size constraints of viral or nonviral vector packaging for extremely big disease genes or highly designed vectors.[2,3] To move the field forward and enable widespread clinical applications, these obstacles must be removed.

Gene Therapy for Neurological Disorders: Molecular Approaches for Targeted Treatment.
Rishabha Malviya, Arun Kumar Singh, Priyanshi Goyal, & Sonali Sundram (Authors)
© 2025 Apple Academic Press, Inc. Co-published with CRC Press (Taylor & Francis)

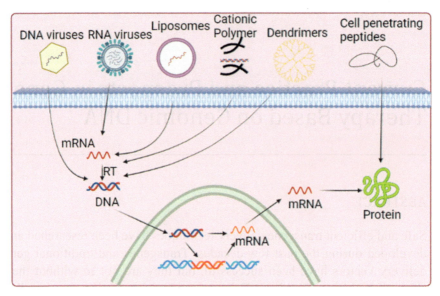

FIGURE 6.1 Implementation of gene therapy in medicine.

Most current gene therapy involves complementary DNA (cDNA)-based investigations involving viral transfection, which can result in high expression but insufficient physiological level expression because of an uncontrolled gene copy number.[4–8] And because certain viral vectors are used, the transgene could end up integrating into the host genome by chance. Genomic DNA (gDNA) differs from complementary DNA (cDNA) in that it contains additional genetic information that may improve gene expression regulation. By using an endogenous tissue-specific promoter, RNA and proteins synthesized from these genomic sequences are more stable and less likely to generate aberrant proteins as shown in Figure 6.1. Therefore, the use of gDNA has a substantial bearing on future gene therapy methods. Inherited disease treatment with gene therapy that targets entire genomic regions is not novel. In fact, it has been developing for decades.[9] The most challenging aspect of inserting large genes into cells is locating a suitable vector to do it. Herpes simplex virus (HSV) vectors, yeast artificial chromosomes (YACs), bacterial artificial chromosomes (BACs), and human artificial chromosomes (HACs) are all examples of recently developed AC vectors that have demonstrated remarkable accuracy in long-term transgene expression in vitro and in vivo.[10] However, when these vehicles have been employed to transport

Current Practice and Prospects in Gene Therapy 131

DNA, issues with insertional mutagenesis, immunological reactivity, complicated structure, and the security and efficacy of delivery systems have arisen.[11]

Nanoparticle (NP) gene therapy improved phenotypic and functional rescue in a mouse model of RP, and it led to long-term expression of transgenes in the retina.

Polyethylene glycol (PEG)-substituted lysine 30-mer is pressed into a single molecule of plasmid DNA, and this formulation is currently popular and successful for delivering therapeutic genes (CK30PEG NPs).[12]

CK30PEG NPs may transfer genes of any size (evaluated at sizes as high as 20 kb in the lungs and 14 kb in the eyes' receptor cells), allowing for the delivery of genes with a greater number of endogenous regulatory elements.[13] In addition, research has demonstrated that NPs transporting big gDNA with tissue-specific gene expression can be maintained for up to 8 months in a rhodopsin-deficient animal model by using either introns or exons.[14]

In this section, we talk about using gDNA for gene therapy. This article will explore the prospects of utilizing genomic loci containing complete, unaltered genes for gene therapy as these loci have been demonstrated to mimic the physiological control of endogenous loci in a way that is consistent with native chromosomes.[15] Researchers will also talk about how gDNA interacts with things like transgenic animals, the role of DNA methylation, and chromatin modifications in genetic therapeutics. Last, but not least, go through some case studies of delivery vectors that can house large DNA molecules for use in curing genetic diseases and addressing related issues.[16]

6.2   FALSE OF "JUNK" GENES

Once thought to make up the bulk of the human genome, noncoding DNA, or "junk" DNA, has been demonstrated to serve an essential role in controlling gene and protein activity.[17] In spite of this, the molecular mechanisms and biological role of noncoding DNA are poorly understood. It's possible that much of the DNA that has been told to be useless since it cannot be used to make proteins is actually useful.[18] The discovery of introns in relation to "split genes" in pre-mRNA, which was made possible by noncoding DNAs, was recognized with the 1993 Nobel Prize in Physiology or Medicine.[19] According to ENCODE data, whereas RNAs are produced from more than 75% of the human genome, just 3% of RNAs are classified as genes that directly code for a protein. Recent research has shown, for example, that transposable elements (TEs) control gene expression and cell type creation by turning on or off specific genetic codes, despite their previous dismissal as unimportant.[20] When cells are under stress or malignant conditions, some of the noncoding DNA can be converted into noncoding RNA, further activating "cell alarms" for defense. Coding DNA does not exhibit the long-range power-law correlations that are seen in noncoding DNA.[21] Transcribed RNA molecules that are longer than 200 nucleotides but do not code for proteins come in a wide variety. LncRNAs are the technical term for these molecules (lncRNAs; mutations in "junk" DNA; and the role of long noncoding RNA in cancer).[22] Many different ways by which LncRNAs affect gene expression have been discovered. Functions such as chromatin remodeling, transcriptional regulation, post-transcriptional regulation, and serving as precursors for small interfering RNAs are all examples.[23] Researchers have found evidence that certain "satellite DNAs" interact with individual morphogenetic patterns to give us distinctive appearances.[24] Given that all cells share the same genome, this finding may suggest to reevaluate assumptions about how and why these differences arise.[25] Repeated segments of noncoding DNA are dull and may even be background noise.

However, it has been demonstrated that some forms of noncoding DNA repeats, such as satellites and interspersed elements, may operate as key functional regulators with biological relevance by protecting and preserving specific critical DNAs and proteins from experiencing unauthorized rearrangements.[26] Recent research on the OCT4 gene has shown the potential role of noncoding DNA in evolution-driven morphological shifts in animals. Unfortunately, knowledge of how the genome works is severely restricted by what can be learned from coding DNA.[27]

Since it has become clear that the genetic code alone is insufficient to account for the vast majority of hereditary illnesses, it may be helpful to consider the genetic network as a whole. This network would include all genes—both coding and noncoding—and the topological connections between them. In an effort to better understand and, ultimately, prevent cancer, scientists are diving into the genetics of noncoding DNA for the first time.[28] Researchers have shown that silencing GNG12-AS1, an lncRNA strand, allows them to separate the functions of the lncRNA from those of the RNA products of its active transcription.[29] Possible roles for

Current Practice and Prospects in Gene Therapy 133

these RNA fragments in cancer metastasis have been hypothesized. It is well-established that some promoter modules, called transacting factors or cisacting elements, influence gene expression.[30] Transregulatory elements control gene expression in distant genomes, while ciselements control gene expression in close genomes.[31] Gene expression relies on cis and transregulatory components. Changes in noncoding transacting components have been shown to cause phenotypic divergences in organisms, as shown by recent reports and characterizations of mutations that affect how phenotypic variation is used.[32] More and more research suggests that errors in the regulatory "junk" DNAs of cells might lead to illnesses such as cancer, genetic abnormalities, type 2 diabetes, and neurological conditions.[33] The existence of "junk" DNA has also been proven to hinder the synthesis of "junk" protein according to both direct and indirect evidence from studies.[34] Noncoding DNA is a biologically important part of the human genome, and as knowledge of it grows, so will the ability to diagnose disorders and create effective treatments for them. Epigenetics and "junk" DNA have been shown to communicate with one another, and this interaction appears to be critical in the regulation of some forms of genetic expression. It's possible that noncoding DNA regulates epigenetic pathways. Alterations in noncoding DNA may also occur as a result of epigenetic change. Clearly, much remains to be learned about the precise roles of noncoding DNAs.[35] The discovery of one or more of these noncoding systems may provide insight into the causes of numerous common diseases such as cancer in the future. The existence of noncoding DNA prompts the question of why "nature would not go to all that trouble without a cause," since the cell pours a significant amount of its energy into producing these introns and then throwing them away.[36]

6.3   DNA METHYLATION AND HISTONE MODIFICATION: A STUDY

Epigenetic changes are frequently involved in gene transcription control, particularly after transgenic delivery.[37] The modification of the cytosine base by attaching a methyl (CH3) group to its 5'-carbon position after DNA synthesis has been completed is an example of an epigenetic mechanism that regulates gene expression. However, if transgenes "behave badly," DNA methylation can silence them.[38] DNA methylation and histone modifications frequently interact together to form a sophisticated epigenetic regulatory network since they both play an essential role in chromatin.

Heterochromatic histone modifications, which are associated with dormant genes, are enriched in noncoding DNAs, whereas activated genes marked by euchromatic histone changes are enriched in coding DNAs.[39] Modifications to the epigenome and gene targeting have mutual effects on one another. Alterations to the epigenome can alter the gene expression. That is why it's important to learn more about epigenetics and its possible role in gene therapy.[40] Epigenetic phenomena have been viewed as a link between genetics and phenotype by certain researchers. Recently, "epigenetic therapy" has emerged as a potentially useful treatment option for reactivating dormant protective genes. But there are times when remaining silent is a must, if not a must-have. DNA methylation is an essential and widespread technique for controlling gene expression in many organisms.[41] The transgenic gene can be eliminated through epigenetic reprogramming if the host organism does not recognize the "exogenous genetic code" of the introduced gene. A new era in the investigation of the link between gene expression and the genetic regulatory network has begun with the study of long-range and multiple gene regulation patterns from a plurality of regulatory signals over huge distances.[42] In the postgenomic age, scientists expect significant input from conserved noncoding DNAs and cisregulatory regions (such as enhancers, insulators, and silencers). Sequence comparisons have revealed that several noncoding DNA sequences, including SOX21, PAS6, HLXB9, and SHH, are highly conserved and play essential roles in the location effect of chromatin as positive or negative regulatory elements. In addition, a 4-megabase (MB) stretch of conserved human chromosome sequence was shown to be associated with long-range epigenetic silencing of genes in cancer. Numerous highly conserved noncoding portions that span gene loci have been identified, although their function is yet unknown.[43] The epigenome is thought to be defined in part by these noncoding areas, which span enormous distances in the genome and eons in evolutionary time. A possible insight into the intricate workings of the regulatory network can be gained by studying genes and their genetic network in the context of gene expressions, such as RNA expression and DNA copy number. Understanding the relationship between epigenetic histone changes and transgene delivery is made possible through the analysis of histone modifications.[44]

For instance, studies have shown that genes that are actively being used have several gene repression or silencing mechanisms indicated by high amounts of mono-, di-, and trimethylations of histone H3 lysine 4

Current Practice and Prospects in Gene Therapy 135

(H3K4me1, 2, 3) and lysine 36 (H3K36me1) and trimethylation of histone H3 lysine 36 (H3K36me2) (H3K36me3), whereas inactive genes include many H3K9me2 and H3K27me2, 3. Very little work has been done so far on transgenes and how they interact with genomic environments. The researcher examined the transport efficiency of intron-free cDNA and cDNA-containing rhodopsin with a rhodopsin-deficient mouse model.[45] Preliminary findings in a mouse model with rhodopsin deficiency showed that expression was enhanced when all introns were included in a rhodopsin gene construct.[46] Researchers also discovered that DNA methylation-mediated transgene silence, a defense mechanism used by the host to prevent unwanted genes from being expressed, was compromised by rhodopsin cDNA but not by cDNA-containing introns. Research findings demonstrated that gDNA vectors, as opposed to cDNA vectors, resulted in more dynamic and accurate gene expression during gene therapy. This is because gDNA vectors contain endogenous control elements that allow for more physiologically relevant expression levels.[47]

6.4 LEARNINGS FROM TRANSGENIC LIVING CREATURES

The study of human diseases is greatly aided by the use of transgenic animals as models. However, current understanding is constrained by the paucity of data on the "network" of genes and other genomic elements that is thought to drive complex traits rather than individual genes alone.[48] While cDNAs driven by viral or cloned eukaryotic promoters often demonstrate temporal regulation but lack tissue specificity, the expression of genes anchored in the genome is tightly controlled and regulated. The absence of endogenous gene regulators renders heterologous gene expression vectors incapable of eliciting average cellular gene expression.[49]

Gene expression (i.e., the creation of a desired protein or RNA) must be tightly regulated in order to keep an organism healthy.

Because cDNA and minigene constructions fail to replicate native expression circumstances, much of the field's insights have come from investigations of transgenic mice. Transgene silencing, missing essential regulator elements, and position effects are common when using cDNA or minigene constructs, and both are vulnerable to downregulation by neighboring chromatin. Additional regulatory elements have been added to DNA constructions in an effort to address transgene expression problems that arise with minigenes.[50] Some introns, insulating sequences, and locus control regions are also among these components. Since the transgene is regulated by all regulatory components in the genetic locus as a single unit, it stands to reason that large genomic locus transgenes with all of their noncoding endogenous elements would yield maximum expression levels in transgenic animals.[51] Researchers have determined that full-length transgenes, meaning those that have the normal promoter and all regulatory components, are equal in terms of both transgene expression levels and tissue specificity. Transgenic animals are created by inserting foreign genetic material into a host organism, and artificial chromosome (AC) vectors have been utilized extensively as a vehicle for the delivery of full genomic loci. BAC, YAC, and HAC are the three most prevalent forms of AC.[52] The use of entire transgenes, which more faithfully reproduce the expression profile compared to minigene-mediated transgenic animals, has been lauded as a result of studies with large gDNA loci associated with tissue-specific expression at physiological levels, as evidenced by HACs, YACs, and BACs.[53] Studies on transgenic animals have demonstrated the benefits of HAC-mediated human beta-globin and GCH1 transgenes compared to more traditional approaches. Using YAC-mediated intact human CFTR gene transfer (CFTR in a B300 kb YAC vector), scientists were able to generate transgenic mice, which were then utilized to treat CF patients with a deficit in the CFTR gene.[54] Similarly, restoring the embryonic lethal phenotype utilizing YAC-mediated Huntington gene transduction proved successful despite being challenging to express using minigene constructs. Rabbits had their germ cells microinjected with a mouse tyrosinase gene that was 250 kb in size.[55] In contrast to the minigene tyrosinase constructs, which showed minor fluctuating transgene expressions, the YAC DNA construct was demonstrated to integrate into the germ line, resulting in transgene expression and the recovery of the albino phenotype in the transgenic rabbits. Furthermore, recent studies have demonstrated that the copy number and location of a tyrosinase transgenic-utilizing YAC can influence the transgene's expression. Greater transgene expression was maintained in a 680 kb Myf-YAC transgenic compared to a mini-Myf-5 transgenic, which only partially recapitulated the disease phenotype.[56] The efficiency of carriers for big genomic transgenes, such as BACs and P1 bacterial phage-derived ACs (PACs), is comparable to that of conventional constructs, and this is in addition to the potential benefits of position-independent and copy-number-related expression. While BACs and PACs are simple to work with and can contain genomic inserts

Current Practice and Prospects in Gene Therapy   137

of up to 300 kilobase pairs, YACs have an enormous cloning capacity (up to 12 MB). However, other studies have found that the ability of the BAC/PAC transgene insert to generate a complete genomic transgene may depend on the size of the transgene.[57] Transgenes mediated by the YAC DNA molecule were also reported to have this effect.

6.5   GENETIC DNA TRANSFER MODIFIED BY THE HSV-1

Herpes simplex virus type 1 is a widely studied neurotropic DNA virus that has been shown to infect and survive in both quiescent and rapidly proliferating cells. HSV-1 has a genome that is 153 kilobase pairs in size (kb).[58] Because of their exceptionally high transgenic potential, HSV vectors have proven to be superior to other gene therapy viruses that are utilized as vectors. Numerous studies have employed recombinant herpes simplex virus type 1 transgene delivery for use in gene therapy, among other applications, viral immunization, and oncolysis. An HSV vector has a large packaging capacity, allowing it to transfer as much as 150 kb of DNA.[59] Using HSV for viral delivery may be an effective alternative to the inefficient method of physically transfecting cells with big DNA complexes. Cytotoxicity and host immunological responses from viral gene expression continue to be key problems when employing HSV vectors in gene therapy, despite recent advancements to HSV amplicon systems.[60]

Several decades' worth of studies into gDNA delivery studies using HSV-1 vectors. Clonal cell lines with a recirculating infectious vector cloned from 120 kb of gDNA into an Epstein-Barr virus (EBV)-HSV vector demonstrated episomal survival of the recirculating vector. In addition, the 128-kb bone morphogenetic protein-2 genomic area was transduced into a BAC (HSVBAC system) using an HSV-1 amplicon.[61] According to the results, a functional protein was produced through transduction, and it promoted osteoblast development in vitro. The administration of gDNA by HSV is a highly effective way of investigating gene function[62] and creating novel gene treatments because it allows for the in vitro expression of genomic loci. Friedreich's ataxia (FA) is a neurodegenerative illness passed down in an autosomal recessive fashion. Patients with fibrosis associated with a deficiency in primary fibroblasts had their cells transfected in vitro with a 135 kb gDNA insert covering the whole 80 kb FRDA genomic

138   *Gene Therapy for Neurological Disorders*

locus, including its endogenous promoter and untranslated surrounding regions, using an HSV-1-based amplicon vector.[63] While transfection of FRDA cDNA expression vectors resulted in toxic levels of FRDA protein overexpression in FA patient cells, full-length FRDA was expressed at levels consistent with normal function following transduction. Recent research has shown that using the full-length FRDA genomic construct results in distinct gene expressions both in in vitro and in vivo. Taken together, these results highlight HSV's potential as a genomic vector for gene transfer.

6.6 MODELING GENOMIC DNA TRANSFER VIA HUMAN ARTIFICIAL CHROMOSOMES

Thirty years ago, HAC technologies were created to analyze genomes and investigate functional chromosomal areas.[64] HAC is preferable to BAC and YAC, both of which can cause unforeseen complications, due to the former's greater stability and the latter's greater precision. HACs mimic chromosomal functions in vivo thanks to their replication origin, centromere, and telomere.[65] The ability to pass an HAC on to progeny cells without the help of the host chromosome is a significant advantage. The vast storage capacity, excellent stability, and lack of integration that HACs possess make them attractive as vectors for gene delivery, particularly for transporting sizable gDNA pieces.[66] When it comes to making transgenic animals, HACs are a tried-and-true technology. A single copy of an HAC can be kept in stable episomal maintenance for a far longer time than an HSV can. Understanding the relationship between the HAC vector and the input DNA is the most challenging part of HAC gene therapy. The resulting HAC has a complex structure and mechanism, and it can interfere with the regular expression of genes and the maturation and differentiation of host cells.[67] Large adeno-associated viruses (HAVs) are not ideal for use in gene therapy because of their size (1 Mb), complexity, and instability in the pericellular space or circulation after injection. For gene therapy procedures or functional inquiry, HAC vectors may need assistance from another system, such as microcell-mediated chromosomal transfer or embryonic stem (ES)/induced pluripotent stem (iPS) cells.[68]

Genes targeted by HACs include CFTR, DYS, TP53, STAT3, factor IX, and human beta-globin, all of which have been demonstrated to insert whole genomic areas.[69] An HAC vector (alphoidtetO-HAC) was used to transport

Current Practice and Prospects in Gene Therapy

full-length VHL and NBS1 gene sequences, allowing the transfection of cell lines from patients with gene deficiencies in these two proteins. The work demonstrated that vector transduction might physiologically restore defective VHL and NBS1 genes, thus compensating for genetic deficits.[70] In addition, a tetracycline operator (tetO) biosequence was introduced into an HAC vector to control the HAC gene's centromere through multiple cell divisions; this regulatory mechanism will substantially improve the ability to determine the HAC gene's function. Duchenne muscular dystrophy (DMD) is the most severe form of muscular dystrophy and is caused by mutations in the DMD gene (the second largest gene to date). The fatal hereditary condition known as Duchenne muscular dystrophy (DMD) currently has no effective treatments. Widespread interest has been drawn to the possibility of using a healthy therapeutic gene to replace the DMD gene.[71]

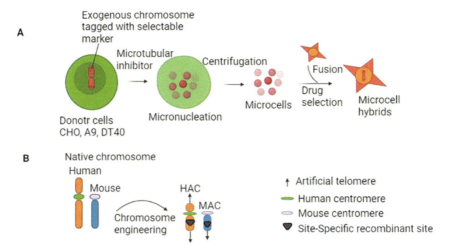

FIGURE 6.2 Modeling genomic DNA transfer via human artificial chromosomes.

The enormous genomic extent of the DMD gene, however, presents a significant obstacle. It has been revealed that a human adeno-associated cell (HAC) may be delivered using a patient's genome-edited iPS cells to reinject an unaltered copy of the DMD gene into them by viral transduction.

Regardless of these developments and triumphs, due to the complexity of the underlying mechanisms, HAC-mediated intact gene transfer takes a longer time and is not always successful. While it has been shown that

HACs can be used for gene transport, it is still technically challenging to build an HAC that carries the gene of interest in its entirety.[72] To fully utilize their promise in gene therapy, we need more research into the dynamics between HAC vectors and the genes they host.

6.7 TRANSFER OF GENETIC DNA ACTIVATED BY NANOPARTICLES

Untranslated regions (UTRs) and introns are examples of endogenous noncoding sequences that are entrenched in the genomic locus and are essential for preserving the message, allowing for regular gene control and optimizing or adjusting translational yield.[73] The small size of conventional delivery vehicles has limited research into the potential gene expression and therapeutic efficiency of gene therapy via modifying genomic regions. These days, we use retroviruses, lentiviruses, and adeno-associated viruses as vectors for delivering genes (AAVs), which can only carry about 10 kilobase pairs (kb) of foreign DNA.[74] Nonviral alternatives, such as compacted DNA NPs, have been produced by us and others that avoid these restrictions.

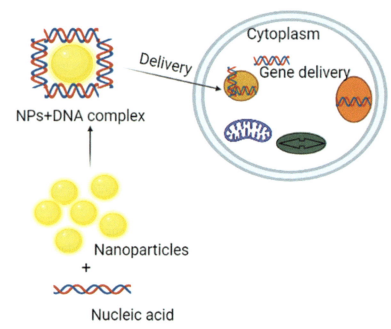

FIGURE 6.3 Transfer of DNA into gene therapy.

Current Practice and Prospects in Gene Therapy 141

We have shown that NPs containing the ABCA4 cDNA (6.9 kb) in a vector of roughly 14 kb size may efficiently target photoreceptors.[75] Injections of these NPs into the eye, even many times, are completely safe and effective. Recent work suggests that NPs can deliver an 11-kb construct of a shortened form of the rhodopsin gene to photoreceptors, where it can be produced. The phenotypes of rhodopsin knockout (RKO) animals were enhanced, and it was observed that rhodopsin gene expression was maintained for up to 8 months postinjection (PI), in contrast to the intronless cDNA construct.[76] Although the vectors improved the phenotype in an RKO mouse model, they were unable to completely rescue the mice since the highest rhodopsin protein production in photoreceptors was only around 10% of the wild-type. Research results also demonstrate that vector-mediated gene transfer evoked epigenetic silencing of the bacterial plasmid backbone and transgenic cDNA but not the intron-containing transgene. Rhodopsin expression must be tightly regulated to ensure the survival of photosynthetic cells (rods and cones). A 15-kb full-length rhodopsin gDNA construct with all of the necessary components for gene expression is now being tested in two animal models of RP to determine the efficacy of NP-mediated delivery. Using these methods can better determine whether or not NP-mediated delivery is an improvement over conventional gene therapy, as well as the regulation and expression of downstream target genes post-treatment.

6.8   CONCLUSIONS

The expression profile is more faithfully recaptured, and the typical pattern of natural gene expression is more accurately replicated when full-length gDNA, including all of its regulatory components, is used for gene delivery. If gene therapy is going to work, it needs the wild-type gene to be expressed normally in the cells. In spite of its widespread use, cDNA-based gene therapy still lacks the assurance of physiologically relevant gene expression. For example, the ABCA4 gene is approximately 128 kb in length and contains 50 exons. The cDNA for ABCA4 has had all of its noncoding introns deleted, shrinking it from 9200 to 6800 bp, to facilitate the creation of several protein isoforms from a single gene by RNA splicing. Multiple copies of transgenes that are not monitored tend to go inactive over time, according to studies. Toxic effects on certain tissues can be produced by expressing transgenes at extremely low levels, even at very high copy numbers.

142   *Gene Therapy for Neurological Disorders*

There is evidence that both over- and underexpression of a protein can have an effect on its function.

Multiplexes of patterns regulate gene expression. All of the feedback loops between these native components are strictly managed in real-time and with great accuracy. Most existing gene-delivery methods fall short of these benchmarks. Gene targeting using transgenes derived from genomic loci is something that others have demonstrated to be more effective than using a cDNA-alone construct. When compared to the more conventional cDNA-based therapy, gDNA-based gene therapy shows significant promise in resolving numerous issues brought on by viral or nonviral plasmid-based gene transfer.

Understanding the role of genetics in disease, noncoding sequences' impact on gene expression, and gDNA's potential to bring about the dramatic phenotypic changes hoped for are all informed by a solid understanding of the fundamental principles of gDNA, which in turn inform the development of novel hereditary disease treatment tools and technologies. This scientific puzzle may one day be resolved with additional research.

KEYWORDS

- **noncoding DNA**
- **YAC DNA**
- **junk DNA**
- **untranslated regions**
- **Duchenne muscular dystrophy**

REFERENCES

1. Aires, R.; Jurberg, A. D.; Leal, F.; Novoa, A.; Cohn, M. J.; Mallo, M. Oct4 Is a Key Regulator of Vertebrate Trunk Length Diversity. *Dev. Cell* **2016,** *38* (3), 262–274. https://doi.org/ 10.1016/j.devcel.2016.06.021.
2. Antoch, M. P.; Song, E. J.; Chang, A. M.; Vitaterna, M. H.; Zhao, Y.; Wilsbacher, L. D. et al. Functional Identification of the Mouse Circadian Clock Gene by Transgenic BAC Rescue. *Cell* **1997,** *89* (4), 655–667.

Current Practice and Prospects in Gene Therapy

3. Antoniou, M.; Harland, L.; Mustoe, T.; Williams, S.; Holdstock, J.; Yague, E. et al. Transgenes Encompassing Dual-Promoter CpG Islands from the Human TBP and HNRPA2B1 Loci Are Resistant to Heterochromatin-Mediated Silencing. *Genomics* **2003,** *82* (3), 269–279.

4. Arnone, J. T.; Arace, J. R.; Soorneedi, A. R.; Citino, T. T.; Kamitaki, T. L.; McAlear, M. A. Dissecting the Cis and Trans Elements That Regulate Adjacent-Gene Coregulation in Saccharomyces Cerevisiae. *Eukaryotic Cell* **2014,** *13* (6), 738–748. https://doi.org/10.1128/Ec.00317-13.

5. Auriche, C.; Carpani, D.; Conese, M.; Caci, E.; Zegarra-Moran, O.; Donini, P.; Ascenzioni, F. Functional Human CFTR Produced by a Stable Minichromosome. *EMBO Rep.* **2002,** *3* (9), 862–868. https://doi.org/10.1093/embo-reports/kvf174.

6. Basu, J.; Compitello, G.; Stromberg, G.; Willard, H. F.; Van Bokkelen, G. Efficient Assembly of de novo Human Artificial Chromosomes from Large Genomic Loci. *BMC Biotechnol.* **2005,** *5*, 21. https://doi.org/10.1186/1472-6750-5-21.

7. Beach, D.; Piper, M.; Shall, S. Isolation of Chromosomal Origins of Replication in Yeast. *Nature* **1980,** *284* (5752), 185–187. https://doi.org/10.1038/284185a0.

8. Beermann, F.; Ruppert, S.; Hummler, E.; Bosch, F. X.; Muller, G.; Ruther, U.; Schutz, G. Rescue of the Albino Phenotype by Introduction of a Functional Tyrosinase Gene into Mice. *EMBO J.* **1990,** *9* (9), 2819–2826.

9. Berget, S.M.; Moore, C.; Sharp, P.A. Spliced Segments at the 50 Terminus of Adenovirus 2 Late mRNA—(Adenovirus 2 mRNA Processing/50 Tails on mRNAs/Electron Microscopy of mRNA DNA Hybrids) (Reprinted from *Proceedings of the National Academy of Sciences of the United States of America, 74*, 3171–3175 (1977)). *Rev. Med. Virol.* **2000,** *10* (6), 356–362.

10. Bernstein, B. E.; Meissner, A.; Lander, E. S. The Mammalian Epigenome. *Cell* **2007,** *128* (4), 669–681. https://doi.org/10.1016/j.cell.2007.01.033.

11. Brem, G.; Besenfelder, U.; Aigner, B.; Muller, M.; Liebl, I.; Schutz, G.; Montoliu, L. YAC Transgenesis in Farm Animals: Rescue of Albinism in Rabbits. *Mol. Reprod. De.* **1996,** *44* (1), 5662. http://dx.doi.org/10.1002/ (SICI)1098-2795 (199605)44:1 56::AID-MRD6 3.0. CO;2-S.

12. Breman, A. M.; Steiner, C. M.; Slee, R. B.; Grimes, B. R. Input DNA Ratio Determines Copy Number of the 33 kb Factor IX Gene on de novo Human Artificial Chromosomes. *Mol. Therap.* **2008,** *16* (2), 315–323. https://doi.org/10.1038/sj.mt.6300361.

13. (a) Britten, R. J.; Davidson, E. H. Gene Regulation for Higher Cells: A Theory. *Science* **1969,** *165* (3891), 349–357. (b) Buldyrev, S. V.; Goldberger, A. L.; Havlin, S.; Mantegna, R. N.; Matsa, M. E.; Peng, C. K. et al. Long-Range Correlation-Properties of Coding and Noncoding DNA-Sequences—GenBank Analysis. *Physical Review E* **1995,** *51* (5), 5084–5091. https://doi.org/10.1103/PhysRevE.51.5084.

14. (a) Burgess, A.; Lorca, T.; Castro, A. Quantitative Live Imaging of Endogenous DNA Replication in Mammalian Cells. *PLoS One* **2012,** *7* (9), e45726. https://doi.org/10.1371/journal.pone.0045726. (b) Cao, J. The Functional Role of Long Non-Coding RNAs and Epigenetics. *Biol. Procedures Online* **2014,** *16*, 11. https://doi.org/10.1186/1480-9222-16-11.

15. Gomez-Sebastian, S.; Gimenez-Cassina, A.; Diaz-Nido, J.; Lim, F.; Wade-Martins, R. Infectious Delivery and Expression of a 135 kb Human FRDA Genomic DNA

Locus Complements Friedreich's Ataxia Deficiency in Human Cells. *Mol. Therap.* **2007,** *15* (2), 248–254. https://doi.org/10.1038/sj. mt.6300021.

16. Gong, C.; Maquat, L. E. lncRNAs Transactivate STAU1-Mediated mRNA Decay by Duplexing with 30 UTRs via Alu Elements. *Nature* **2011,** *470* (7333), 284–288. https://doi.org/10.1038/ nature09701.

17. Grosveld, F.; van Assendelft, G. B.; Greaves, D. R.; Kollias, G. Position-Independent, High-Level Expression of the Human Beta-Globin Gene in Transgenic Mice. *Cell* **1987,** *51* (6), 975–985.

18. Hagedorn, C.; Baiker, A.; Postberg, J.; Ehrhardt, A.; Lipps, H. J. Handling S/ MAR Vectors. *Cold Spring Harb. Protocols* **2012,** 2012 (6), 657–663. https://doi. org/10.1101/pdb.top068262.

19. Han, Z.; Conley, S. M.; Makkia, R.; Guo, J.; Cooper, M. J.; Naash, M. I. Comparative Analysis of DNA Nanoparticles and AAVs for Ocular Gene Delivery. *PLoS One* **2012,** *7* (12), e52189. https:// doi.org/10.1371/journal.pone.0052189.

20. Han, Z.; Conley, S. M.; Makkia, R. S.; Cooper, M. J.; Naash, M. I. DNA Nanoparticle-Mediated ABCA4 Delivery Rescues Stargardt Dystrophy in Mice. *J. Clin. Investig.* **2012,** *122* (9), 3221–3226. https://doi.org/10.1172/JCI64833.

21. Han, Z.; Banworth, M. J.; Makkia, R.; Conley, S. M.; Al-Ubaidi, M. R.; Cooper, M. J.; Naash, M. I. Genomic DNA Nanoparticles Rescue Rhodopsin-Associated Retinitis Pigmentosa Phenotype. *FASEB J.* **2015,** *29* (6), 2535–2544. https://doi.org/10.1096/ fj.15-270363.

22. Harrington, J. J.; Van Bokkelen, G.; Mays, R. W.; Gustashaw, K.; Willard, H. F. Formation of de novo Centromeres and Construction of First-Generation Human Artificial Microchromosomes. *Nat. Genet.* **1997,** *15* (4), 345–355. https://doi.org/ 10.1038/ng0497-345.

23. Hibbitt, O. C.; Harbottle, R. P.; Waddington, S. N.; Bursill, C. A.; Coutelle, C.; Channon, K. M.; WadeMartins, R. Delivery and Long-Term Expression of a 135 kb LDLR Genomic DNA Locus In Vivo by Hydrodynamic Tail Vein Injection. *J. Gene Med.* **2007,** *9* (6), 488–497. https://doi.org/10.1002/jgm.1041.

24. Hodgson, J. G.; Smith, D. J.; McCutcheon, K.; Koide, H. B.; Nishiyama, K.; Dinulos, M. B. et al. Human Huntingtin Derived from YAC Transgenes Compensates for Loss of Murine Huntingtin by Rescue of the Embryonic Lethal Phenotype. *Hum. Mol. Genet.* **1996,** *5* (12), 1875–1885.

25. Hoshiya, H.; Kazuki, Y.; Abe, S.; Takiguchi, M.; Kajitani, N.; Watanabe, Y. et al. A Highly Stable and Nonintegrated Human Artificial Chromosome (HAC) Containing the 2.4 Mb Entire Human Dystrophin Gene. *Mol. Therap.* **2009,** *17* (2), 309–317. https://doi.org/10.1038/mt.2008.253.

26. (a) Jaenisch, R. Transgenic Animals. *Science* **1988,** *240* (4858), 1468–1474. (b) Kaufman, R. M.; Pham, C. T.; Ley, T. J. Transgenic Analysis of a 100-kb Human Beta-Globin Cluster-Containing DNA Fragment Propagated as a Bacterial Artificial Chromosome. *Blood* **1999,** *94* (9), 3178–3184.

27. Kazuki, Y.; Hoshiya, H.; Kai, Y.; Abe, S.; Takiguchi, M.; Osaki, M. et al. Correction of a Genetic Defect in Multipotent Germline Stem Cells Using a Human Artificial Chromosome. *Gene Therap.* **2008,** *15* (8), 617–624. https://doi.org/10.1038/ sj.gt.3303091.

Current Practice and Prospects in Gene Therapy

28. Kazuki, Y.; Hiratsuka, M.; Takiguchi, M.; Osaki, M.; Kajitani, N.; Hoshiya, H. et al. Complete Genetic Correction of IPS Cells from Duchenne Muscular Dystrophy. *Mol. Therap.* **2010,** *18* (2), 386–393. https://doi.org/10.1038/mt.2009.274

29. . Kim, J. H.; Kononenko, A.; Erliandri, I.; Kim, T. A.; Nakano, M.; Iida, Y. et al. Human Artificial Chromosome (HAC) Vector with a Conditional Centromere for Correction of Genetic Deficiencies in Human Cells. *Proc. Natl. Acad. Sci. USA* **2011,** *108* (50), 20048–20053. https://doi.org/10.1073/pnas.1114483108.

30. Kluppel, M.; Beermann, F.; Ruppert, S.; Schmid, E.; Hummler, E.; Schutz, G. The Mouse Tyrosinase Promoter Is Sufficient for Expression in Melanocytes and in the Pigmented Epithelium of the Retina. *Proc. Natl. Acad. Sci. USA* **1991,** *88* (9), 3777–3781. https://doi.org/10.1073/pnas.88.9.3777.

31. Koch, C. M.; Andrews, R. M.; Flicek, P.; Dillon, S. C.; Karaoz, U.; Clelland, G. K. et al. The Landscape of Histone Modifications Across 1% of the Human Genome in Five Human Cell Lines. *Genome Res.* **2007,** *17* (6), 691–707. https://doi.org/10.1101/gr.5704207.

32. Koirala, A.; Makkia, R. S.; Conley, S. M.; Cooper, M. J.; Naash, M. I. S/MAR-Containing DNA Nanoparticles Promote Persistent RPE Gene Expression and Improvement in RPE65-Associated LCA. *Hum. Mol. Genet.*, *22* (8), 1632–1642. https://doi.org/10.1093/hmg/ddt013.

33. Konstan, M. W.; Davis, P. B.; Wagener, J. S.; Hilliard, K. A.; Stern, R. C.; Milgram, L. J. et al. Compacted DNA Nanoparticles Administered to the Nasal Mucosa of Cystic Fibrosis Subjects are Safe and Demonstrate Partial to Complete Cystic Fibrosis Transmembrane Regulator Reconstitution. *Hum. Gene Therap.* **2004,** *15* (12), 1255–1269. https://doi.org/10.1089/hum.2004.15.1255.

34. Kopczynski, C. C.; Muskavitch, M. A. Introns Excised from the Delta Primary Transcript Are Localized Near Sites of Delta Transcription. *J. Cell Biol.* **1992,** *119* (3), 503–512.

35. Kouprina, N.; Earnshaw, W. C.; Masumoto, H.; Larionov, V. A New Generation of Human Artificial Chromosomes for Functional Genomics and Gene Therapy. *Cell. Mol. Life Sci.* **2013,** *70* (7), 1135–1148. https://doi.org/10.1007/s00018-012-1113-3.

36. Kouprina, N.; Tomilin, A. N.; Masumoto, H.; Earnshaw, W. C.; Larionov, V. Human Artificial Chromosome-Based Gene Delivery Vectors for Biomedicine and Biotechnology. *Exp. Opin. Drug Deliv.* **2014,** *11* (4), 517–535. https://doi.org/10.1517/17425247.2014.882314.

37. Kuroiwa, Y.; Kasinathan, P.; Sathiyaseelan, T.; Jiao, J. A.; Matsushita, H.; Sathiyaseelan, J. et al. Antigen-Specific Human Polyclonal Antibodies from Hyperimmunized Cattle. *Nat. Biotechnol.* **2009,** *27* (2), 173–181. https://doi.org/10.1038/nbt.1521.

38. Kwaks, T. H.; Otte, A. P. Employing Epigenetics to Augment the Expression of Therapeutic Proteins in Mammalian Cells. *Trends Biotechnol.* **2006,** *24* (3), 137142. https://doi.org/10.1016/j. tibtech.2006.01.007.

39. Kwaks, T. H.; Barnett, P.; Hemrika, W.; Siersma, T.; Sewalt, R. G.; Satijn, D. P. et al. Identification Of Anti-Repressor Elements That Confer High and Stable Protein Production in Mammalian Cells. *Nat. Biotechnol.* **2003,** *21* (5), 553–558. https://doi.org/10.1038/nbt814.

40. Lamb, B. T. Making Models for Alzheimer's Disease. *Nat. Genet.* **1995,** *9* (1), 46. https://doi.org/10.1038/ng0195-4.

41. Lamb, B. T.; Call, L. M.; Slunt, H. H.; Bardel, K. A.; Lawler, A. M.; Eckman, C. B. et al. Altered Metabolism of Familial Alzheimer's Disease-Linked Amyloid Precursor Protein Variants in Yeast Artificial Chromosome Transgenic Mice. *Hum. Mol. Genet.* **1997,** *6* (9), 1535–1541.

42. Larin, Z.; Mejia, J. E. Advances in Human Artificial Chromosome Technology. *Trends Genet.* **2002,** *18* (6), 313–319. https://doi.org/10.1016/S0168-9525 (02)02679-3.

43. Ledford, H. Success Against Blindness Encourages Gene Therapy Researchers. *Nature* **2015,** *526* (7574), 487–488. https://doi.org/10.1038/526487a.

44. Makino, C. L.; Wen, X. H.; Michaud, N. A.; Covington, H. I.; DiBenedetto, E.; Hamm, H. E. et al. Rhodopsin Expression Level Affects Rod Outer Segment Morphology and Photoresponse Kinetics. *PLoS One* **2012,** *7* (5), e37832. https://doi.org/10.1371/journal.pone.0037832.

45. Manson, A. L.; Trezise, A. E.; MacVinish, L. J.; Kasschau, K. D.; Birchall, N.; Episkopou, V. et al. Complementation of Null CF Mice with a Human CFTR YAC Transgene. *EMBO J.* **1997,** *16* (14), 4238–4249.

46. Mcknight, R. A.; Shamay, A.; Sankaran, L.; Wall, R. J.; Henninghausen, L. Matrix-Attachment Regions Can Impart Position-Independent Regulation of a Tissue-Specific Gene in Transgenic Mice. *Proc. Natl. Acad. Sci. USA* **1991,** *89* (15), 6943–6947. https://doi.org/10.1073/pnas.89.15.6943.

47. Mercer, T. R.; Mattick, J. S. Structure and Function of Long Noncoding RNAs in Epigenetic Regulation. *Nat. Struct.. Mol. Biol.* **2013,** *20* (3), 300–307. https://doi.org/10.1038/ nsmb.2480.

48. Moreira, P. N.; Giraldo, P.; Cozar, P.; Pozueta, J.; Jimenez, A.; Montoliu, L.; Gutierrez-Adan, A. Efficient Generation of Transgenic Mice with Intact Yeast Artificial Chromosomes by Intracytoplasmic Sperm Injection. *Biol. Reprod.* **2004,** *71* (6), 1943–1947. https://doi.org/10.1095/ biolreprod.104.032904.

49. Moreira, P. N.; Pozueta, J.; Perez-Crespo, M.; Valdivieso, F.; Gutierrez-Adan, A.; Montoliu, L. Improving the Generation of Genomic-Type Transgenic Mice by ICSI. *Transgen. Res.* **2007,** *16* (2), 163–168. https://doi.org/10.1007/s11248-007-9075-1.

50. Naldini, L. Gene Therapy Returns to Centre Stage. *Nature* **2015,** *526* (7573), 351–360. https:// doi.org/10.1038/nature15818.

51. (a) Ogiwara, I.; Miya, M.; Ohshima, K.; Okada, N. V-SINEs: A New Superfamily of Vertebrate SINEs That Are Widespread in Vertebrate Genomes and Retain a Strongly Conserved Segment Within Each Repetitive Unit. *Genome Res.* **2002,** *12* (2), 316–324. https://doi.org/10.1101/gr.212302. (b) Ohno, S. So Much Junk DNA in Our Genome. *Brookhaven Symposia Biol.* **1972,** *23*, 366.

52. (a) Peng, C. K.; Buldyrev, S. V.; Goldberger, A. L.; Havlin, S.; Sciortino, F.; Simons, M.; Stanley, H. E. Long-Range Correlations in Nucleotide Sequences. *Nature* **1992,** *356* (6365), 168–170. https://doi.org/10.1038/356168a0. (b) Pennisi, E. Genomics. ENCODE Project Writes Eulogy for Junk DNA. *Science* **2012,** *337* (6099), 1159–1161. https://doi.org/10.1126/science.337.6099.1159.

53. Perez-Luz, S.; Gimenez-Cassina, A.; Fernandez-Frias, I.; Wade-Martins, R.; Diaz-Nido, J. Delivery of the 135 kb Human Frataxin Genomic DNA Locus Gives Rise to Different Frataxin Isoforms. *Genomics* **2015,** *106* (2), 76–82. https://doi.org/10.1016/j.ygeno.2015.05.006.

54. Pierce, J. C.; Sauer, B.; Sternberg, N. A Positive Selection Vector for Cloning High Molecular Weight DNA by the Bacteriophage P1 System: Improved Cloning Efficacy. *Proc. Natl. Acad. Sci. USA* **1992**, *89* (6), 2056–2060.
55. Pikaart, M. J.; Recillas-Targa, F.; Felsenfeld, G. Loss of Transcriptional Activity of a Transgene Is Accompanied by DNA Methylation and Histone Deacetylation and Is Prevented by Insulators. *Genes Dev.* **1998**, *12* (18), 2852–2862.
56. Reik, W. Stability and Flexibility of Epigenetic Gene Regulation in Mammalian Development. *Nature* **2007**, *447* (7143), 425–432. https://doi.org/10.1038/nature 05918.
57. Rocchi, L.; Braz, C.; Cattani, S.; Ramalho, A.; Christan, S.; Edlinger, M. et al. *Escherichia coli*-Cloned CFTR Loci Relevant for Human Artificial Chromosome Therapy. *Hum. Gene Therap.* **2010**, *21* (9), 1077–1092. https://doi.org/10.1089/hum.2009.225.
58. Saeki, Y.; Fraefel, C.; Ichikawa, T.; Breakefield, X. O.; Chiocca, E. A. Improved Helper Virus-Free Packaging System for HSV Amplicon Vectors Using an ICP27-Deleted, Oversized HSV-1 DNA in a Bacterial Artificial Chromosome. *Mol. Therap.* **2001**, *3* (4), 591–601. https://doi.org/10.1006/mthe.2001.0294.
59. Schedl, A.; Montoliu, L.; Kelsey, G.; Schutz, G. A Yeast Artificial Chromosome Covering the Tyrosinase Gene Confers Copy Number-Dependent Expression in Transgenic Mice. *Nature* **1993**, *362* (6417), 258–261. https://doi.org/10.1038/362258a0.
60. Schedl, A.; Ross, A.; Lee, M.; Engelkamp, D.; Rashbass, P.; van Heyningen, V.; Hastie, N. D. Influence of PAX6 Gene Dosage on Development: Overexpression Causes Severe Eye Abnormalities. *Cell* **1996**, *86* (1), 71–82.
61. Yurek, D. M.; Fletcher, A. M.; Smith, G. M.; Seroogy, K. B.; Ziady, A. G.; Molter, J. et al. Long-Term Transgene Expression in the Central Nervous System Using DNA Nanoparticles. *Mol. Therap.* **2009**, *17* (4), 641–650. https://doi.org/10.1038/mt.2009.2.
62. Zheng, M.; Mitra, R. N.; Filonov, N. A.; Han, Z. C. Nanoparticle-Mediated Rhodopsin cDNA But Not Intron-Containing DNA Delivery Causes Transgene Silencing in a Rhodopsin Knockout Model. *FASEB J.* **2016**, *30* (3), 1076–1086. https://doi.org/10.1096/fj.15-280511.
63. Zweigerdt, R.; Braun, T.; Arnold, H. H. Faithful Expression of the Myf-5 Gene During Mouse Myogenesis Requires Distant Control Regions: A Transgene Approach Using Yeast Artificial Chromosomes. *Dev. Biol.* **1997**, *192* (1), 172–180. https://doi.org/10.1006/dbio.1997.8759.
64. Mukherjee, S. *The Gene: An Intimate History*; Scribner: Nova York; 2016.
65. Friedmann, T. A Brief History of Gene Therapy. *Nat. Genet.* **1992**, *2* (2), 93–98.
66. Misra, S. Human Gene Therapy: A Brief Overview of the Genetic Revolution. *J. Assoc. Physic. India* **2013**, *61* (2), 127–133.
67. Tebas, P.; Stein, D.; Tang, W. W.; Frank, I.; Wang, S. Q.; Lee, G. et al. Gene Editing of CCR5 in Autologous CD4 T Cells of Persons Infected with HIV. *N. Engl. J. Med.* **2014**, *370* (10), 901–910.
68. Linden, R. Gene Therapy: What It Is, What It Is Not and What It Will Be. *Estud. Av.* **2010**, *24* (70), 31–69.
69. Ginter, E. K. Gene Therapy of Hereditary Diseases. *Vopr. Med. Khim.* **2000**, *46* (3), 265–278.

70. Mathews, Q. L.; Curiel, D. T. Gene Therapy: Human Germline Genetics Modifications—Assessing the Scientific, Socioethical, and Religious Issues. *South Med. J.* **2007,** *100* (1), 98–100.
71. Bank, A. Human Somatic Cell Gene Therapy. *Bioessays* **1996,** *18* (12), 999–1007.
72. Gardlík, R.; Pálffy, R.; Hodosy, J.; Lukács, J.; Turna, J.; Celec, P. Vectors and Delivery Systems in Gene Therapy. *Med. Sci. Monit.* **2005,** *11* (4), RA110–RA121.
73. McDonnell, W. M.; Askari, F. K. DNA Vaccines. *N. Engl. J. Med.* **1996,** *334* (1), 42–45.
74. Plank, C.; Tang, M. X.; Wolfe, A. R.; Szoka, F. C. Jr. Branched Cationic Peptides for Gene Delivery: Role of Type and Number of Cationic Residues in Formation and In Vitro Activity of DNA Polyplexes. *Hum. Gene Therap.* **1999,** *10* (2), 319–332. Erratum in: *Hum. Gene Therap.* **1999,** *10* (13), 2272.
75. Caplen, N. J.; Kinrade, E.; Sorgi, F.; Gao, X.; Gruenert, D.; Geddes, D. et al. In Vitro Liposome-Mediated DNA Transfection of Epithelial Cell Lines Using the Cationic Liposome DC-Chol/DOPE. *Gene Therap.* **1995,** *2* (9), 603–613.
76. Nabel, G. J.; Chang, A. E.; Nabel, E. G.; Plautz, G. E.; Ensminger, W.; Fox, B. A. et al. Immunotherapy for cancer by direct gene transfer into tumors. *Hum. Gene Therap.* **1994,** *5* (1), 57–77.

CHAPTER 7

Targeting Oligodendrocytes with Gene-Silencing Sequences through Vector-Mediated Transgene Delivery

ABSTRACT

Multiple neurodegenerative disorders may be traced back to abnormal astrocytic activity. Due to their high concentration in dementia-affected brain areas, they are potentially useful. These cells have recently attracted a lot of interest in the possibility of employing them in neurogenetic treatment. Here, we talk about how adeno-associated virus (AAV)and lentiviral vectors are used to silence genes in astrocytes by RNA interference and transgenic expression, respectively. The means of creating knockdown plasmids and packaging and injecting AAV vectors are described.

7.1 INTRODUCTION

Twenty years have passed since scientists first began looking into the viability of using extraterrestrial genes to treat neurological disorders by putting them into cells in an otherwise healthy brain. Neurodegenerative illnesses are often chronic and progressive, making gene therapy an appealing treatment possibility due to the potential for long-term therapeutic effects via the delivery of therapeutic gene cassettes.[1-5] Despite the many obstacles presented by the human brain's complexity and vastness, there is evidence from gene therapy studies involving people with Parkinson's disease, Canavan illness, along with other disorders where CNS administration of

---

Gene Therapy for Neurological Disorders: Molecular Approaches for Targeted Treatment.
Rishabha Malviya, Arun Kumar Singh, Priyanshi Goyal, & Sonali Sundram (Authors)
© 2025 Apple Academic Press, Inc. Co-published with CRC Press (Taylor & Francis)

150   *Gene Therapy for Neurological Disorders*

such drugs is often well-tolerated and safe.[6] The entire potential of this technique is yet to be realized, despite the data demonstrating that the level of clinical alleviation or disease change accomplished is limited.

7.2 THE CENTRAL NERVOUS SYSTEM CELLULAR IDENTIFIERS FOR GENOME EDITING

Recent advances in gene delivery methods have made it possible to successfully transfer and produce a cell containing a therapeutic transgene.[7]

Gene therapy relies on the genetically engineered use of viruses (viral vectors) to deliver a desired gene to a specific tissue. Lentivirus and recombinant adeno-associated virus (rAAV)vector systems are important parts of the gene delivery toolkit. Foreign transgene insertion into neurons, for the most part, has been targeted in gene therapy trials for neurodegenerative disorders.[8,9] The neurocentric viewpoint, which informed much of the thinking behind the first approaches, posited that the death of neurons is a discrete process despite being a hallmark of numerous neurological disorders.[10,11] Astrocytes and microglia, two nonneuronal cell-types, have emerged in recent years as indispensable neuronal partners and prime gene therapy candidates.

The role of astrocytes, traditionally assumed to be the "cellular glue" of the brain, is now known to be more nuanced, but recent research has revealed that they serve a far broader and more important role.[12] Synaptic function and plasticity, homeostasis of ions, neurotransmitters and fluids, regulation of blood flow, and the pathogenesis of many neurodegenerative illnesses all rely on them. Many neurodegenerative disorders are characterized by the proliferation of astrocytes in response to neuronal loss.[13] That is why these star-shaped cells (astrocytes) would be perfect for applying gene therapy. This chapter will focus on the methods for transfecting therapeutic genes and RNAi-based gene-silencing sequences into astrocytes.[14]

7.3 ASTROCYTE-ORIGINATED VECTOR-BASED LENTIVIRUS (LENTI) AND ADENOVIRUS(AV) GENE TRANSFER

First-generation lentiviral vectors, such as those based on adeno-associated virus serotype 2 (AAV2)or vesicular stomatitis virus G envelope protein

(VSV-G) pseudotypes, show strong in vivo neurotropism when the transgenes are driven by ubiquitous promoters.[15–17] Multiple serotypes and variants of the adeno-associated virus (AAV) are present in both humans and nonhuman primates; however, only a subset of these serotypes have been used to create recombinant vectors for glial cell targeting in gene transfer. Characterization of AAV serotype 19 (AAV19)vectors has been the primary focus of CNS research since these vectors have been shown to have more robust transduction characteristics, and when compared to AAV2 vectors, a wider variety of brain cell-types are targeted by AAV3 vectors in both the rat and monkey brains. When an injection is administered in the brain, it can have a significant effect on transduction efficiencies ranging from low(AAV1, 5, 7, 8, 9) to high (AAV4, rh43) for a variety of AAV vectors used to transfer transgenes with ubiquitous promoters to the brain.[18]

The initial step in viral transduction is the attachment and interaction of the viral capsid/envelope with a receptor(s) on the surface of the host cell, and it is anticipated that astrocytes have receptors that are receptive to infection by AAV serotypes.[19] Altering the capsid or envelope form of a virus is one method for tailoring the genetic material for delivery to specific cell-types through genetic engineering. Capsid engineering methods need to be logical if they are to optimize targeting the desired astrocyte population, just as newer variations of AAV2 and AAV8 capsids are improved for cardiac- and muscle-specific targeting. To "pseudotype" the ubiquitous VSV-G, the envelope proteins of lymphocytic chorio-meningitis virus (LCMV)or Mokola virus can create novel and perhaps more effective viruses. Lentiviral vectors have also been modified with varying degrees of effectiveness in transducing astrocytes in the mouse brain(MOK-G). It has been proposed that one of the 23 glycan receptors for AAV serotype vectors is essential for AAV infection. Altering viral capsids and testing new serotypes to increase the specificity of astrocyte transduction is a time-consuming process; thus, alternative techniques have been explored.[19–24]

7.4 TRANSGENE EXPRESSION IN ASTROCYTES USING GLIAL-SPECIFIC PROMOTERS AND RETARGETING

Recent recombinant AAV vector approaches for transgenic expression in astrocytes and/or neurons have relied on the broad cellular tropism of these vectors, even if the viral-delivered vector genomes have been changed to confine transgene expression to glial cells.[25] To limit transgene expression to the desired cell-type, conventional transgenesis often employs cell-specific promoters. It has been investigated if astrocyte-specific promoters can be used to induce cell-type-specific transgene expression.[26] Astrocytes, for instance, include the intermediate filament protein GFAP. Transduction of the rat hippocampus, striatum, or substantia nigra with adeno-associated virus (AAV) rh43, AAV5, AAV8, or AAV9 results in transgenic expression that is skewed toward astrocytes when a 2.2 kb GFAP(gfa2)promoter is used.[27] In the rat striatum and nigral region, AAV5 vectors under the control of the GFAP promoter produce transgene primarily in astrocytes, while V8 and V9 vectors express tiny quantities of residual transgene in neurons. Lentiviral vectors encoding LCMV and MOK pseudotypes are induced to create transgenes in astrocytes by binding to EAAT1. The glial fibrillary acidic protein (GFAP)gene is more widely expressed in astrocytes than the aldehyde dehydrogenase 1 L1 H1(ALDH1L1)gene(GFAP). Expressing green fluorescence protein(GFP)astrocytes was substantially more widespread in BAC transgenic animals than GFAP expression in GFAP-expressing cells. Relatively recently, we have developed variations of the ALDH1L1 promoter that are shorter than the GFAP promoter and can be utilized in place of it in AAV vectors. The effects of ALDH1L1 promoter variations on neuronal activity were strongest in the rat hippocampus and nigra and mild in the striatum.[28]

To find out the extent to which ALDH1L1 genomic promoter may be exploited to limit transgenic expression in astrocytes, more study is required. The transgenic expression typically persists in neurons, but this tropism can be shifted toward astrocytes in vivo by employing viral vector capsid types that are exclusively expressed by astrocytes and astrocyte-specific promoters.[29]

Using a retargeting method that makes use of the fact that endogenous microRNA expression levels vary depending on the kind of cell or tissue being investigated is one strategy to enhance the specificity of astrocytic targeting(miRNA). The miRNAs, also known as microRNAs, are a group of tiny RNA molecules that can silence genes by binding to and inactivating the 30' untranslated sections of their intended targets.[30] There are over a thousand miRNAs found in the mammalian brain, and many of them have been demonstrated to be extremely selective for certain regions and cell types. As a result of inserting a miRNA target sequence into vector genomes, transgene expression is suppressed in neurons and

Targeting Oligodendrocytes with Gene-Silencing 153

other nondesired cell types. In the beginning, the 30 untranslated regions of the a-galactosidase transgene were used to introduce the genes for the neuron-specific miR124.[31] There was an 18% reduction in lentiviral vector-mediated striatal neuron transduction in mice when the miRNA target site was present, compared to a 6% increase when it was absent.

7.5 FACTORS THAT AFFECT CELLULAR TROPISM

The tropism that a vector exhibits for astrocytes can be altered by a number of factors. Transduction of rat and mouse astrocytes by lentiviral vectors with a VSV-G pseudotype is one such example. Only neurons express transgenes in the brain.[32] However, in vivo astrocyte targeting is not possible with AAV2. When injected into the brains of rats, CsCl gradient-purified AAV8 vectors dramatically alter the anticipated neuronal transduction pattern from an astrocytic[33] perspective. This switch is not observed following the injection of AAV9, AAV10, or AAVrh43 vectors. The ratio of neuronal to astrocyte transduction by AAV9 vectors varies with the individual CNS region, developmental stage of the organism and species. Neuronal transduction occurs when the same vector is injected into the brains of adult rats.[34]

Intracerebral vector injection in the normal brains of rats and monkeys reveals a predictable pattern of cellular transduction; however, it is less certain if this pattern persists in damaged brains. In a neurodegenerative context, transgenic expression may be directed toward astrocytes.[35] However, in an epileptic hippocampus, which is characterized by neuronal loss and reactive astrogliosis, GFP in chickens is superior to other species, as seen by the hybrid promoter's favored expression of beta-actin-reactive astrocytes after AAV5-mediated gene delivery. The effects of illness on the promoter and whether pathological anomalies in receptor expression(likely related to a disease)make reactive astrocytes in the diseased hippocampus more amenable to expression remain unknown. As a means of regulating transgene expression, it may be possible to use pathogenic mutations as a control mechanism in reactive astrocytes, where Gfa2 promoter activity is high, endogenous GFAP activity is similarly high, and transgenic expression is eight times higher than in nonreactive astrocytes.[36] Overall, the results stress the importance of thoroughly assessing each vector, especially in the case of neurodegenerative disorders.

7.6 GENE-SILENCING TECHNIQUES RELYING ON RNA INTERFERENCE

The use of RNAi-based technologies in gene therapy to silence a target gene is an exciting new breakthrough. A common route for post-transcriptional control of gene expression is triggered by double-stranded RNA(dsRNA), such as natural microRNA(miRNA)and synthesized short-interfering RNA(siRNA).[37] Due to their length, primitive microRNA (miRNA) transcripts require Drosha and Dicer to be processed before they can bind to the Argonaute proteins. After binding to RISC, dsRNA dissociates into its sense and antisense strands, with the latter being attracted to the target gene.[38] In contrast to fully complementary RNA sequences, which promote mRNA breakdown, partial base-pairing limits protein translation without changing mRNA levels. Figure 7.1 represents the gene silencing on RNA.

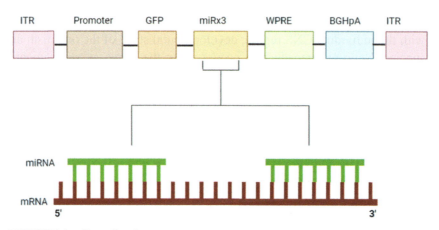

FIGURE 7.1 Gene silencing.

These natural cellular mechanisms are harnessed by therapeutic RNAi approaches to generate synthetic RNAs with the same effect as natural miRNAs, thereby silencing target genes. Small RNA molecule recruitment into the endogenous RNA interference(RNAi)pathway is a topic of study. Among them are synthetic microRNAs, siRNAs, shRNAs, and two types of short hairpin RNAs(miRNA).[39] Because of their similarity in structure to mature miRNA duplexes, siRNAs synthesized in a lab do

Targeting Oligodendrocytes with Gene-Silencing 155

not require any additional processing before being functionally active in a cell. Short-lived gene silencing in vivo is one of the primary drawbacks of using siRNA because of its susceptibility to rapid nuclease degradation.

The development of shRNA has allowed for the persistent silence of a gene of interest, which may be required to cure a neurodegenerative disease. Since shRNA is structurally identical to pre-miRNA, it can be carried by viral vectors in the form of expression cassettes. Together, they make sense and no sense.[40] When two RNA molecules with complementary base pairs anneal, a hairpin loop is formed. This process requires the U6 or H1 promoter of RNA polymerase III. The shRNA's hairpin loop is snipped by the cytoplasmic enzyme Dicer, yielding a siRNA that can be employed by the RISC to mediate interference activity.[41]

Applying RNAi-based techniques to neurodegenerative illnesses where genetic alterations give a gain of function traits will have the greatest influence on pathogenesis. The majority of the preclinical data used to guide the application of RNAi therapies comes from efforts to treat expanded repeat disorders.[42] The gene in HD patients that produces the huntingtin protein is one of the most promising possibilities for gene silencing or gene correction. Particularly, a dominant pathogenic gain of function for the huntingtin protein is caused by the amplification of a CAG repeat in exon 1 of the huntingtin gene. These abnormal protein clumps in the nucleus and cytoplasm lead to neuronal malfunction and, eventually, neuronal cell death, most often in the caudate–putamen region of the brain. Studies in transgenic mice have shown improvement in HD-related neuro-pathological and motor problems when small interfering RNA(siRNA)and short hairpin RNA(shRNA)are used to target areas in the N-terminus of human huntingtin. After gene expression cassettes encoding huntingtin-specific small hairpin RNA(shRNA) were delivered by adeno-associated virus(AAV), lentiviral, and adeno-associated virus (AAV), the cellular and regional distribution of shRNA could be monitored using green fluorescent protein(GFP)reporter genes(AAV).[43] Through robust and long-lasting GFP expression, we see that presymptomatic transgenic HD striatal huntingtin mRNA and protein levels are lowered by 28% and 78%, respectively. The expression of DARPP-32, encephalin, and proenkephalin can all be normalized by knocking down mutant huntingtin. If neuronal aggregates can be reduced or eliminated, motor abilities can improve, and the beginning of some motor traits, like the inability to clasp one's own rear limbs, can be delayed.[44]

In a rat model of fast-onset HD, we reduced mutant huntingtin mRNA by 80% and mutant huntingtin protein by 50% by utilizing an AAV vector to overexpress exon 1 of huntingtin containing 70 CAG repeats. Due to a dramatic decrease in mutant huntingtin mRNA expression, 919 out of every 1,000 striatal neurons were protected in this HD model, whereas only 60 out of every 1,000 were protected in control rats. Six months after AAV-shRNA therapy, the mRNA and protein levels of wild-type huntingtin were lowered by 28 and 45%, respectively, in the striatum of nonhuman primates.[45] These results point to the possible therapeutic benefits of RNAi-based gene silencing. Gene expression analysis in striatal tissue reveals that normal huntingtin-associated molecular pathways may be altered by gene silencing. However, more work needs to be done in the field of shRNA design, particularly in the assessment of allele-specific shRNA.[46]

Oversaturation of endogenous miRNA pathways may occur if shRNA synthesis is not well-controlled, which might lead to a shortage of exportin-5-mediated nuclear export, a severe bottleneck. Toxic effects on cells may come from gene deregulation caused by low amounts of endogenous miRNA. Even though shRNA's nonspecific toxicity can be mitigated by proper sequence selection and dose management, doing so in vivo in the absence of a suitable gene regulatory mechanism is difficult.[47]

7.7 SIGNIFICANT EXPANSION IN THE USE OF ARTIFICIAL MIRNA

Alternative RNAi-triggering molecules, known as artificial miRNA shuttles, have been investigated; these molecules are modeled after the stem-loop structure of natural miRNAs. While the mature miRNA duplex in the stem has been replaced by sequences specific to a particular target transcript, the natural recognition sequences for Drosha and Dicer cleavage have been preserved. Generated by RNA polymerase II-based expression systems, synthetic miRNAs' longer transcripts can further regulate tissue selectivity. After discovering that overexpressing shRNA in transgenic mouse models resulted in substantial neurotoxicity, researchers began exploring synthetic miRNA with the hope of treating HD.[48] Striatum of CAG140 knock-in HD mice showed significant neurotoxicity after receiving two shRNA-targeting mRNA sections of huntingtin that are conserved between humans and animals, while a third benign shRNA had the same effect on huntingtin gene suppression. When a mismatch control shRNA was used to see whether toxicity could be generated without huntingtin knockdown, it was observed that toxicity occurred regardless of the silencing activity.[49] These identical sequences expressed in a synthetic miRNA backbone were nontoxic and retained their silencing effectiveness. Safety assessments of artificial miRNA to knockdown huntingtin after administration to the putamen of nonhuman primates confirmed these findings.[50] These results suggest that when utilizing the same inhibitory sequences as shRNAs, synthesized miRNAs have a higher safety profile without losing silencing efficacy as shown in Figure 7.2.[51]

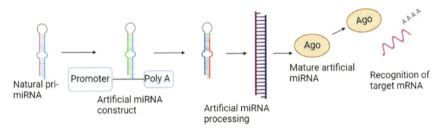

FIGURE 7.2 Formation of artificial miRNA.

Research into these miRNA approaches has been expanded to include testing in nonhuman primate models. There was no obvious neuronal toxicity, inflammatory reactions, or motor abnormalities after 6 weeks of gene therapy using an AAV vector to deliver a synthetic miRNA targeting a miR-30 scaffold sequence conserved among mice, rhesus monkeys, and humans in the huntingtin gene. The miRNA sequence employed to silence huntingtin may cause some offtarget silence and species-specific harm according to recent studies.[52] The potential toxicity of these sequences may hinder preclinical safety testing in rodents and nonhuman primates. How much information can be taken from studies on the consequences of chronic gene silencing on human neuron patients is not understood. All in all, results support the notion that synthetic miRNA can be employed to efficiently silence target genes in neuronal populations.[53]

7.8 DIRECTED DELIVERY FROM SYNTHETIC RNA TO THE ASTROCYTES

Using cell-specific promoters for the transcribed-direct synthesis of artificial miRNA in a targeted population of cells is one benefit of adopting an artificial miRNA platform. Evidence suggests that adenosine acts as an endogenous anticonvulsant in the brain; hence, suppression of the astrocytic enzyme adenosine kinase(ADK)was chosen as a technique for epileptic gene therapy. Adenosine deaminase(ADK)is an enzyme that controls the quantity of endogenous adenosine in the body and is only expressed in astrocytes.[54] Since ADK helps reduce tonic adenosine levels, its presence in seizure-prone brain areas lowers the seizure threshold. Adenosine deaminase(ADK)activity-releasing cell transplantation in the mouse brain reduces seizures in kindling models and spontaneous seizures. Antisense transfer against ADK in astrocytes using adeno-associated viral 8(AAV8) effectively eliminates spontaneous seizures in mice. In this research, we employed AAV9 vectors to rapidly deliver synthetic miRNA-targeting ADK to the astrocytes of the hippocampus.[55–58]

Finally, some transgenic expression was still selectively localized to neurons.

MiR-ADK reduced ADK protein levels by 90% at the vector dosage utilized, which was correlated with shorter kainate-induced seizure durations in miRADK vector-injected rats compared to controls.[59–62] According to findings, the GFAP promoter may stimulate the creation of miRNA sequences at high enough levels to significantly reduce ADK expression.[63–65]

Here, we detail the processes utilized to package AAV vectors and inject them into research participants, as well as the methods developed for silencing genes using artificial microRNAs.

7.9 CONCLUSIONS

Careful consideration of vector titers is required for effective transgene delivery in astrocytes from the rat brain. Glutamate synthetase is the central enzyme in the biosynthesis of glutamate and glutamine(GS), which can be transduced using AAV vectors with GFP expression. Findings suggest that GS expression levels in CA1 astrocytes may be almost totally suppressed by 3.331010 genome copies injected per gram of vector. The researcher's results are consistent with this finding. Hippocampal network hyperexcitability would rise further if reactive gliosis caused impairments in neural inhibition. Since glutamate participates in synaptic transmission and is involved in excitotoxic cell damage, it is critical that its management is not jeopardized.

Targeting Oligodendrocytes with Gene-Silencing

KEYWORDS

- gene silencing
- adeno-associated virus
- astrocytes
- microglia
- genome editing
- Lentivirus
- gene transfer

REFERENCES

1. Bak, M.; Silahtaroglu, A.; Moller, M.; Christensen, M.; Rath, M. F.; Skryabin, B. et al. MicroRNA Expression in the Adult Mouse Central Nervous System. *RNA* **2008,** *14* (3), 432–444. https://doi.org/10.1261/rna.783108.
2. Barres, B. A. The Mystery and Magic of Glia: A Perspective on Their Roles in Health and Disease. *Neuron* **2008,** *60* (3), 430–440. https://doi.org/10.1016/j.neuron.2008.10.013.
3. Bartel, D. P. MicroRNAs: Genomics, Biogenesis, Mechanism, and Function. *Cell* **2004,** *116* (2), 281–297.
4. Bartel, D. P.; Chen, C. Z. Micromanagers of Gene Expression: The Potentially Widespread Influence of Metazoan microRNAs. *Nat. Rev. Genet.* **2004,** *5* (5), 396–400. https://doi.org/ 10.1038/nrg1328.
5. Bartlett, J. S.; Samulski, R. J.; McCown, T. J. Selective and Rapid Uptake of Adeno-Associated Virus Type 2 in Brain. *Hum. Gene Therap.* **1998,** *9* (8), 1181–1186. https://doi.org/10.1089/ hum.1998.9.8–1181.
6. Berry, G. E.; Asokan, A. Cellular Transduction Mechanisms of Adeno-Associated Viral Vectors. *Curr. Opin. Virol.* **2016,** *21,* 5460. https://doi.org/10.1016/j.coviro.2016.08.001.
7. Boison, D. Engineered Adenosine-Releasing Cells for Epilepsy Therapy: Human Mesenchymal Stem Cells and Human Embryonic Stem Cells. *Neurotherapeutics* **2009,** *6* (2), 278–283. https://doi.org/ 10.1016/j.nurt.2008.12.001.
8. Boison, D.; Scheurer, L.; Tseng, J. L.; Aebischer, P.; Mohler, H. Seizure Suppression in Kindled Rats by Intraventricular Grafting of an Adenosine Releasing Synthetic Polymer. *Exp. Neurol.* **1999,** *160* (1), 164–174. https://doi.org/10.1006/exnr.1999.7209.
9. Cahoy, J. D.; Emery, B.; Kaushal, A.; Foo, L. C.; Zamanian, J. L.; Christopherson, K. S. et al. A Transcriptome Database for Astrocytes, Neurons, and Oligodendrocytes: A New Resource for Understanding Brain Development and Function. *J. Neurosci.* **2008,** *28* (1), 264–278. https://doi.org/10.1523/JNEUROSCI.4178–07.2008.

10. Cai, X.; Hagedorn, C. H.; Cullen, B. R. Human microRNAs Are Processed from Capped, Polyadenylated Transcripts That Can Also Function as mRNAs. *RNA* **2004,** *10* (12), 1957–1966.

11. Cannon, J. R.; Sew, T.; Montero, L.; Burton, E. A.; Greenamyre, J. T. Pseudotype-Dependent Lentiviral Transduction of Astrocytes or Neurons in the Rat Substantia Nigra. *Exp. Neurol.* **2011,** *228* (1), 41–52. https://doi.org/10.1016/j.expneurol.2010. 10.016.

12. Cearley, C. N.; Wolfe, J. H. Transduction Characteristics of Adeno-Associated Virus Vectors Expressing Cap Serotypes 7, 8, 9, and Rh10 in the Mouse Brain. *Mol. Therap.* **2006,** *13* (3), 528–537.

13. Choudhury, S. R.; Hudry, E.; Maguire, C. A.; Sena-Esteves, M.; Breakefield, X. O.; Grandi, P. Viral Vectors for Therapy of Neurologic Diseases. *Neuropharmacology.* https://doi.org/10.1016/j.neuropharm.2016.02.013.

14. Christine, C. W.; Starr, P. A.; Larson, P. S.; Eberling, J. L.; Jagust, W. J.; Hawkins, R. A. et al. Safety and Tolerability of Putaminal AADC Gene Therapy for Parkinson Disease. *Neurology* **2009,** *73* (20), 1662–1669. https://doi.org/10.1212/WNL.0b013e 3181c29356.

15. Colin, A.; Faideau, M.; Dufour, N.; Auregan, G.; Hassig, R.; Andrieu, T. et al. Engineered Lentiviral Vector Targeting Astrocytes In Vivo. *Glia* **2009,** *57* (6), 667–679. https://doi.org/10.1002/ glia.20795.

16. Davidson, B. L.; Stein, C. S.; Heth, J. A.; Martins, I.; Kotin, R. M.; Derksen, T. A. et al. Recombinant Adeno-Associated Virus Type 2, 4, and 5 Vectors: Transduction of Variant Cell Types and Regions in the Mammalian Central Nervous System. *Proc. Natl. Acad. Sci. USA* **2000,** *97* (7), 3428–3432. https://doi.org/10.1073/pnas. 050581197.

17. (a) Dragunow, M. Adenosine: The Brain'S Natural Anticonvulsant. *Trends Pharmacol. Sci.* **1986,** *7*, 128–130. (b) Dragunow, M. Adenosine and Seizure Termination. *Ann. Neurol.* **1991,** *29* (5), 575. https://doi.org/10.1002/ana.410290524.

18. Drinkut, A.; Tereshchenko, Y.; Schulz, J. B.; Bahr, M.; Kugler, S. Efficient Gene Therapy for Parkinson's Disease Using Astrocytes as Hosts for Localized Neurotrophic Factor Delivery. *Mol. Therap.* **2012,** *20* (3), 534–543. https://doi.org/ 10.1038/mt.2011.249.

19. Drouet, V.; Perrin, V.; Hassig, R.; Dufour, N.; Auregan, G.; Alves, S. et al. Sustained Effects of Nonallele-Specific Huntingtin Silencing. *Ann. Neurol.* **2009,** *65* (3), 276–285.

20. Eberling, J. L.; Jagust, W. J.; Christine, C. W.; Starr, P.; Larson, P.; Bankiewicz, K. S.; Aminoff, M. J. Results from a Phase I Safety Trial of hAADC Gene Therapy for Parkinson Disease. *Neurology* **2008,** *70* (21), 1980–1983.

21. Foust, K. D.; Nurre, E.; Montgomery, C. L.; Hernandez, A.; Chan, C. M.; Kaspar, B. K. Intravascular AAV9 Preferentially Targets Neonatal Neurons and Adult Astrocytes. *Nat. Biotechnol.* **2009,** *27* (1), 59–65. DOI: 10.1038/nbt.1515.

22. Gray, S. J.; Matagne, V.; Bachaboina, L.; Yadav, S.; Ojeda, S. R.; Samulski, R. J. Preclinical Differences of Intravascular AAV9 Delivery to Neurons and Glia: A Comparative Study of Adult Mice and Nonhuman Primates. *Mol. Therap.* **2011,** *19* (6), 1058–1069. https://doi.org/10.1038/mt.2011.72.

23. Grimm, D.; Streetz, K. L.; Jopling, C. L.; Storm, T. A.; Pandey, K.; Davis, C. R. et al. Fatality in Mice Due to Oversaturation of Cellular microRNA/Short Hairpin RNA Pathways. *Nature* **2006,** *441* (7092), 537–541.

24. Grondin, R.; Kaytor, M. D.; Ai, Y.; Nelson, P. T.; Thakker, D. R.; Heisel, J. et al. Six-Month Partial Suppression of Huntingtin Is Well Tolerated in the Adult Rhesus Striatum. *Brain* **2012,** *135* (4), 1197–1209.

25. Hamby, M. E.; Sofroniew, M. V. Reactive Astrocytes as Therapeutic Targets for CNS Disorders. *Neurotherapeutics* **2010,** *7* (4), 494506. https://doi.org/10.1016/j.nurt.2010.07.003.

26. Harper, S. Q.; Staber, P. D.; He, X.; Eliason, S. L.; Martins, I. H.; Mao, Q. et al. RNA Interference Improves Motor and Neuropathological Abnormalities in a Huntington's Disease Mouse Model. *Proc. Natl. Acad. Sci. USA* **2005,** *102* (16), 5820–5825.

27. He, M.; Liu, Y.; Wang, X.; Zhang, M. Q.; Hannon, G. J.; Huang, Z. J. Cell-Type-Based Analysis of microRNA Profiles in the Mouse Brain. *Neuron* **2012,** *73* (1), 35–48. https://doi.org/10.1016/j. neuron.2011.11.010.

28. Huang, B.; Schiefer, J.; Sass, C.; Landwehrmeyer, G. B.; Kosinski, C. M.; Kochanek, S. High Capacity Adenoviral Vector-Mediated Reduction of Huntingtin Aggregate Load In Vitro and In Vivo. *Hum. Gene Therap.* **2007,** *18* (4), 303–311.

29. Huber, A.; Padrun, V.; Deglon, N.; Aebischer, P.; Mohler, H.; Boison, D. Grafts of Adenosine Releasing Cells Suppress Seizures in Kindling Epilepsy. *Proc. Natl. Acad. Sci. USA* **2001,** *98* (13), 7611–7616. https://doi.org/10.1073/pnas.131102898.

30. Jakobsson, J.; Georgievska, B.; Ericson, C.; Lundberg, C. Lesion-Dependent Regulation of Transgene Expression in the Rat Brain Using a Human Glial Fibrillary Acidic Protein-Lentiviral Vector. *Eur. J. Neurosci.* **2004,** *19* (3), 761–765.

31. Judge, A. D.; Bola, G.; Lee, A. C. H.; MacLachlan, I. Design of Noninflammatory Synthetic siRNA Mediating Potent Gene Silencing In Vivo. *Mol. Therap.* **2006,** *13* (3), 494–505.

32. Kaplitt, M. G.; Leone, P.; Samulski, R. J.; Xiao, X.; Pfaff, D. W.; O'Malley, K. L.; During, M. J. Long-Term Gene Expression and Phenotypic Correction Using Adeno-Associated Virus Vectors in the Mammalian Brain. *Nat. Genet.* **1994,** *8* (2), 148154. https://doi.org/10.1038/ng1094–148.

33. Kay, C.; Skotte, N. H.; Southwell, A. L.; Hayden, M. R. Personalized Gene Silencing Therapeutics for Huntington Disease. *Clin. Genet.* **2014,** *86* (1), 29–36. https://doi.org/10.1111/cge.12385.

34. Kay, C.; Collins, J. A.; Skotte, N. H.; Southwell, A. L.; Warby, S. C.; Caron, N. S. et al. Huntingtin Haplotypes Provide Prioritized Target Panels for Allele-Specific Silencing in Huntington Disease Patients of European Ancestry. *Mol. Therap.* **2015,** *23* (11), 1759–1771. https://doi.org/ 10.1038/mt.2015.128.

35. Klein, R. L.; Dayton, R. D.; Tatom, J. B.; Henderson, K. M.; Henning, P. P. AAV8, 9, Rh10, Rh43 Vector Gene Transfer in the Rat Brain: Effects of Serotype, Promoter and Purification Method. *Mol. Therap.* **2007,** *16* (1), 89–96.

36. Lawlor, P. A.; Bland, R. J.; Mouravlev, A.; Young, D.; During, M. J. Efficient Gene Delivery and Selective Transduction of Glial Cells in the Mammalian Brain by AAV Serotypes Isolated from Nonhuman Primates. *Mol. Therap.* **2009,** *17* (10), 1692–1702. DOI: 10.1038/mt.2009.170.

37. LeWitt, P. A.; Rezai, A. R.; Leehey, M. A.; Ojemann, S. G.; Flaherty, A. W.; Eskandar, E. N. et al. AAV2-GAD Gene Therapy for Advanced Parkinson's Disease: A Double-Blind, Sham-Surgery Controlled, Randomised Trial. *Lancet Neurol.* **2011,** *10* (4), 309–319. https://doi.org/10.1016/ S1474–4422 (11)70039–4.

38. Lee, Y.; Messing, A.; Su, M.; Brenner, M. GFAP Promoter Elements Required for Region-Specific and Astrocyte-Specific Expression. *Glia* **2008,** *56* (5), 481–493. https://doi.org/10.1002/glia.20622.

39. Leone, P.; Shera, D.; McPhee, S. W.; Francis, J. S.; Kolodny, E. H.; Bilaniuk, L. T. et al. Long-Term Follow-Up After Gene Therapy for Canavan Disease. *Sci. Transl. Med.* **2012,** *4* (165), 165–163. https://doi.org/10.1126/scitranslmed.3003454.

40. Li, C.; Diprimio, N.; Bowles, D. E.; Hirsch, M. L.; Monahan, P. E.; Asokan, A. et al. Single Amino Acid Modification of Adeno-Associated Virus Capsid Changes Transduction and Humoral Immune Profiles. *J. Virol.* **2012,** *86* (15), 7752–7759. https://doi.org/10.1128/JVI.00675–12.

41. Luthi-Carter, R.; Hanson, S. A.; Strand, A. D.; Bergstrom, D. A.; Chun, W.; Peters, N. L. et al. Dysregulation of Gene Expression in the R6/2 Model of Polyglutamine Disease: Parallel Changes in Muscle and Brain. *Hum. Mol. Genet.* **2002,** *11* (17), 1911–1926.

42. Machida, Y.; Okada, T.; Kurosawa, M.; Oyama, F.; Ozawa, K.; Nukina, N. rAAV-Mediated shRNA Ameliorated Neuropathology in Huntington Disease Model Mouse. *Biochem. Biophys. Res. Commun.* **2006,** *343* (1), 190–197.

43. McBride, J. L.; Boudreau, R. L.; Harper, S. Q.; Staber, P. D.; Monteys, A. M.; Martins, I. et al. Artificial miRNAs Mitigate shRNA-Mediated Toxicity in the Brain: Implications for the Therapeutic Development of RNAi. *Proc. Natl. Acad. Sci. USA* **2008,** *105* (15), 5868–5873.

44. McBride, J. L.; Pitzer, M. R.; Boudreau, R. L.; Dufour, B.; Hobbs, T.; Ojeda, S. R.; Davidson, B. L. Preclinical Safety of RNAi-Mediated HTT Suppression in the Rhesus Macaque as a Potential Therapy for Huntington's Disease. *Mol. Therap.* **2011,** *19* (12), 2152–2162.

45. Monteys, A. M.; Wilson, M. J.; Boudreau, R. L.; Spengler, R. M.; Davidson, B. L. Artificial miRNAs Targeting Mutant Huntingtin Show Preferential Silencing In Vitro and In Vivo. *Mol. Therap. Nucl. Acids* **2015,** *4*, e234. https://doi.org/10.1038/mtna.2015.7.

46. Mudannayake, J. M.; Mouravlev, A.; Fong, D. M.; Young, D. Transcriptional Activity of Novel ALDH1L1 Promoters in the Rat Brain Following AAV Vector-Mediated Gene Transfer. *Mol. Therap. Methods Clin. Dev.* **2016,** *3*, 16075. https://doi.org/10.1038/mtm.2016.75.

47. Naldini, L.; Blomer, U.; Gage, F. H.; Trono, D.; Verma, I. M. Efficient Transfer, Integration, and Sustained Long-Term Expression of the Transgene in Adult Rat Brains Injected with a Lentiviral Vector. *Proc. Natl. Acad. Sci. USA* **1996,** *93* (21), 11382–11388.

48. Ortinski, P. I.; Dong, J.; Mungenast, A.; Yue, C.; Takano, H.; Watson, D. J. et al. Selective Induction of Astrocytic Gliosis Generates Deficits in Neuronal Inhibition. *Nat. Neurosci.* **2010,** *13* (5), 584–591. https://doi.org/10.1038/nn.2535.

49. Paddison, P. J.; Caudy, A. A.; Bernstein, E.; Hannon, G. J.; Conklin, D. S. Short Hairpin RNAs (shRNAs) Induce Sequence-Specific Silencing in Mammalian Cells. *Genes Dev.* **2002,** *16* (8), 948–958.

Targeting Oligodendrocytes with Gene-Silencing 163

50. (a) Paxinos, G.; Watson, C. *The rat brain in stereotaxic coordinates*; Academic Press: San Diego, 1986. (b) Pekny, M.; Pekna, M.; Messing, A.; Steinhauser, C.; Lee, J. M.; Parpura, V. et al. Astrocytes: A Central Element in Neurological Diseases. Acta Neuropathologica **2016,** *131* (3), 323345. https://doi.org/10.1007/s00401-015-1513-1. (c) Pillay, S.; Meyer, N. L.; Puschnik, A. S.; Davulcu, O.; Diep, J.; Ishikawa, Y. et al. An Essential Receptor for Adeno-Associated Virus Infection. *Nature* **2016,** *530* (7588), 108–112. https://doi.org/10.1038/nature16465.

51. Pulicherla, N.; Shen, S.; Yadav, S.; Debbink, K.; Govindasamy, L.; Agbandje-McKenna, M.; Asokan, A. Engineering Liver-Detargeted AAV9 Vectors for Cardiac and Musculoskeletal Gene Transfer. *Mol. Therap.* **2011,** *19* (6), 1070–1078. https://doi.org/10.1038/mt.2011.22.

52. Ren, G.; Li, T.; Lan, J. Q.; Wilz, A.; Simon, R. P.; Boison, D. Lentiviral RNAi-Induced Downregulation of Adenosine Kinase in Human Mesenchymal Stem Cell Grafts: A Novel Perspective for Seizure Control. *Exp. Neurol.* **2007,** *208* (1), 26–37. https://doi.org/10.1016/j.expneurol.2007.07.016.

53. Rodriguez-Lebron, E.; Denovan-Wright, E. M.; Nash, K.; Lewin, A. S.; Mandel, R. J. Intrastriatal rAAV-Mediated Delivery of Anti-Huntingtin shRNAs Induces Partial Reversal of Disease Progression in R6/1 Huntington's Disease Transgenic Mice. *Mol. Therap.* **2005,** *12* (4), 618–633.

54. Ross, C. A.; Tabrizi, S. J. Huntington's Disease: From Molecular Pathogenesis to Clinical Treatment. *Lancet Neurol.* **2011,** *10* (1), 83–98. https://doi.org/10.1016/S1474–4422 (10)70245–3.

55. Seifert, G.; Schilling, K.; Steinhauser, C. Astrocyte Dysfunction in Neurological Disorders: A Molecular Perspective: Nature Reviews. *Neuroscince* **2006,** *7* (3), 194–206.

56. Shevtsova, Z.; Malik, J. M.; Michel, U.; Bahr, M.; Kugler, S. Promoters and Serotypes: Targeting of Adeno-Associated Virus Vectors for Gene Transfer in the Rat Central Nervous System In Vitro and In Vivo. *Exp. Physiol.* **2005,** *90* (1), 53–59. https://doi.org/10.1113/expphysiol.2004.028159.

57. Srivastava, A. In Vivo Tissue-Tropism of Adeno-Associated Viral Vectors. *Curr. Opin. Virol.* **2016,** *21*, 75–80. https://doi.org/10.1016/j.coviro.2016.08.003.

58. Su, M.; Hu, H.; Lee, Y.; d'Azzo, A.; Messing, A.; Brenner, M. Expression Specificity of GFAP Transgenes. *Neurochem. Res.* **2004,** *29* (11), 2075–2093.

59. Theofilas, P.; Brar, S.; Stewart, K. A.; Shen, H. Y.; Sandau, U. S.; Poulsen, D.; Boison, D. Adenosine Kinase as a Target for Therapeutic Antisense Strategies in Epilepsy. *Epilepsia* **2011,** *52* (3), 589–601. https://doi.org/10.1111/j.1528–1167.2010.02947.x.

60. Wang, C.; Wang, C. M.; Clark, K. R.; Sferra, T. J. Recombinant AAV Serotype 1 Transduction Efficiency and Tropism in the Murine Brain. *Gene Therap.* **2003,** *10* (17), 1528–1534. https://doi.org/ 10.1038/sj.gt.3302011.

61. Weinberg, M. S.; Blake, B. L.; Samulski, R. J.; McCown, T. J. The Influence of Epileptic Neuropathology and Prior Peripheral Immunity on CNS Transduction by rAAV2 and rAAV5. *Gene Therap.* **2011,** *18* (10), 961–968. https://doi.org/10.1038/gt.2011.49.

62. Wiznerowicz, M.; Szulc, J.; Trono, D. Tuning Silence: Conditional Systems for RNA interference. *Nat. Methods* **2006,** *3* (9), 682–688.

63. Wu, Z.; Asokan, A.; Samulski, R. J. Adeno-Associated Virus Serotypes: Vector Toolkit for human gene therapy. *Mol. Therap.* **2006,** *14* (3), 316–327.

64. Yang, Y.; Vidensky, S.; Jin, L.; Jie, C.; Lorenzini, I.; Frankl, M.; Rothstein, J. D. Molecular Comparison of GLT1 1 and ALDH1L1 1 Astrocytes In Vivo in Astroglial Reporter Mice. *Glia* **2011,** *59* (2), 200–207. https://doi.org/10.1002/glia.21089.

65. Young, D.; Fong, D. M.; Lawlor, P. A.; Wu, A.; Mouravlev, A.; McRae, M. et al. Adenosine Kinase, Glutamine Synthetase and EAAT2 as Gene Therapy Targets for Temporal Lobe Epilepsy. *Gene Therap.* **2014,** *21* (12), 1029–1040. https://doi.org/10.1038/gt.2014.82.

CHAPTER 8

Astrocytes: Genetic Treatment Targets for Alzheimer's Disease

ABSTRACT

Amyloid plaques and neurofibrillary tangles, both of which accumulate in dead neurons, are hallmarks of Alzheimer's disease (AD), the most prevalent form of dementia. Symptoms, such as dementia and death, are mostly caused by neuronal degeneration; nonetheless, other types of brain cells also have an impact on the progression of the illness. In this chapter, we look closely at astrocytes and their role in both normal brain dysfunction and the onset of Alzheimer's disease. Moreover, cutting-edge viral gene transfer techniques permit effective and selective transduction of astrocytes to explore astrocyte-specific processes that identify intervention targets. We conclude by discussing a variety of in vitro and animal results that lend credence to the concept that if astrocytes were selectively targeted, the disease's progression may be slowed or stopped altogether.

8.1 INTRODUCTION

Memory loss, mental deterioration, behavioral and emotional changes, and mortality are all hallmarks of a degenerative neurological ailment known as Alzheimer's disease (AD). As the most common form of dementia, Alzheimer's disease (AD) affects 47 million people worldwide.[1–3] The already high societal price tag of AD is expected to rise further as the world's population ages.

Gene Therapy for Neurological Disorders: Molecular Approaches for Targeted Treatment.
Rishabha Malviya, Arun Kumar Singh, Priyanshi Goyal, & Sonali Sundram (Authors)
© 2025 Apple Academic Press, Inc. Co-published with CRC Press (Taylor & Francis)

Over a century ago, Alois Alzheimer originally defined Alzheimer's disease (AD), focusing on three pathologic markers: First, there is the amyloid plaque, which may lead to neuronal morphological abnormalities and reactive glial cells (Alzheimer, 1911). Researchers have learned a lot about Alzheimer's disease in the last century, but these pathological traits are still important to understanding its cause and progression.[4]

Amyloid plaques are extracellular aggregations of insoluble proteins that are widely dispersed and caused by Alzheimer's disease (AD). Amyloid precursor protein (APP) is a transmembrane amyloid protein broken into A and beta-secretase to generate this protein. To put it succinctly, neurons are the primary cell-type responsible for A production. The steady-state concentration of A in ISF is maintained through a finely tuned balancing act between A production and clearance following their secretion from APP.[5] Mutations in either APP or the enzymes responsible for digesting APP have been linked to the familial, Mendelian form of AD, which results in an overproduction of A and the subsequent onset of the illness. When A is present in large enough quantities, it forms fibrils, the building blocks of amyloid plaques. These fibrils have a highly organized, pleated sheet structure.[6]

Histological analysis of Alzheimer's disease in brain tissue reveals morphological abnormalities, such as dystrophic neurites and neurofibrillary tangles (NFTs), in the neurons there. Dystrophic neurites, also known as massive varicosities, form in axons and dendrites close to plaques. They lose synapses and have aberrant calcium signaling. Additionally, prior to neuronal death, clumps of hyperphosphorylated tau form inclusions called NFTs.[7]

It's important to keep in mind that the level of dementia in Alzheimer's patients does not seem to correspond with the number of amyloid plaques in their brains.[8] Tau aggregates in postmortem brains or tau-binding tracers in positron emission tomography (PET) imaging provide a more precise correlation between cognitive decline and NFT load. Because amyloid deposition occurs decades before cognitive decline and neural disease reflects the late impacts of amyloid buildup, this is probably the case. Thus, A and tau are expected to engage in a nuanced reciprocal relationship that leads to neuronal malfunction, death, and severe dementia.[9]

While there has been more focus on neuronal dysfunction, evidence is growing to suggest that glial cells impact the development of numerous diseases in significant ways.[10] When amyloid plaques are present, both

Astrocytes: Genetic Treatment Targets 167

microglia and astrocytes play a role in their shape and increase their production of neuroinflammatory mediators.[11] Amyloid plaques and reactive astrocytes are often found in close proximity to one another through hypertrophied processes that extend into the plaques; this phenomenon is known as the "peripheral encapsulation" phenotype.[12] Evidence from targeted transcriptome profiling suggests the activation of genes and pathways that may have a role in either preventing or reversing illness manifestations, including onset and development. The idea of compartmentalization, which allows the same molecular pathways to drive distinct actions in distinct cell types, has also recently been proposed.[13–15] Common signaling pathways may induce various responses in distinct cell types, including those involved in the astrocytic processes critical for AD. Therefore, targeted intervention is challenging using traditional pharmacological techniques.[16]

Human therapeutic studies using viral-mediated gene transfer have increased during the last decade. These results show that viruses may be controlled to alter gene expression in specific subsets of tissues and cell types.[17] Numerous animal research studies have shown that the transduction of astrocytes is feasible, and these methods might be used in human medicine. Throughout the course of Alzheimer's illness, astrocytes play a critical role in brain function, and the focus in this chapter is on the several ways in which viral-mediated gene transfer might be used to treat these cells specifically.[18]

8.2 ASTROCYTES' IMPORTANCE IN DISEASE AND HEALTH

Since the cells looked like stars when stained with silver, they were mistakenly labeled "astrocytes" in the 19th century.[19] Through these rudimentary descriptions of histology, we saw that while neurons' lengthy projections allowed them to make connections over great distances, astrocytes' more traditional domains and cellular processes were limited to shorter hops.[20–22] Factoring in these results, several researchers have proposed that neurons serve as the brain's computing units, while astrocytes provide the tissue that holds the brain (thus the name "glia," from the Greek for "glue"). Over the past few decades, neuron research has exploded in popularity.[23]

These star-shaped cells, called astrocytes, have been getting a lot of attention as of late. Once thought to just offer neurons structural support, in recent years, astrocytes are having a potential significance in the brain in a plethora of complex mental operations.[24–28]

The astrocytic domain and distribution have been re-evaluated in light of recent genetically encoded protein labeling and dye insertion. Although they look like sponges, astrocytes really inhabit highly ordered and nonoverlapping territories that tile the whole brain, refuting earlier results that claimed that astrocytes were randomly scattered cells arranged in a star pattern.[29]

Astrocytes are able to interact directly with their surrounding neuronal cells and vascular structures and extend large processes within their own astrocytic domain, which then ramify into smaller and smaller processes.[30] Synapses, along with the tiny arterioles and capillaries they encase, are surrounded by astrocytes' proximal processes. By establishing and maintaining these connections, astrocytes are able to influence neuronal activity, control neurovascular coupling, and support the condition of the blood-brain barrier (BBB). Outside or on the outskirts of each astrocytic domain, astrocytes connect with one another via extensive intercellular gap junctions formed by fine processes that extend from neighboring astrocytes.[31] Astrocytes use gap junctions to generate connected syncytia, which aid in the transfer of ions and tiny molecules across huge brain areas.

Although astrocytes have traditionally been thought to be unable to generate action potentials, recent in vivo investigations utilizing Ca21 indicators have shown that, in response to brain activity and blood flow, transient Ca21 waves propagate across astrocytes via gap junctions. The activity of astrocytes on neurons and blood vessels may be grounded in the dynamic signaling revealed by Ca21 waves, although their significance is not entirely understood.[32] Ca21 waves in astrocytes have been observed both starting in one cell and spreading to nearby cells. As a result, it is possible that the organization (or disorganization) of calcium signaling is crucial for the coordination of astrocytic activity on neuronal and vascular networks spanning enormous spatial and temporal ranges.[33]

8.3 ASTROCYTE–NEURON SYMBIOSIS AND MULTILATERAL SYNAPSE

Synapses and astrocytic processes are closely linked. The position of the astrocyte in close proximity to axon terminals and postsynaptic dendritic spines is essential. This structure, called a tripartite synapse, may be found in almost every region of the brain. The synaptic connection between

Astrocytes: Genetic Treatment Targets 169

neurons relies heavily on astrocytes, which serve a pivotal role in maintaining a precisely controlled extracellular environment.[34] Numerous transmembrane transporters are expressed by astrocytes to aid in the transport and regulation of tiny molecules such as Na+, K+, neurotransmitters, and others. Unlike neurons, which also have similar equipment, astrocytes can rapidly buffer spatial information over wider areas thanks to their intercellular syncytia. Although small in the context of the whole brain, abrupt changes in the concentration of individual ions inside a synapse may require this system to function properly.[35–38] The effective glutamate absorption provided by astrocytes helps maintain a low enough concentration of synaptic neurotransmitters to prevent excessive neurotransmission over time. Through their interactions with both synapses and blood vessels, astrocytes are also able to regulate the balance between neural activity and regional blood flow.[39] This allows for the dynamic supply of energy and the elimination of waste, helping the brain's synapses to maintain stability when they fire. Astrocytes are the fuel cells for neurons. An important example ischolesterol, but another is the exchange of carbon atoms. Transport of lactate, a carbon source generated from glucose, from astrocytes to neurons across intercellular domains is facilitated by the astrocyte–neuron lactate shuttle. Since cholesterol is found in high concentrations in the membranes of dendritic spines and axons, these cell bodies require a steady supply of the lipid. ApoE and ApoI are cholesterol-carrying lipoproteins that transport cholesterol from the cells that make it to do with the central nervous system to peripheral cells.[40]

Growing data suggests that astrocytes regulate synapses through their perineuronal astrocytic processes. At synapses, traditional neurotransmitters released by astrocytes control long-term potentiation (LTP) and long-term depression (LTD). Additionally, they may secrete trophic substances such as thrombospondins, which promote the development of new synapses. Synapses may be eliminated in two ways: via phagocytosis or indirectly when astrocytes stimulate the neuronal synthesis of C1q, which marks synapses for clearance by microglia.[41]

8.4 ASTROCYTES AND THE BLOOD-BRAIN AND LYMPHATIC BORDERS

Due to its high energy requirements, the brain's metabolic processes, including nutrition exchange and waste elimination, must be lightning fast.[42] However, numerous peripheral components, such as circulating cells and big chemicals, must be tightly prevented from entering the brain. When it's functioning properly, the BBB strictly controls who gets in and who does not. However, immune cells need to enter the body after severe assaults (the elimination of disease-causing microbes and the repair of tissue damage caused by a variety of traumatic or ischemic events). Consequently, the neurovascular unit's (NCU neurons) astrocytes, pericytes, and endothelial cells play a crucial role in controlling the conversation between the brain and the arteries as shown in Figure 8.1.[43–45]

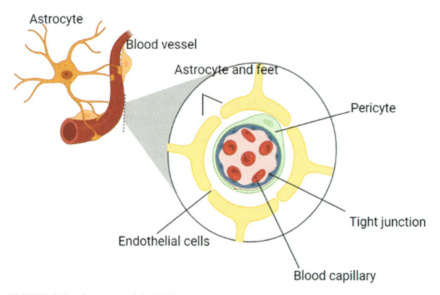

FIGURE 8.1 Structure of the BBB.

Individual astrocytes, with their territorial arrangement, are in a prime position to coordinate interactions with neighboring synapses and vascular structures. In addition to coordinating with pericytes and smooth muscle cells to control blood flow, astrocytes also coordinate with endothelial cells to control permeability.[46] The transcellular barriers formed by cerebrovascular endothelial cells are more stringent than those formed by peripheral endothelial cells. Glia limitans is the name given to the continuous wall of endfeet formed by astrocytes positioned along endothelial cells. Factors expressed by the astrocyte endfeet regulate junction and transporter protein expression in endothelial cells.[47–49] In the event of an infection, astrocytes

Astrocytes: Genetic Treatment Targets 171

release cytokines that break down the blood-brain barrier (BBB) and chemokines that entice leukocytes from the periphery to enter the brain. As the protective effect wears off, astrocytes release chemicals that cause the BBB to close again. When the BBB is being dynamically updated to meet current needs, this regulation looks to be of utmost importance.[50]

The brain parenchyma does not have a well-developed lymphatic system like other areas of the body, yet it has been shown that the leptomeninges contain lymphatic capillaries, which make fluid and protein clearance more difficult.[51] New research has uncovered an alternate pathway for brain fluid drainage. Levels of expression of AQP-4, a transmembrane water channel, are quite high in astrocytes, the cells that form the endfeet that surround the arteries in the brain and create the perivascular space. This creates a paravascular route for the transport of CSF and ISF.[52] Toxic compounds, such as amyloid-β, are cleared at reduced rates by up to 70% when AQP-4 is knocked out, highlighting the importance of this so-called "glymphatic system" to interstitial solute turnover.[53]

8.5 ASTROCYTOSIS OCCURS USUALLY WHEN THE CENTRAL NERVOUS SYSTEM IS INJURED

When the brain is injured, astrocytes respond in a predictable way by changing their morphology (process hypertrophy) and gene expression. A transcriptional study revealed an upregulation of glial fibrillary acidic protein (GFAP) and vimentin, two intermediate filament proteins.[54] This cellular component of neuroinflammation is called astrocytosis and occurs everywhere. There is a spectrum of astrocytosis that varies depending on the kind and extent of the damage.

Individual astrocytic domains are preserved with modest damage, whereas GFAP expression is increased in situations when damage is less extensive, for example, a contained infection or moderate nonpenetrating trauma.[55] These modifications may return to normal if the insult ceases. Hypertrophy of GFAP processes, overexpression of GFAP, astrocyte proliferation, and disruption of cellular domains characterize astrocytosis, which occurs in response to severe damage such as penetrating or virulent infection. Reactive astrocytes, in conjunction with invading peripheral cells, may create a glial scar when the insult comprises specific lesions (such as in a penetrating trauma or stroke), effectively sealing off the damaged region from further infection.[56]

Since ancient times, researchers have speculated that astrocytosis might worsen cellular damage processes. In spite of this, it is becoming more and more apparent that the morphologic abnormalities displayed by astrocytes are simply a small representation of a much larger transcriptional change that may vary according to the damage type.[57-60] The transcript profiles of astrocytes are affected differently by ischemia and LPS, yet they share certain alterations in gene expression. So, it's possible that there is a group of genes that is always at work in driving astrocytosis, whereas other sets of genes may only be expressed in certain situations. Recent studies have indicated a favorable function for astrocytosis in specific settings, when the expression of damage-induced genes by astrocytes is inhibited, hence increasing injury and worsening neurologic outcomes. For a long time, the idea that astrocytosis contributes negatively to brain function has been supported by the fact that activated astrocytes emit proinflammatory signaling molecules and that glial scars form barriers that limit axonal regeneration following acute damage. Astrocytic secretion of cytokines, chemokines, and complement proteins has been linked to neurotoxicity.[61]

Nonetheless, there is mounting evidence that astrocytosis can improve recovery outcomes. Two of astrocytosis' most obvious and consequential roles are to decrease central nervous system (CNS) inflammation and the quantity of chondroitin sulfate proteoglycans (CSPGs) produced in the glial scar, which inhibit axon development.[62] There is mixed evidence about whether or not astrocytic responses help or impede neurodegeneration. Therefore, it is essential to investigate the role of astrocytosis in the context of distinct CNS illnesses at the level of individual molecular pathways. During the damage response, astrocytes indirectly affect neuronal function by modulating the activity of cells that are not astrocytes. Neuroinflammation is a chain reaction that begins when the central nervous system is injured; it involves many different cell types, some of which move in from the periphery. While multiple cell types must work together, astrocytes are essential in coordinating their efforts.[63] Restricting the access of circulating leukocytes into brain tissue is one way in which the BBB helps maintain the central nervous system's immunological integrity.[64]

Aside from playing a role in peripheral inflammatory reactions, astrocytes also regulate inflammation within the central nervous system. Chemokines such as MIP-1, which are produced by active microglia, may be drawn to an injury site by astrocytes.[65]

Astrocytes: Genetic Treatment Targets 173

The recent discovery that astrocyte-secreted chemicals can reduce microglial activation signs suggests that astrocytes play a crucial role in controlling microglial reactions to CNS damage. Astrocytes are special in that they can independently communicate with neurons and affect how those cells behave.[66] The production of thrombospondins upon being injured by astrocytes may be beneficial since they aid in synaptic survival and recovery. As an added bonus, astroglia can be activated by signaling molecules secreted by other cells. Microglia have recently been found to induce a classic neurotoxic astrocytosis phenotype through the simultaneous production of IL-1, TNF, and C1q. It is possible that different astrocytosis phenotypes exist and that astrocytes can be directed to these distinct states by varying signaling molecule mixtures that are released.[67]

8.6 ROLE OF ASTROCYTES IN THE PROGRESSION OF ALZHEIMER'S DISEASE

One of the earliest pathogenic features of Alzheimer's disease is the activation of astrocytes and other glia surrounding amyloid plaques. Hypertrophy, structural alterations, and a rise in several inflammatory cytokines and intracellular signaling cascades are all hallmarks of the reactive phenotype of astrocytes.[68] It's fascinating to think about how the lengthy processes of activated astrocytes intercalate deeply into amyloid plaques. Astrocyte reactivity is not yet fully understood, nor is it fully recognized how it contributes to the onset of disease.[69] However, it is well-known that astrocytes in Alzheimer's patients' brains not only take on a reactive phenotype but also gradually stop carrying out their vital tasks in maintaining brain homeostasis. The accumulation of amyloid is associated with a cascade of dysregulation of gene clusters in human brain astrocytes, as shown by transcriptome microarrays.[70] Astrocytic senescence biomarkers and the release of inflammatory cytokines are both indicators that exposure to A hastens the emergence of a senescent phenotype.[71] How significant is the loss of healthy astrocyte functions due to reactive astrocytosis in the progression of plaque disease and neurodegeneration, and is there any way to stop it? Recent studies on astrocytosis in Alzheimer's disease have tried to investigate whether or not inhibiting astrocyte reactivity can decrease the progression of neurodegeneration. Astrocytosis is characterized by the overexpression of connecting intermediate filaments (such as GFAP, vimentin, and others) leading to cellular enlargement. Both GFAP and Vim gene deletions have the same effect on astrocyte inactivation.[72] However, when both genes are removed, central nervous system (CNS) injury no longer causes astrocytes to develop hypertrophic morphological changes. The investigation examined whether inhibiting astrocytosis in an AD mouse model would have any effect on amyloid plaque development. Knocking down the genes for GFAP and Vim in young APP/PS1 mice had no apparent effect on the astrocytes. However, astrocytosis-associated astrocytic morphological changes did not occur when amyloid plaques appeared in the brain at older ages. Interactions between astrocytic processes and amyloid were drastically reduced when knocking out intermediate filaments, indicating that this infiltration into plaques is dependent on intermediate filaments. Dystrophic neurites and amyloid plaque burden were also amplified in GFAP/Vim-null mice by a factor of two. The expression levels of a panel of important inflammatory mediators (IL-1b, IL-6, IL-10, TNF-β, TGF-β, and iNOS) hardly budged after GFAP and vimentin deletion, which is intriguing. Deletion of intermediate filament genes had no effect on the expression of enzymes involved in APP processing (ADAM10, ADAM17, presenilin-1, memapsin-2, nicastrin, APH-1b, and PEN2) or A degradation (neprilysin (NEP), endothelin-converting enzyme (IDE), matrix metalloproteinase-9 (MMP-9), and matrix metalloproteinase-2 (MMP-2).[73]

In light of the fact that astrocyte reactivity can be differentiated from other typical neuroinflammatory alterations, it appears to benefit from the presence of these intermediate filaments. Plaque load was not altered in another investigation using the same gene modifications in a distinct line of APP mice.[74] However, they displayed lower expression of neural support genes and reproduced changes in astrocyte shape. These results demonstrate the role of astrocytosis in the progression of Alzheimer's disease and show the intricacy of the activated phenotype in relation to inflammation and normal astrocyte function. The following are examples of alterations that occur during reactivity that may speed up disease, whereas others (such as the overexpression of intermediate filaments) appear protective.[75] Targeting specific pathways and subsets of cells within this complex network is expected to be crucial to the effectiveness of future medicines. Here, we discuss the three studies that have progressed the furthest in the therapeutic pipeline for astrocyte-targeted gene therapy for AD and review some of the specific astrocyte functions that are disrupted during AD and

Astrocytes: Genetic Treatment Targets 175

how they might be rescued with virally delivered gene therapy to prevent or reverse neurodegeneration.[76]

8.7 TENDERNESS

Firstly, astrocytosis in AD is mostly known in terms of its link to inflammation. Numerous signaling pathways and cytokines are mobilized in AD neuroinflammation caused by astrocytes, active microglia, and dead neurons. Janus kinase/STAT3, calcineurin/nuclear factor A/T, and nuclear factor (NF)-B are only a few examples.[77]

Neurodegeneration is believed to be caused by plaques because they stimulate astrocytes and other glial cells to produce more inflammatory and cytotoxic substances (this is known as the "inflammatory hypothesis"). Inflammation arises due to a continuous give-and-take between proinflammatory and anti-inflammatory factors. Long-term plaque-induced inflammation may cause a shift in the relative advantages of different inflammatory mediators.[78] Thus, it has been difficult to identify specific treatment targets for inflammation within this complex and ever-evolving network of interactions. Different cell types secrete different cytokines at different sites and at different phases of illness, and these cytokines have a wide range of distinct effects. Intracellular targets in signaling cascades may, like their extracellular counterparts, participate in both beneficial and harmful pathways.[79]

The advancement of targeted cell sorting calls for a more comprehensive assessment of gene expression patterns across cell types in pathologies. One study showed that a significant elevation of inflammatory genes in astrocytes is to blame for the impairment of many astrocytic processes seen in AD, such as cholesterol synthesis and synaptic support (much more so than in microglia).[80] Researchers discovered that cystatin F, a regulator of IL-1 and TNF-β, was the most dramatically elevated gene in astrocytes. Potential exists for targeting this protein as a therapeutic strategy to decrease inflammation.[81] It is interesting that the authors noted an increase in Il-1, TNF-β, and complement cascade members because these variables have been linked to the development of AD.[82] For instance, the knowledge that mutations in the Il-1 genes are recognized as genetic risk factors for AD and that Il-1 induces excessive neuronal A production has been known for some time. It is possible that members of the tumor necrosis factor

(TNF) family play more than one role in Alzheimer's disease, including promoting neuronal death and inhibiting the production of glutamate by astrocytes.[83]

Complement, in the meantime, is associated with an absorption by astrocytes, the tagging of amyloid-damaged synapses for eventual astrocyte pruning, and the mitigation of A-induced dendritic damage. According to these results, inflammation is linked to several changes in astrocyte activity, such as protein clearance and synaptic support. Because of this, it's probable that lowering inflammation would not have a particularly positive effect on health in the long run.[84]

Supporting this notion is the fact that pharmaceutical attempts to diminish neuroinflammation on a large scale in the treatment of AD have thus far been unsuccessful. Early epidemiological research found that nonsteroidal anti-inflammatory drugs (NSAIDs) could delay the onset of Alzheimer's disease. However, results from recent randomized controlled studies of NSAIDs for treating mild to moderate AD have been mixed.[85] Fenamate NSAIDs, which particularly target the NLRP3 inflammasome that facilitates IL-1 activation, have recently been found to decrease neuroinflammation and memory problems in two separate animal models of Alzheimer's disease (AD). Once again, the importance of specificity in targeting the intricate web of inflammatory cascades thought to be involved in AD is highlighted by the fact that gene therapy is well-suited to isolating a particular node of inflammatory signaling and a specific cell population. As an example of a promising gene therapy target in a preclinical mouse model of Alzheimer's disease, we examine the astrocytic CN/NFAT signaling pathway.[86]

8.8 CLEARANCE OF AB AND AMYLOID

The pathogenesis of Alzheimer's disease relies heavily on A's accumulation in the brain's interstitial spaces. This indicates that the ratio of production to clearance is an important element in predicting health. The brain is filled with astroglial cells with particularly advantageous positions at synapses and the BBB, raising the possibility that they are pivotal in clearance and metabolism.[87]

The accumulation of these in the brain is thought to play a role in the pathophysiology of Alzheimer's disease as fibrils in astrocytes, as was shown in early studies.[88] In addition, preliminary evidence was presented by the authors suggesting that astrocytes consume the aggregates released by dying neurons. It has since been demonstrated that soluble A is taken up by astrocytes and that these cells mediate its internal and external clearance.[89–94]

The levels of An in ISF are thought to be regulated through direct absorption by astrocytesaccording to a number of studies. Receptors for apolipoprotein E, or ApoE, have been discovered as mediators of uptake as shown in Figure 8.2. The low-density lipoprotein receptor (LDLR), the very low-density lipoprotein receptor (VLDLR), and the low-density lipoprotein receptor-related protein 1 (LRP1) are all examples.[95] A is absorbed less when LDLR is deleted, but endolysosomal trafficking and clearance of A are improved when LDLR levels are raised. At the same time, LRP1's relevance has been established.[96] Knocking down LRP1 in astrocytes worsens plaque development in APP/PS1 rats by reducing A absorption and decreasing the expression of adegrading enzymes in culture. It's possible that ApoE acts as a chaperone, allowing A to more easily connect to lipoprotein receptors. Human astrocyte binding and uptake of A are influenced by its size, shape, and the presence of other amyloid-related proteins including ApoE. It would appear that endolysosomal breakdown mechanisms are predominantly responsible for clearance following absorption. Now, we discuss studies that used viral gene therapy to enhance lysosomal clearance of A in a monkey model of the disease.[97]

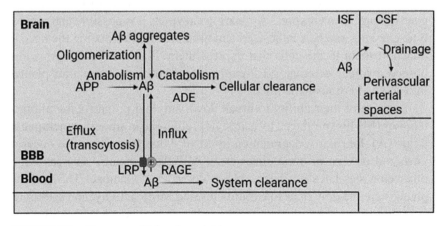

FIGURE 8.2 Clearance of Aβ and amyloid.
Source: Adapted from Ref. [119]

Proteolysis plays a role in A's degradation after it has been taken up by cells. It has been suggested that a number of enzymes play a role in mediating this process, with each enzyme having a preference for either an intracellular or extracellularly localized version of the A isoform.[98–102] A increases the expression of genes encoding receptors for internalizing A, as well as other enzymes, including matrix metalloproteinase-9 (MMP-9), a protein involved in neuron excitability (NEP), and insulin breakdown (IDE).[103] On the other hand, research shows that enzymes appear to operate at close to full capacity, suggesting that the absence of even a single enzyme may lead to a rise in A levels.[104] Therefore, age-related oxidative damage, in conjunction with other environmental variables, may limit the activity of proteolytic enzymes, resulting in a net accumulation of A. With pharmacological inhibition of NEP, endogenous A accumulates in plaques and is eliminated from the body at a slower rate compared to NEP-sufficient animals. The deletion of one or both copies of the NEP gene in the J9 mouse strain, which displays low expression of human APP, leads to elevated levels of A in plasma and brain ISF, the development of hippocampal plaques, and amyloid angiopathy. In one study, NEP was successfully delivered to individual neurons in the hippocampus of both wild-type and APP transgenic mice via an adeno-associated virus 5 (AAV5) vector.[105–110] Both significant increases in A catabolism and NEP expression were observed in presynaptic terminals and cytoplasmic compartments. Although NEP is primarily a neuronal enzyme and is not present in astrocytes, this study demonstrates the value of utilizing viral gene therapy to overexpress A-clearing enzymes. It is possible that proteolytic enzymes can be synthesized and used locally, eliminating the need to transport them to the cells that express them. Plaque reduction was also observed after secretory NEP-expressing fibroblasts were transplanted into aged APP transgenic mice.[111]

Because of their ability to break down amyloid-β, matrix metalloproteinases (MMPs) produced by astrocytes represent an attractive therapeutic target (A). Fibrillar A degradation by MMP-9 has been shown to occur in vitro and in vivo in brain slices from APP/PS1 animals, whereas many other enzymes have not been able to do so.[112–114] Compact ThS-positive plaques are the only ones to exhibit elevated MMP activity, and astrocytes surrounding amyloid plaques are the only ones to show MMP-9 immunoreactivity. A-degrading activity is also present in the astrocyte-conditioned medium (ACM), but it is inhibited by MMP-2/9 inhibitors and is absent

Astrocytes: Genetic Treatment Targets 179

in ACM from MMP-2/9 mutant animals.[115,117] These knockout mice also have higher A levels than wild-type controls. This data lends credence to the idea that age-related plaques in the brain reach a steady state in size throughout time as a result of a constant equilibrium between plaque creation and removal. As seen, the clearance-inhibition ratio may change if astrocytes overexpress A-degrading enzymes like MMP-9.[118] Not only is overexpression not limited to native enzymes, but it can also be used to distribute novel synthetic enzymes that break down amyloid spread throughout the brain and force them to form plaques by infiltrating on their own. Thus, viral gene therapy might be effective in preventing protein aggregation and subsequent neurodegeneration by targeting proteolytic clearance.

8.9 CONCLUSIONS

Despite the fact that Alzheimer's disease (AD) has traditionally been examined from a neuron-centric perspective, additional research has shown that cells besides neurons, such as astrocytes, play a crucial role in disease development. According to the findings of the research team, modifying astrocytotic mechanisms helps Alzheimer's disease animal models. Astrocytic cells can be protected from developing AD by using viral gene therapy to reduce inflammatory cascades and restore degradative pathways. Astrocytic targets for viral gene delivery include receptors implicated in responsiveness, cholesterol synthesis, synaptic maintenance, and neuronal trophic support. Since the astrocytic roles of humans may be more subtle, further study is needed before these results can be applied to them. The relationship between astrocytosis, amyloidosis, and tau pathology in human disease must first be better understood before it can be determined whether targeting inflammation, neurotransmitter homeostasis, BBB integrity, or any of the other astrocytic functions discussed earlier would provide the most therapeutic benefits. Last but not least, understanding the dynamic changes in astrocyte activities that occur over the course of the long prodromal phase of AD is essential for preventing and, perhaps, reversing disease progression. Through the development of new AAV serotypes, LV envelope proteins, and astrocyte-specific promoters, viral gene transfer can now be directed specifically toward astrocytes. Increased viral transduction in the CNS can also be attributed to better delivery by pharmacologic and mechanical modification of the blood-brain barrier and the central endothelium barrier. Developments such as these are especially crucial because of the intricacy of AD therapy brought about by the need to target specific anatomical locations and cell types.

Transduction must be restricted to the specific brain regions and cell types that are of interest. Astrocytes are in a prime position to provide therapeutic benefit to broad sections of the brain afflicted by AD because of their widespread distribution and extensive interactions with synapses and the BBB. Considered collectively, these findings lend credence to the theory that blocking or reversing the progression of disease by focusing on astrocytic populations is a viable option.

KEYWORDS

- **Alzheimer's disease**
- **glial cells**
- **neurofibrillary tangles**
- **astrocytes**
- **glial fibrillary acidic protein**
- **blood brain barrier**

REFERENCES

1. Corder, E.; Saunders, A.; Strittmatter, W.; Schmechel, D.; Gaskell, P.; Small, G. et al. Gene Dose of Apolipoprotein E Type 4 Allele and the Risk of Alzheimer's Disease in Late Onset Families. *Science* **1993,** *261* (5123), 921–923. https://doi.org/10.1126/science.8346443.
2. Cornell-Bell, A. H.; Finkbeiner, S. M.; Cooper, M. S.; Smith, S. J. Glutamate Induces Calcium Waves in Cultured Astrocytes: Long-Range Glial Signaling. *Science* **1990,** 247 (4941), 470–473. Danbolt, N. C. Glutamate Uptake. *Progress Neurobiol.* **2001,** *65* (1), 1105.
3. Dani, J. W.; Chernjavsky, A.; Smith, S. J. Neuronal Activity Triggers Calcium Waves in Hippocampal Astrocyte Networks. *Neuron* **1992,** *8* (3), 429–440.
4. Daniels, M. J.; Rivers-Auty, J.; Schilling, T.; Spencer, N. G.; Watremez, W.; Fasolino, V. et al. Fenamate NSAIDs Inhibit the NLRP3 Inflammasome and Protect Against

Alzheimer's Disease in Rodent Models. *Nat. Commun.* **2016,** *7,* 12504. https://doi.org/10.1038/ncomms12504.

5. Dashkoff, J.; Lerner, E. P.; Truong, N.; Klickstein, J. A.; Fan, Z.; Mu, D. et al. Tailored Transgene Expression to Specific Cell Types in the Central Nervous System After Peripheral Injection with AAV9: Molecular Therapy. *Methods Clin. Dev.* **2016,** *3,* 16081. https://doi.org/10.1038/ mtm.2016.81.

6. De Strooper, B.; Karran, E. The Cellular Phase of Alzheimer's Disease. *Cell* **2016,** *164* (4), 603615. https://doi.org/10.1016/j.cell.2015.12.056.

7. Debernardi, R.; Pierre, K.; Lengacher, S.; Magistretti, P. J.; Pellerin, L. Cell-Specific Expression Pattern of Monocarboxylate Transporters in Astrocytes and Neurons Observed in Different Mouse Brain Cortical Cell Cultures. *J. Neurosci. Res.* **2003,** *73* (2), 141–155. https://doi.org/10.1002/ jnr.10660.

8. Delekate, A.; Fuchtemeier, M.; Schumacher, T.; Ulbrich, C.; Foddis, M.; Petzold, G. C. Metabotropic P2Y1 Receptor Signalling Mediates Astrocytic Hyperactivity In Vivo in an Alzheimer's Disease Mouse Model. *Nat. Commun.* **2014,** *5,* 5422. https://doi.org/10.1038/ncomms6422.

9. Derouiche, A.; Frotscher, M. Astroglial Processes Around Identified Glutamatergic Synapses Contain Glutamine Synthetase: Evidence for Transmitter Degradation. *Brain Res.* **1991,** *552* (2), 346–350.

10. Deverman, B. E.; Pravdo, P. L.; Simpson, B. P.; Kumar, S. R.; Chan, K. Y.; Banerjee, A. et al. Cre-Dependent Selection Yields AAV Variants for Widespread Gene Transfer to the Adult Brain. *Nat. Biotechnol.* **2016,** 17. https://doi.org/10.1038/nbt.3440.

11. Dietschy, J. M.; Turley, S. D. Thematic Review Series: Brain Lipids. Cholesterol Metabolism in the Central Nervous System During Early Development and in the Mature Animal. *J. Lipid Res.* **2004,** *45* (8), 1375–1397. https://doi.org/10.1194/jlr.R400004-JLR200.

12. Dowell, J. A.; Johnson, J. A.; Li, L. Identification of Astrocyte Secreted Proteins with a Combination of Shotgun Proteomics and Bioinformatics. *J. Proteome Res.* **2009,** *8* (8), 4135–4143. https://doi.org/10.1021/pr900248y.

13. Drinkut, A.; Tereshchenko, Y.; Schulz, J. B.; Bahr, M.; Kugler, S. Efficient Gene Therapy for Parkinson's Disease Using Astrocytes as Hosts for Localized Neurotrophic Factor Delivery. *Mol. Therap.* **2012,** *20* (3), 534–543. https://doi.org/10.1038/mt.2011.249.

14. Eleftheriadou, I.; Dieringer, M.; Poh, X. Y.; Sanchez-Garrido, J.; Gao, Y.; Sgourou, A. et al. Selective Transduction of Astrocytic and Neuronal CNS Subpopulations by Lentiviral Vectors Pseudotyped with Chikungunya Virus Envelope. *Biomaterials* **2017,** *123,* 114. https://doi.org/10.1016/j.biomaterials.2017.01.023.

15. Farris, W.; Schutz, S. G.; Cirrito, J. R.; Shankar, G. M.; Sun, X.; George, A. et al. Loss of Neprilysin Function Promotes Amyloid Plaque Formation and Causes Cerebral Amyloid Angiopathy. *Am. J. Pathol..* **2007,** *171* (1), 241–251. https://doi.org/10.2353/ajpath.2007.070105.

16. Abbott, N. J.; Ronnback, L.; Hansson, E. Astrocyte-Endothelial Interactions at the Blood-Brain Barrier. *Nat. Rev. Neurosci.* **2006,** *7* (1), 41–53. https://doi.org/10.1038/nrn1824.

17. Aisen, P. S.; Schafer, K. A.; Grundman, M.; Pfeiffer, E.; Sano, M.; Davis, K. L. et al. Effects of Rofecoxib or Naproxen vs Placebo on Alzheimer Disease Progression: A Randomized Controlled Trial. *JAMA, J. Am. Med. Assoc.* **2003,** *289* (21), 2819–2826. https://doi.org/10.1001/jama.289.21.2819.

18. Akiyama, H.; Barger, S.; Barnum, S.; Bradt, B.; Bauer, J.; Cole, G. M. et al. Inflammation and Alzheimer's Disease. *Neurobiol. Aging* **2000**, *21* (3), 383–421. (b) Alzheimer, A. U¨ ber eigenartige Krankheitsfa¨lle des spa¨teren Alters. *Zbl Ges Neurol. Psychiatry* **1911**, *4*, 356–385.

19. Anderson, M. A.; Ao, Y.; Sofroniew, M. V. Heterogeneity of Reactive Astrocytes. *Neurosci. Lett.* **2014**, *565*, 23–29. https://doi.org/10.1016/j.neulet.2013.12.030.

20. Anderson, M. A.; Burda, J. E.; Ren, Y.; Ao, Y.; O'Shea, T. M.; Kawaguchi, R. et al. Astrocyte Scar Formation Aids Central Nervous System Axon Regeneration. *Nature* **2016**, *532* (7598), 195–200. https://doi.org/10.1038/nature17623.

21. (a) Andriezen, W. L. The Neuroglia Elements in the Human Brain. *Br. Med. J.* **1893**, *2* (1700), 227–230. (b) Aryal, M.; Arvanitis, C. D.; Alexander, P. M.; McDannold, N. Ultrasound-Mediated Blood-Brain Barrier Disruption for Targeted Drug Delivery in the Central Nervous System. *Adv. Drug Deliv. Rev.* **2014**, *72*, 94109. https://doi.org/10.1016/j.addr.2014.01.008.

22. Attwell, D.; Buchan, A. M.; Charpak, S.; Lauritzen, M.; Macvicar, B. A.; Newman, E. A. Glial and Neuronal Control of Brain Blood Flow. *Nature* **2010**, *468* (7321), 232–243. https://doi.org/10.1038/ nature09613.

23. Bankiewicz, K. S.; Eberling, J. L.; Kohutnicka, M.; Jagust, W.; Pivirotto, P.; Bringas, J. et al. Convection-Enhanced Delivery of AAV Vector in Parkinsonian Monkeys; In Vivo Detection of Gene Expression and Restoration of Dopaminergic Function Using Pro-Drug Approach. *Exp. Neurol,* **2000**, *164*, 214. https://doi.org/10.1006/exnr.2000.7408.

24. Bartus, R. T.; Baumann, T. L.; Brown, L.; Kruegel, B. R.; Ostrove, J. M.; Herzog, C. D. Advancing Neurotrophic Factors as Treatments for Age-Related Neurodegenerative Diseases: Developing and Demonstrating "Clinical Proof-of-Concept" for AAV-Neurturin (CERE-120) in Parkinson's Disease. *Neurobiol. Aging* **2013**, *34* (1), 3561. https://doi.org/10.1016/j.neurobiolaging.2012.07.018.

25. Basak, J. M.; Verghese, P. B.; Yoon, H.; Kim, J.; Holtzman, D. M. Low-Density Lipoprotein Receptor Represents an Apolipoprotein E-Independent Pathway of Abeta Uptake and Degradation by Astrocytes. *J. Biol. Chem.* **2012**, *287* (17), 13959–13971. https://doi.org/10.1074/jbc. M111.288746.

26. Bateman, R. J.; Munsell, L. Y.; Morris, J. C.; Swarm, R.; Yarasheski, K. E.; Holtzman, D. M. Human Amyloid-Beta Synthesis and Clearance Rates as Measured in Cerebrospinal Fluid In Vivo. *Nat. Med.* **2006**, *12* (7), 856–861. https://doi.org/ 10.1038/nm1438.

27. Bateman, R. J.; Xiong, C.; Benzinger, T. L.; Fagan, A. M.; Goate, A.; Fox, N. C. et al. Clinical and Biomarker Changes in Dominantly Inherited Alzheimer's Disease. *N. Engl. J. Med.* **2012**, *367* (9), 795–804. https://doi.org/10.1056/ NEJMoa1202753.

28. Bezzi, P.; Carmignoto, G.; Pasti, L.; Vesce, S.; Rossi, D.; Rizzini, B. L. et al. Prostaglandins Stimulate Calcium-Dependent Glutamate Release in Astrocytes. *Nature* **1998**, *391* (6664), 281–285. https://doi.org/10.1038/34651.

29. Bhat, R.; Crowe, E. P.; Bitto, A.; Moh, M.; Katsetos, C. D.; Garcia, F. U. et al. Astrocyte Senescence as a Component of Alzheimer's Disease. *PLoS One* **2012**, *7* (9), e45069. https://doi. org/10.1371/journal.pone.0045069.

30. Bialas, A. R.; Stevens, B. TGF-Beta Signaling Regulates Neuronal C1q Expression and Developmental Synaptic Refinement. *Nat. Neurosci.* **2013**, *16* (12), 1773–1782. https://doi.org/10.1038/ nn.3560.

Astrocytes: Genetic Treatment Targets

31. Braak, H.; Braak, E. Neuropathological Stageing of Alzheimer-Related Changes. *Acta Neuropathol.* **1991,** *82* (4), 239–259.

32. Brier, M. R.; Gordon, B.; Friedrichsen, K.; McCarthy, J.; Stern, A.; Christensen, J. et al. Tau and Abeta Imaging, CSF Measures, and Cognition in Alzheimer's Disease. *Sci. Transl. Med.* **2016,** *8* (338). https://doi.org/10.1126/scitranslmed.aaf2362, 338ra366.

33. Bu, G. Apolipoprotein E and Its Receptors in Alzheimer's Disease: Pathways, Pathogenesis and Therapy. *Nat. Rev. Neurosci.* **2009,** *10* (5), 333–344. https://doi.org/10.1038/nrn2620.

34. Bush, T. G.; Puvanachandra, N.; Horner, C. H.; Polito, A.; Ostenfeld, T.; Svendsen, C. N. et al. Leukocyte Infiltration, Neuronal Degeneration, And Neurite Outgrowth After Ablation of Scarforming, Reactive Astrocytes in Adult Transgenic Mice. *Neuron* **1999,** *23* (2), 297–308.

35. Bushong, E. A.; Martone, M. E.; Jones, Y. Z.; Ellisman, M. H. Protoplasmic Astrocytes in CA1 Stratum Radiatum Occupy Separate Anatomical Domains. *J. Neurosci.* **2002,** *22* (1), 183–192.

36. Cahoy, J. D.; Emery, B.; Kaushal, A.; Foo, L. C.; Zamanian, J. L.; Christopherson, K. S. et al. A Transcriptome Database for Astrocytes, Neurons, and Oligodendrocytes: A New Resource for Understanding Brain Development and Function. *J. Neurosci.* **2008,** *28* (1), 264–278. https://doi.org/10.1523/JNEUROSCI.4178-07.2008.

37. Cannon, J. R.; Sew, T.; Montero, L.; Burton, E. A.; Greenamyre, T. Pseudotype-Dependent Lentiviral Transduction of Astrocytes or Neurons in the Rat Substantia Nigra. *Exp. Neurol.* **2011,** *228*, 4152. https://doi.org/10.1016/j.expneurol.2010.10.016. Pseudotype-dependent.

38. Cantarella, G.; Di Benedetto, G.; Pezzino, S.; Risuglia, N.; Bernardini, R. TRAIL-Related Neurotoxicity Implies Interaction with the WNT Pathway in Human Neuronal Cells In Vitro. *J. Neurochem.* **2008,** *105* (5), 1915–1923. https://doi.org/10.1111/j.1471-4159.2008.05291.x.

39. Carpentier, A.; Canney, M.; Vignot, A.; Reina, V.; Beccaria, K.; Horodyckid, C.; Hoang-xuan, K. Clinical Trial of Blood-Brain Barrier Disruption by Pulsed Ultrasound. *Sci. Transl. Med.* **2016,** *8* (343), 343re2. DOI: 10.1126/scitranslmed.aaf6086.

40. Christine, C. W.; Starr, P. A.; Larson, P. S.; Eberling, J. L.; Jagust, W. J.; Hawkins, R. A. et al. Safety and Tolerability of Putaminal AADC Gene Therapy for Parkinson Disease. *Neurology* **2009,** *73* (20), 1662–1669. https://doi.org/10.1212/WNL.0b013e3181c29356.

41. Christopherson, K. S.; Ullian, E. M.; Stokes, C. C.; Mullowney, C. E.; Hell, J. W.; Agah, A. et al. Thrombospondins Are Astrocyte-Secreted Proteins That Promote CNS Synaptogenesis. *Cell* **2005,** *120* (3), 421–433. https://doi.org/10.1016/j.cell.2004.12.020.

42. Chung, W. S.; Clarke, L. E.; Wang, G. X.; Stafford, B. K.; Sher, A.; Chakraborty, C. et al. Astrocytes Mediate Synapse Elimination Through MEGF10 and MERTK Pathways. *Nature* **2013,** *504* (7480), 394–400. https://doi.org/10.1038/nature12776.

43. Chung, W. S.; Verghese, P. B.; Chakraborty, C.; Joung, J.; Hyman, B. T.; Ulrich, J. D. et al. Novel Allele-Dependent Role for APOE in Controlling the Rate of Synapse Pruning by Astrocytes. *Proc. Natl. Acad. Sci. USA* **2016,** *113* (36), 10186–10191. https://doi.org/10.1073/pnas.1609896113.

44. Cideciyan, A. V.; Aleman, T. S.; Boye, S. L.; Schwartz, S. B.; Kaushal, S.; Roman, A. J. et al. Human Gene Therapy for RPE65 Isomerase Deficiency Activates the Retinoid Cycle of Vision **2008,** *105* (39), 15112–15117. https://doi.org/10.1073/pnas.0807027105.

45. Burn, L.; Gutowski, N.; Whatmore, J.; Giamas G.; Pranjol, M. Z. I. The Role of Astrocytes in Brain Metastasis at the Interface Of Circulating Tumour Cells and the Blood Brain Barrier. *Front. Biosci.* (Landmark Ed) **2021,** *26*(9), 590–601. https://doi.org/10.52586/4969

46. Faulkner, J. R.; Herrmann, J. E.; Woo, M. J.; Tansey, K. E.; Doan, N. B.; Sofroniew, M. V. Reactive Astrocytes Protect Tissue and Preserve Function After Spinal Cord Injury. *J. Neurosci.* **2004,** *24* (9), 2143–2155. https://doi.org/10.1523/JNEUROSCI.3547-03.2004.

47. Foust, K. D.; Nurre, E.; Montgomery, C. L.; Hernandez, A.; Chan, C. M.; Kaspar, B. K. Intravascular AAV9 Preferentially Targets Neonatal Neurons and Adult Astrocytes. *Nat. Biotechnol.* **2009,** *27*, 5965. https://doi.org/10.1038/nbt.1515.

48. Furman, J. L.; Sama, D. M.; Gant, J. C.; Beckett, T. L.; Murphy, M. P.; Bachstetter, A. D. et al. Targeting Astrocytes Ameliorates Neurologic Changes in a Mouse Model of Alzheimer's Disease. *J. Neurosci.* **2012,** *32* (46), 16129–16140. https://doi.org/10.1523/ JNEUROSCI.2323-12.2012.

49. Giannakopoulos, P.; Herrmann, F. R.; Bussiere, T.; Bouras, C.; Kovari, E.; Perl, D. P. et al. Tangle and Neuron Numbers, But Not Amyloid Load, Predict Cognitive Status in Alzheimer's Disease. *Neurology* **2003,** *60* (9), 1495–1500.

50. Giaume, C.; McCarthy, K. D. Control of Gap-Junctional Communication in Astrocytic Networks. *Trends Neurosci.* **1996,** *19* (8), 319–325.

51. Gong, J. S.; Kobayashi, M.; Hayashi, H.; Zou, K.; Sawamura, N.; Fujita, S. C. et al. Apolipoprotein E (ApoE) Isoform-Dependent Lipid Release from Astrocytes Prepared from Human ApoE3 and ApoE4 Knock-in Mice. *J. Biol. Chem.* **2002,** *277* (33), 29919–29926. https://doi.org/10.1074/jbc.M203934200.

52. Haim, L. B.; Carrillo-de Sauvage, M. A.; Ceyzeriat, K.; Escartin, C. Elusive Roles for Reactive Astrocytes in Neurodegenerative Diseases. *Front. Cell. Neurosci.* **2015,** *9*, 278. https://doi. org/10.3389/fncel.2015.00278.

53. Haj-Yasein, N. N.; Vindedal, G. F.; Eilert-Olsen, M.; Gundersen, G. A.; Skare, O.; Laake, P. et al. Glial-Conditional Deletion of Aquaporin-4 (Aqp4) Reduces Blood-Brain Water Uptake and Confers Barrier Function on Perivascular Astrocyte Endfeet. *Proc. Natl. Acad. Sci. USA* **2011,** *108* (43), 17815–17820. https://doi.org/10.1073/pnas.1110655108.

54. Hardy, J.; Selkoe, D. J. The Amyloid Hypothesis of Alzheimer's Disease: Progress and Problems on the Road to Therapeutics. *Science* **2002,** *297* (5580), 353–356. https://doi.org/10.1126/science.1072994.

55. Haughey, N. J.; Mattson, M. P. Alzheimer's Amyloid β-Peptide Enhances ATP/Gap Junction Mediated Calcium-Wave Propagation in Astrocytes. *NeuroMol. Med.* **2003,** *3* (3), 173–180. https://doi.org/10.1385/nmm:3:3:173.

56. Hawkins, B. T.; Davis, T. P. The Blood-Brain Barrier/Neurovascular Unit in Health and Disease. *Pharmacol. Rev.* **2005,** *57* (2), 173–185. https://doi.org/10.1124/pr.57.2.4.

57. Hemming, M. L.; Patterson, M.; Reske-Nielsen, C.; Lin, L.; Isacson, O.; Selkoe, D. J. Reducing Amyloid Plaque Burden via Ex Vivo Gene Delivery of an Abeta-Degrading

Astrocytes: Genetic Treatment Targets

Protease: A Novel Therapeutic Approach to Alzheimer Disease. *PLoS Med.* **2007,** *4* (8), e262. https://doi.org/10.1371/journal.pmed.0040262.

58. Hoshi, A.; Yamamoto, T.; Shimizu, K.; Ugawa, Y.; Nishizawa, M.; Takahashi, H.; Kakita, A. Characteristics of Aquaporin Expression Surrounding Senile Plaques and Cerebral Amyloid Angiopathy in Alzheimer Disease. *J. Neuropathol. Exp. Neurol.* **2012,** *71* (8), 750–759. https://doi.org/10.1097/NEN.0b013e3182632566.

59. Hu, J.; Liu, C. C.; Chen, X. F.; Zhang, Y. W.; Xu, H.; Bu, G. Opposing Effects of Viral Mediated Brain Expression of Apolipoprotein E2 (apoE2) and apoE4 on apoE Lipidation and Abeta Metabolism in apoE4-Targeted Replacement Mice. *Mol. Neurodegen.* **2015,** *10*, 6. https://doi.org/ 10.1186/s13024-015-0001-3.

60. Hu, Y.-C. Baculovirus Vectors for Gene Therapy. *Adv. Virus Res.* **2006,** *68*, 287–320. https://doi.org/10.1016/S0065-3527 (06)68008-1.

61. Iliff, J. J.; Wang, M.; Liao, Y.; Plogg, B. A.; Peng, W.; Gundersen, G. A. et al. A Paravascular Pathway Facilitates CSF Flow Through the Brain Parenchyma and the Clearance of Interstitial Solutes, Including Amyloid Beta. *Sci. Transl. Med.* **2012,** *4*, 147. https://doi.org/10.1126/scitranslmed.3003748,147ra111.

62. Iram, T.; Trudler, D.; Kain, D.; Kanner, S.; Galron, R.; Vassar, R. et al. Astrocytes from Old Alzheimer's Disease Mice Are Impaired in Abeta Uptake and in Neuroprotection. *Neurobiol. Dis.* **2016,** *96*, 8494. https://doi.org/10.1016/j.nbd.2016.08.001.

63. Iwata, N.; Tsubuki, S.; Takaki, Y.; Watanabe, K.; Sekiguchi, M.; Hosoki, E. et al. Identification of the Major Abeta1-42-Degrading Catabolic Pathway in Brain Parenchyma: Suppression Leads to Biochemical and Pathological Deposition. *Nat. Med.* **2000,** *6* (2), 143–150. https://doi.org/10.1038/72237.

64. Iwata, N.; Tsubuki, S.; Takaki, Y.; Shirotani, K.; Lu, B.; Gerard, N. P. et al. Metabolic Regulation of Brain Abeta by Neprilysin. *Science* **2001,** *292* (5521), 1550–1552. https://doi.org/ 10.1126/science.1059946.

65. Jacob, C. P.; Koutsilieri, E.; Bartl, J.; Neuen-Jacob, E.; Arzberger, T.; Zander, N. et al. Alterations in Expression of Glutamatergic Transporters and Receptors in Sporadic Alzheimer's Disease. *J. Alzheimer's Dis.* **2007,** *11*, 97–116.

66. Jakobsson, J.; Lundberg, C. Lentiviral Vectors for Use in the Central Nervous System. *Mol. Therap.* **2006,** *13*, 484–493. https://doi.org/10.1016/j.ymthe.2005.11.012.

67. Jo, S.; Yarishkin, O.; Hwang, Y. J.; Chun, Y. E.; Park, M.; Woo, D. H. et al. GABA from Reactive Astrocytes Impairs Memory in Mouse Models of Alzheimer's Disease. *Nat. Med.* **2014,** *20* (8), 886–896. https://doi.org/10.1038/nm.3639.

68. Jung, E. S.; An, K.; Hong, H. S.; Kim, J. H.; Mook-Jung, I. Astrocyte-Originated ATP Protects Abeta (1-42)-Induced Impairment of Synaptic Plasticity. *J. Neurosci.* **2012,** *32* (9), 3081–3087. https://doi.org/10.1523/JNEUROSCI.6357-11.2012.

69. Jurevics, H.; Morell, P. Cholesterol for Synthesis of Myelin Is Made Locally, Not Imported Into Brain. *J. Neurochem.* **1995,** *64* (2), 895–901.

70. Kacem, K.; Lacombe, P.; Seylaz, J.; Bonvento, G. Structural Organization of the Perivascular Astrocyte End Feet and Their Relationship with the Endothelial Glucose Transporter: A Confocal Microscopy Study. *Glia* **1998,** *23* (1), 110.

71. Kamphuis, W.; Kooijman, L.; Orre, M.; Stassen, O.; Pekny, M.; Hol, E. M. GFAP and Vimentin Deficiency Alters Gene Expression in Astrocytes and Microglia in Wild-Type Mice and Changes the Transcriptional Response of Reactive Glia in Mouse Model for Alzheimer's Disease. *Glia* **2015,** *63* (6), 1036–1056. https://doi.org/10.1002/glia.22800.

72. Kang, J.; Jiang, L.; Goldman, S. A.; Nedergaard, M. Astrocyte-Mediated Potentiation of Inhibitory Synaptic Transmission. *Nat. Neurosci.* **1998,** *1* (8), 683–692. https://doi.org/10.1038/ 3684.

73. Kanninen, K.; Heikkinen, R.; Malm, T.; Rolova, T.; Kuhmonen, S.; Leinonen, H. et al. Intrahippocampal Injection of a Lentiviral Vector Expressing Nrf2 Improves Spatial Learning in a Mouse Model of Alzheimer's Disease. *Proc. Natl. Acad. Sci. USA* **2009,** *106,* 16505–16510. https://doi.org/10.1073/pnas.0908397106.

74. Karwoski, C. J.; Lu, H. K.; Newman, E. A. Spatial Buffering of Light-Evoked Potassium Increases by Retinal Muller (Glial) Cells. *Science* **1989,** *244* (4904), 578–580.

75. Kim, J.; Jiang, H.; Park, S.; Eltorai, A. E.; Stewart, F. R.; Yoon, H. et al. Haploinsufficiency of Human APOE Reduces Amyloid Deposition in a Mouse Model of Amyloid-Beta Amyloidosis. *J. Neurosci.* **2011,** *31* (49), 18007–18012. https://doi.org/10.1523/ JNEUROSCI.3773-11.2011.

76. Kim, J.; Eltorai, A. E.; Jiang, H.; Liao, F.; Verghese, P. B.; Kim, J. et al. Anti-apoE Immunotherapy Inhibits Amyloid Accumulation in a Transgenic Mouse Model of Abeta Amyloidosis. *J. Exp. Med.* **2012,** *209* (12), 2149–2156. https://doi.org/10.1084/ jem.20121274.

77. Koistinaho, M.; Lin, S.; Wu, X.; Esterman, M.; Koger, D.; Hanson, J. et al. Apolipoprotein E Promotes Astrocyte Colocalization and Degradation of Deposited Amyloid-Beta Peptides. *Nat. Med.* **2004,** *10* (7), 719–726. https://doi.org/10.1038/ nm1058.

78. Kordower, J. H.; Bloch, J.; Ma, S. Y.; Chu, Y.; Palfi, S.; Roitberg, B. Z. et al. Lentiviral Gene Transfer to the Nonhuman Primate Brain. *Exp. Neurol.* **1999,** *160,* 116. https://doi.org/10.1006/exnr.1999.7178.

79. Kraft, A. W.; Hu, X.; Yoon, H.; Yan, P.; Xiao, Q.; Wang, Y. et al. Attenuating Astrocyte Activation Accelerates Plaque Pathogenesis in APP/PS1 Mice. *FASEB J.* **2013,** *27* (1), 187–198. https://doi.org/10.1096/fj.12-208660.

80. Kuchibhotla, K. V.; Lattarulo, C. R.; Hyman, B. T.; Bacskai, B. J. Synchronous Hyperactivity and Intercellular Calcium Waves in Astrocytes in Alzheimer Mice. *Science* **2009,** *323* (5918), 1211–1215. https://doi.org/10.1126/science.1169096.

81. Kucukdereli, H.; Allen, N. J.; Lee, A. T.; Feng, A.; Ozlu, M. I.; Conatser, L. M. et al. Control of Excitatory CNS Synaptogenesis by Astrocyte-Secreted Proteins Hevin and SPARC. *Proc. Natl. Acad. Sci. USA* **2011,** *108* (32), E440–E449. https://doi.org/10.1073/pnas.1104977108.

82. Kulijewicz-Nawrot, M.; Sykova, E.; Chvatal, A.; Verkhratsky, A.; Rodriguez, J. J. Astrocytes and Glutamate Homoeostasis in Alzheimer's Disease: A Decrease in Glutamine Synthetase, But Not in Glutamate Transporter-1, in the Prefrontal Cortex. *ASN Neuro* **2013,** *5* (4), 273–282. https://doi.org/10.1042/ AN20130017.

83. Lawlor, P. a, Bland, R. J.; Mouravlev, A.; Young, D.; During, M. J. Efficient Gene Delivery and Selective Transduction of Glial Cells in the Mammalian Brain by AAV Serotypes Isolated from Nonhuman Primates. *Mol. Therap.* **2009,** *17,* 1692–1702. https://doi.org/10.1038/mt.2009.170.

84. Lee, Y.; Messing, A.; Su, M.; Brenner, M. GFAP Promoter Elements Required for Region-Specific and Astrocyte-Specific Expression. *Glia* **2008,** *56,* 481–493. https://doi.org/10.1002/glia.20622.

Astrocytes: Genetic Treatment Targets 187

85. Leoni, V. The Effect of Apolipoprotein E (ApoE) Genotype on Biomarkers of Amyloidogenesis, Tau Pathology and Neurodegeneration in Alzheimer's Disease. *Clin. Chem. Lab. Med.* **2011,** *49* (3), 375–383. https://doi.org/10.1515/CCLM.2011.088.

86. Li, C.; Zhao, R.; Gao, K.; Wei, Z.; Yin, M. Y.; Lau, L. T. et al. Astrocytes: Implications for Neuroinflammatory Pathogenesis of Alzheimer's Disease. *Curr. Alzheimer Res.* **2011,** *8* (1), 6780. https://doi.org/10.2174/156720511794604543.

87. Li, L.; Lundkvist, A.; Andersson, D.; Wilhelmsson, U.; Nagai, N.; Pardo, A. C. et al. Protective Role of Reactive Astrocytes in Brain Ischemia. *J. Cereb. Blood Flow Metabol.* **2008,** *28* (3), 468–481. https://doi.org/10.1038/sj.jcbfm.9600546.

88. Lian, H.; Yang, L.; Cole, A.; Sun, L.; Chiang, A. C.; Fowler, S. W. et al. NFkappaB-Activated Astroglial Release of Complement C3 Compromises Neuronal Morphology and Function Associated with Alzheimer's Disease. *Neuron* **2015,** *85* (1), 101–115. https://doi.org/10.1016/j. neuron.2014.11.018.

89. Liao, F.; Hori, Y.; Hudry, E.; Bauer, A. Q.; Jiang, H.; Mahan, T. E. et al. Anti-ApoE Antibody Given After Plaque Onset Decreases Abeta Accumulation and Improves Brain Function in a Mouse Model of Abeta Amyloidosis. *J. Neurosci.* **2014,** *34* (21), 7281–7292. https://doi.org/ 10.1523/JNEUROSCI.0646-14.2014.

90. Liauw, J.; Hoang, S.; Choi, M.; Eroglu, C.; Choi, M.; Sun, G. H. et al. Thrombospondins 1 and 2 Are Necessary for Synaptic Plasticity and Functional Recovery After Stroke. *J. Cereb. Blood Flow Metabol.* **2008,** *28* (10), 1722–1732. https://doi.org/ 10.1038/ jcbfm.2008.65.

91. Lidar, Z.; Mardor, Y.; Jonas, T.; Pfeffer, R.; Faibel, M.; Nass, D. et al. Convection-Enhanced Delivery of Paclitaxel for the Treatment of Recurrent Malignant Glioma: A Phase I/II Clinical Study. *J. Neurosurg.* **2004,** *100*, 472–479. https://doi.org/10.3171/ jns.2004.100.3.0472.

92. Liddelow, S. A.; Guttenplan, K. A.; Clarke, L. E.; Bennett, F. C.; Bohlen, C. J.; Schirmer, L. et al. Neurotoxic Reactive Astrocytes Are Induced by Activated Microglia. *Nature* **2017,** *541* (7638), 481–487. https://doi.org/10.1038/nature21029.

93. Lin, C. L.; Kong, Q.; Cuny, G. D.; Glicksman, M. A. Glutamate Transporter EAAT2: A New Target for the Treatment of Neurodegenerative Diseases. *Fut. Med. Chem.* **2012,** *4* (13), 1689–1700. https://doi.org/10.4155/fmc.12.122.

94. Liu, C. C.; Hu, J.; Zhao, N.; Wang, J.; Wang, N.; Cirrito, J. R. et al. Astrocytic LRP1 Mediates Brain Abeta Clearance and Impacts Amyloid Deposition. *J. Neurosci.* **2017,** *37* (15), 4023–4031. https://doi.org/10.1523/JNEUROSCI.3442-16.2017.

95. Livet, J.; Weissman, T. A.; Kang, H.; Draft, R. W.; Lu, J.; Bennis, R. A. et al. Transgenic Strategies for Combinatorial Expression of Fluorescent Proteins in the Nervous System. *Nature* **2007,** *450* (7166), 5662. https://doi.org/10.1038/nature06293.

96. Lomakin, A.; Teplow, D. B.; Kirschner, D. A.; Benedek, G. B. Kinetic Theory of Fibrillogenesis of Amyloid Beta-Protein. *Proc. Natl. Acad. Sci. USA* **1997,** *94* (15), 79427947.

97. Louboutin, J.-P. P.; Chekmasova, A. A.; Marusich, E.; Chowdhury, J. R.; Strayer, D. S. Efficient CNS Gene Delivery by Intravenous Injection. *Nat. Methods* **2010,** *7*, 905–907. https://doi.org/ 10.1038/nmeth.1518.

98. Louveau, A.; Smirnov, I.; Keyes, T. J.; Eccles, J. D.; Rouhani, S. J.; Peske, J. D. et al. Structural and Functional Features of Central Nervous System Lymphatic Vessels. *Nature* **2015,** *523* (7560), 337–341. https://doi.org/10.1038/nature14432.

99. Lucca, U.; Tettamanti, M.; Forloni, G.; Spagnoli, A. Nonsteroidal Antiinflammatory Drug-Use in Alzheimer's Disease. *Biol. Psychiatry* **1994,** *36* (12), 854–856. https://doi.org/10.1016/ 0006-3223 (94)90598-3.

100. Machler, P.; Wyss, M. T.; Elsayed, M.; Stobart, J.; Gutierrez, R.; von Faber-Castell, A. et al. In Vivo Evidence for a Lactate Gradient from Astrocytes to Neurons. *Cell Metabol.* **2016,** *23* (1), 94102. https://doi.org/10.1016/j.cmet.2015.10.010.

101. Mandel, R. J. CERE-110, an Adeno-Associated Virus-Based Gene Delivery Vector Expressing Human Nerve Growth Factor for the Treatment of Alzheimer's Disease. *Curr. Opin. Mol. Therap.* **2010,** *12* (2), 240–247.

102. Maragakis, N. J.; Rothstein, J. D. Glutamate Transporters: Animal Models to Neurologic Disease. *Neurobiol. Dis.* **2004,** *15* (3), 461–473. https://doi.org/10.1016/j.nbd.2003.12.007.

103. Masliah, E. Deficient Glutamate Transport Is Associated with Neurodegenerationin Alzheimer's Disease. *Ann. Neurol.* **1996,** *40* (5), 759–766.

104. Masliah, E.; Alford, M.; Mallory, M.; Rockenstein, E.; Moechars, D.; Van Leuven, F. Abnormal Glutamate Transport Function in Mutant Amyloid Precursor Protein Transgenic Mice. *Exp. Neurol.* **2000,** *163* (2), 381–387. https://doi.org/10.1006/exnr.2000.7386.

105. Mawuenyega, K. G.; Sigurdson, W.; Ovod, V.; Munsell, L.; Kasten, T.; Morris, J. C. et al. Decreased Clearance of CNS Beta-Amyloid in Alzheimer's Disease. *Science* **2010,** *330* (6012), 1774. https://doi.org/10.1126/science.1197623.

106. McCarty, D. M.; Dirosario, J.; Gulaid, K.; Muenzer, J.; Fu, H. Mannitol-Facilitated CNS Entry of rAAV2 Vector Significantly Delayed the Neurological Disease Progression in MPS IIIB Mice. *Gene Therap.* **2009,** 113. https://doi.org/10.1038/gt.2009.85.

107. Merienne, N.; Le Douce, J.; Faivre, E.; Deglon, N.; Bonvento, G. Efficient Gene Delivery and Selective Transduction of Astrocytes in the Mammalian Brain Using Viral Vectors. *Front. Cell. Neurosci.* **2013,** *7*, 106. https://doi.org/10.3389/fncel.2013.00106.

108. Merlini, M.; Meyer, E. P.; Ulmann-Schuler, A.; Nitsch, R. M. Vascular Beta-Amyloid and Early Astrocyte Alterations Impair Cerebrovascular Function and Cerebral Metabolism in Transgenic arcAbeta Mice. *Acta Neuropathol.* **2011,** *122* (3), 293–311. https://doi.org/10.1007/s00401-011-0834-y.

109. Meyer-Luehmann, M.; Spires-Jones, T. L.; Prada, C.; Garcia-Alloza, M.; de Calignon, A.; Rozkalne, A. et al. Rapid Appearance and Local Toxicity of Amyloid-Beta Plaques in a Mouse Model of Alzheimer's Disease. *Nature* **2008,** *451* (7179), 720–724. https://doi.org/10.1038/ nature06616.

110. Min, K. J.; Yang, M. S.; Kim, S. U.; Jou, I.; Joe, E. H. Astrocytes Induce Hemeoxy-genase-1 Expression in Microglia: A Feasible Mechanism for Preventing Excessive Brain Inflammation. *J. Neurosci.* **2006,** *26* (6), 1880–1887. https://doi.org/10.1523/JNEUROSCI.3696-05.2006.

111. Mingozzi, F.; High, K. A. Therapeutic In Vivo Gene Transfer for Genetic Disease Using AAV: Progress and Challenges. *Nat. Rev. Genet.* **2011,** *12* (5), 341–355. https://doi.org/10.1038/ nrg2988.

112. Mothet, J. P.; Pollegioni, L.; Ouanounou, G.; Martineau, M.; Fossier, P.; Baux, G. Glutamate Receptor Activation Triggers a Calcium-Dependent and SNARE Protein-Dependent Release of the Gliotransmitter Dserine. *Proc. Natl. Acad. Sci. USA* **2005,** *102* (15), 5606–5611. https://doi.org/10.1073/pnas.0408483102.

Astrocytes: Genetic Treatment Targets 189

113. (a) Mrak, R. E.; Sheng, J. G.; Griffin, W. S. Glial Cytokines in Alzheimer's Disease: Review and Pathogenic Implications. *Hum. Pathol.* **1995,** *26* (8), 816–823. (b) Mudannayake, J. M.; Mouravlev, A.; Fong, D. M.; Young, D. Transcriptional Activity of Novel ALDH1L1 Promoters in the Rat Brain Following AAV Vector-Mediated Gene Transfer. *Mol. Therap: Methods Clin. Dev.* **2016,** *3*, 16075. https://doi.org/10.1038/mtm.2016.75.

114. Mulder, S. D.; Veerhuis, R.; Blankenstein, M. A.; Nielsen, H. M. The Effect of Amyloid Associated Proteins on the Expression of Genes Involved in Amyloid-Beta Clearance by Adult Human Astrocytes. *Exp. Neurol.* **2012,** *233* (1), 373–379. https://doi.org/10.1016/j. expneurol.2011.11.001.

115. Nagele, R. G.; D'Andrea, M. R.; Lee, H.; Venkataraman, V.; Wang, H.-Y. Astrocytes accumulate Aβ42 and give rise to astrocytic amyloid plaques in Alzheimer disease brains. Brain Research, *971* (2), 197–209. https://doi.org/10.1016/s0006-8993 (03)02361-8.

116. Nagy, J. I.; Li, W.; Hertzberg, E. L.; Marotta, C. A. Elevated Connexin43 Immuno-reactivity at Sites of Amyloid Plaques in Alzheimer's Disease. *Brain Res.* **1996,** *717* (1–2), 173–178. https:// doi.org/10.1016/0006-8993 (95)01526-4.

117. Nielsen, H. M.; Veerhuis, R.; Holmqvist, B.; Janciauskiene, S. Binding and Uptake of A Beta1-42 by Primary Human Astrocytes In Vitro. *Glia* **2009,** *57* (9), 978–988. https://doi.org/10.1002/ glia.20822.

118. Nielsen, H. M.; Mulder, S. D.; Belien, J. A.; Musters, R. J.; Eikelenboom, P.; Veerhuis, R. Astrocytic A Beta 1-42 Uptake Is Determined by A Beta-Aggregation State and the Presence of Amyloidassociated Proteins. Glia **2010,** 58 (10), 1235–1246. https://doi. org/10.1002/glia.21004.

119. Yoon, S., & Jo, S.A. (2012). Mechanisms of Amyloid-β Peptide Clearance: Potential Therapeutic Targets for Alzheimer's Disease. Biomolecules & Therapeutics, 20, 245 - 255.

CHAPTER 9

Clinical Studies of Gene Therapy for the Treatment of Neurodegenerative Disorders

ABSTRACT

A resurgence in gene therapy is occurring. Particularly promising for the treatment of neurodegenerative diseases are gene-based therapies, here encompassing all forms of genome modification where conventional pharmacologic methods have largely failed intriguingly because of their dual promises of 'long-term correction' and targeting disease etiology. An example of such a therapeutic intervention and a foundation for further development is provided by the recent success related to the application of viruses as carriers for therapeutic genes to treat spinal muscular atrophy, which improved motor function and survival with a single intravenous injection. The main causes of the newfound confidence are the creation concerns regarding the potential use of genome engineering techniques to modify disease circuits and the use of viral vectors to spread genes throughout the central nervous system in previously unfeasible ways, even though hurdles still exist. One might foresee a day when gene-based treatments will be a part of a clinician's toolkit. Surely, spinal muscular atrophy is not the only neurodegenerative illness that can be treated with gene therapy. This chapter's objective is to provide a forward-looking look at this rapidly developing field while highlighting developments in gene therapy for treating neurodegenerative diseases.

Gene Therapy for Neurological Disorders: Molecular Approaches for Targeted Treatment.
Rishabha Malviya, Arun Kumar Singh, Priyanshi Goyal, & Sonali Sundram (Authors)
© 2025 Apple Academic Press, Inc. Co-published with CRC Press (Taylor & Francis)

9.1 INTRODUCTION

Because of their complex and multicausal origin, neurological illnesses continue to provide a significant challenge for medical professionals.[1,2] Treating diseases of the neurological system is difficult because of the BBB, the slowness of nerve tissue regeneration, and the complexity of the CNS. The traditional, continuous therapy and surgical interventions are still challenging. Numerous potentially significant compounds with high molecular weights and lipophilicity are specifically prohibited from entering the BBB.[1-4] These compounds require the use of osmotic micropumps, intracerebroventricular injections, or intracerebral injections. Additionally, neurons behave as convolutions with the ability to receive and send signals or information that is physically and physiologically different from any other human body cells.[1,2,5] A novel treatment approach called gene therapy has emerged as a desirable means of delivering genetic material. With the use of a transgene that can be turned on and off at will, can replace the faulty gene, and governs how the disease environment is expressed, gene therapy treats disorders.[6] Initial findings were so encouraging that numerous researchers submitted plans for first- and second-stage trials for various neurological illnesses. Recent advancements, such as neuroimaging, have aided clinical evaluation by assessing an accurate understanding of the anatomical-functional relationship.[7,8] In fact, several preclinical and clinical studies are required to show that gene therapy is effective in treating CNS illnesses.[9,10] It's also important to remember that gene therapy is a technique that requires the optimization of a number of variables, including the choice of an appropriate vector, transgene, and delivery method. Due to the complexity of neural tissue, not only does the host immune system interact with the vector and transgene, but gene therapy for neurodegenerative diseases is also challenging to perform. Additionally, a treatment plan based on gene therapy involves difficulties like ensuring that the therapeutic agent is delivered as effectively as possible. This can be achieved by either intracerebral administration or by channeling growth factors or therapeutics that promote growth factor production into the brain parenchyma.[11] Growth factors have shown promise in preclinical investigations, but they should proceed through all stages of clinical trials since they should be administered cautiously. Growth factors function through appropriate molecular pathways, in contrast to other neuroprotective drugs, and restore, protect, and generate

Clinical Studies of Gene Therapy

neurons as well as their functionality. The effects of growth factors, despite having a shorter half-life, can persist for days to months after growth factor deactivation by activating the corresponding receptors that set off a chain of events that directs second messengers to activate transcription factors.[12] Two other significant techniques should be addressed. One is a combination of gene and stem cell treatment, which may be effective in treating neurodegenerative diseases by altering the transplanted cells' production of ectopic proteins.[13] One instance of this is the administration of to a neurotrophin called dopaminergic neurons that were damaged by PD and benefited from glial cell line-derived neurotrophic factor (GDNF).[14] And by using neurotrophic gene therapy, the efficacy of grafts derived from human pluripotent stem cells can be improved. We talk about the numerous gene therapy options and vectors in this topic, as well as the preclinical and clinical research done to treat the various neurological illnesses.

9.2 TACTICS FOR GENE THERAPY

The two gene therapy techniques that are utilized to transfer genes are ex vivo and in vivo. A new gene is inserted into an organism during in vivo gene therapy which uses a viral or plasmid vector to be introduced into the body of a patient. The gene is currently undergoing refinement through the use of the CRISPR technology.[15,16] Modifying cells outside of the body, or "ex vivo," is what happens during gene therapy before they are transplanted into the patient either as a permanent graft for the purpose of replacing dead cells or as a temporary graft to give therapeutic proteins.[17–19] Nonspecific gene expression, targeted insertional mutagenesis, gene silencing, and immunological reactions to the vector are among the complications of in vivo gene therapy.[20] The intensive production of therapeutic molecules required by cellular CNS cells may make them particularly vulnerable to the stresses of gene therapy. Out-of-body gene therapy does not directly expose the patient to the vector; instead, modified cells are characterized before being administered to the patient.[21] Ex vivo gene therapy appears to have a bright future thanks to recent developments. By using a patient's own tissue or cells (from their blood or skin), scientists can create iPSC, which is one example of an NSC approach.[22,23] In addition to producing the necessary or advantageous protein, tissues can form as a result of cell differentiation that is suitable for therapy, like oligodendrocytes or astrocytes. Mesenchymal stem cells and fibroblasts have substantial problems with ex vivo gene therapy because the foreign genes cannot properly integrate with the nervous system.[24–26] Researchers explore MSCs for tissue repair, angiogenesis-promoting cytokines, growth factors, and immunomodulatory action.[27,28] Since MSCs cannot cross the BBB, they cannot reach the brain, and they also have a short shelf-life; therefore, continued administration is required for long-lasting benefits. Neural progenitor cells (NPCs) or NSCs can develop in many parts of the brain. The brain's NPCs have limited self-renewal and give rise to astrocytes and neurons.[29] In the right conditions, the NSC has the potential to develop into oligodendrocytes, astrocytes, or neurons.[30] One type of cell that can profit from ex vivo gene therapy is human embryonic stem cells; however, their ethical use has been questioned.[31,32] The moral issues of using embryonic stem cells are also avoided by using iPSCs, which can also be used for autologous CNS transplantation.[33,34] Nonviral approaches appear. In addition to using gene therapy ex vivo, dormant cells can nonetheless express proteins for extended periods of time.[35,36] Recent developments have made it possible to use gene editing methods like CRISPR-Cas9, TALEN, and ZFN.[37] The methods are based on precise gene knock-ins to target harbor loci, which are made possible by double-stranded breaks at specific genomic sites.[38,39] These gene editing techniques can be used and show promise for the treatment of genetic diseases like HD and hereditary versions of ALS and PD.[40]

9.3 UTILIZING VECTORS IN GENE TREATMENT

The process of introducing a transgene into a vector is complicated, and vectors need to have certain characteristics,[41–43] such as:

- The vector must enable simple recombinant technology modification and propagation in appropriate hosts.
- The vector should have a high capacity for cloning and little invasiveness. The vector should not be able to alter the host genome in an unintended or uncontrolled way, and it should allow for the adaption, guaranteeing adequate regulation of transgenic expression in space and time.

Clinical Studies of Gene Therapy 195

- The transgene chosen must only express itself in the intended cells.
- Immunogenicity must not be caused by the vector (it should not contain any immune-stimulating genes).
- The vector needs to support continuous, long-term expression of a working gene without affecting the progeny of the cell.

As a matter of fact, both viral and nonviral vectors are frequently used. Carrier lipids, such as liposomes, synthetic macromolecules, and cationic polymers, containing particular ligands for cell surface receptors can all be examples of these. Viral vectors are a practical means of delivering and expressing host-cell genetic material. In the field of neurovirology, lentiviruses (LVs), AAV, HSV1, and retroviruses (RVs) are among the most often used and studied viruses (CNS). Cells can be infected in a natural way.[44–46] Nevertheless, there are many considerations to make while using viral vectors, such as (1) the viral genome's interaction with the host genome; (2) virus-gene interactions or viral tropism and antigenicity, potential toxicity, and tumorigenicity; (3) the capacity to mass-produce viral vectors for effective transduction; and (4) the ability to mass-produce viruses. Adenovirus, it turns out, is one of the most effective vectors for the CNS since it can safely and effectively divide dormant cells in methods like in vivo and in vitro.[47] Adenoviruses, for instance, can accommodate vast areas and cause cytotoxicity by the viral capsid and infection when the E1 and E3 sections are removed. They are brain cells despite the fact that they are poorly adapted to the host's genome and transduce often. Furthermore, RV only infects dividing cells, and insertional mutagenesis may result from RV integrating into the host cells' DNA.[48,49]

9.4 IN VIVO STUDY FOR NEUROLOGICAL DISEASE

A novel method for DNA transposition utilizing science[50] was reported on the CRISPR-associated transposon (CAST), while Nature[51] published an article on the topic. The bacterial CRISPR/Cas system is enlisted by Tn7-like transposons through the use of CAST.[52] After being altered, transposons with a similar structure to Tn7 can be utilized to insert DNA with high accuracy. Unlike the standard gene knock-in method, CAST can transport cargo genes up to 10 kilobase pairs in size efficiently without the need for DSBs.[53]

196   *Gene Therapy for Neurological Disorders*

9.4.1 ALZHEIMER'S DISEASE

Alzheimer's disease (AD) is characterized by the development of neuro-fibrillary tangles (NFTs), the accumulation of senile plaques (SPs), and the death are hallmarks.[54] Amyloid-beta protein deposition in the brain also contributes to the disease. The amyloid cascade theory has been the mainstay of Alzheimer's disease (AD) pathophysiology studies for the last 20 years. The identification of mutations in the APP (on chromosome 21), PSEN1 (on chromosome 14), and PSEN2 (on chromosome 1) has changed this picture and has profoundly changed research approaches.[54–56]

After GWAS, many SNPs, the risk gene ApoE4, and additional locations associated with AD were discovered. Future editing targets for these genes could be the proteins they encode, which are involved in a number of biological processes related to AD.

Numerous risk loci have been identified thanks to recent GWAS.[58–61] The following genes have been proven to operate beyond a doubt: ApoE, ABCA7, BIN1, TREM2, SORL1, ADAM10, SPI1, and CR1. In a number of disease models, ApoE4 in particular has undergone significant characterization.[62] A recent study found that when exposed to Klotho hormone in its biological form, people with ApoE4 had a decreased probability of developing AD. Additionally, it was proposed that a heterozygous KL-VS (KLVSHET+) genotype was associated with a lower AD and A protein load.[63] Another clinical investigation, however, discovered no link between KL-VS, a Klotho variant, and patient cognitive decline.[64] The likely function of ApoE4 in AD was later examined from a number of perspectives. The phenotype caused by ApoE4 may be related to REST, a key regulator of brain development.[65] Furthermore, the ApoE4 genotype may regulate metabolism in light of the failure of energy metabolism in AD patients.

Additionally, gender differences have been connected to these metabolic alterations.[66] One benefit is that ApoE4 and its allele, ApoE3, differ by just one nucleotide. As a result, it is possible to cause single nucleotide alterations, particularly when using the PE method. The genomic region known as TREM2 is present in both AD and PD.

In TREM2-deficient mice, severe neurodegeneration has been seen, to which microglial activation may be related.[67] Another in vivo experiment showed transformative significance for clinical care. In APP transgenic mice, A pathogenesis was successfully improved by researchers[68] (see Table 9.1).

Clinical Studies of Gene Therapy 197

The genetic basis of the clinical symptoms of AD has also been studied. For instance, CHRFAM7A inhibits TALEN-transfected pluripotent stem cells (iPSCs) expressing cholinergic receptors.[69] Researchers found that PSENLIN2 is linked to more amyloid protein buildup than PSENLIN1.[70] However, CRISPR-based editing of the APP C-terminus successfully reduced the production of A protein in iPSCs.[71] In APP transgenic mice, phosphorylation of Threonine 205 (T205) similarly suppressed the A protein-related behavior. p38, a postsynaptic form of the MAPK protein kinase (MAPK), is hypothesized as having a hand in command.[72] A Caenorhabditis elegans genetic model has revealed the existence of additional epigenetically dysregulated sites. In a second study, C. elegans mimicking the age-related decreases in touch sensitivity was linked to phosphorylation of threonine 231 (T231) and acetylation of lysines 274 (K274) and 281 (K281) in abnormal brain architecture.[73]

Other risk loci were discovered by GWAS that have not been confirmed in animal or cell-based studies yet, in addition to those that have been thoroughly studied. Peripheral tissues, including skin tissue, have been examined in studies worth counting. Nonetheless, one must ascertain the role these newly discovered AD genes play in disease pathogenesis.[74]

9.4.2 PARKINSON'S DISEASE

Aggregation of the protein β-synuclein characterizes serious PD, a chronic, progressive neurological ailment that typically affects older people. Patients with hereditary mutations in LRRK2, PARK2, DJ-1, PINK1, and SNCA have been the focus of numerous investigations.[75] The presence of SNCA is a strong predictor of an increased chance of developing sporadic Parkinson's disease (PD) associated with β-synuclein expression.[76] A53T SNCA triplication and mutation alters β-synuclein-mediated nucleocytoplasmic trafficking.[77] In CRISPR-edited iPSCs, this regulation has been further verified.[78] According to reports, rs12411216, a different recently identified β-syn SNP location, controls how glucocerebrosidase works, promoting the protein-syn distribution.[79] A PD cell model has been developed using a more efficient SCNA β-specific CRISPR technique.[80] To further downregulate transcription and expression, a special CRISPR-based lentiviral vector has been developed to precisely methylate intron 1 of SNCA.[81] A separate study found that cell lines with low SNCA levels showed resistance to Lewy pathology.[82]

Additionally identified as potential therapeutic targets are P13, PINK, and PARKIN due to their roles in the control of mitochondrial activity. The impact of the effect of PARKIN mutation on PD-relative protein expression in iPSC lines has been studied by a number of labs.[83] According to reports, both toxin-induced and genetic PD models have neuroprotective effects when P13 expression is reduced. On the other hand, it has been demonstrated that overexpressing P13 helps PD animals that have been exposed to toxins develop their phenotypes.[84] Through cytogenetic analysis, several researchers have suggested resources for building a model of PD stem cells involving LRRK2.[85] Another TALEN-derived LRRK2 iPSC model can serve as a model.[86] In an interesting work, Nigral dopaminergic neurons had the PARKIN, DJ-1, and ATP13A2 genes deleted using CRISPR/Cas (DN). Researchers revealed that oxidative stress was the prevalent source of dysregulation in isogenic cell lines by integrating transcriptome and proteome data.[87] Regular clinical typing may be useless now that we know more about the molecular pathways of PD. It is necessary to differentiate between PD subtypes more precisely, and understanding the molecular basis of these diseases may open up new therapeutic possibilities that might be used to treat every single NDD illness.

Parkinson's disease impairment (PD) is potentially attributable to a novel DNAJC6 mutation in human embryonic stem cells.[88] Additionally, LIN28A knockout mice have shown behavioral abnormalities associated with PD.[89] Recently, multiple GWAS for PD have been undertaken, similar to those for AD.[90,91] If these revealed that mutations can aid in clinical prediction, more research utilizing cell and animal models is necessary.

9.4.3 HUNTINGTON'S DISEASE

An inherited neurological disorder called Huntington's disease causes uncontrollable dancing movements and progressive declines in behavior and cognition. It is frequently accompanied by disability and early mortality. When it comes to pathology, neuronal loss and astrocytosis, as well as imaging show significant brain shrinkage, while HD is distinct. Genetic mutations, clinical symptoms, and family history are the key factors used to confirm a diagnosis.

HD is linked to the Huntington's disease gene (HTT) exon 1 duplication of CAG trinucleotides.[92] On HTT, normal CAG repetitions are in the

Clinical Studies of Gene Therapy 199

range of 27; when the number of CAG repetitions is more than 39, full penetration has been achieved.[93] The proteins made by the mutated HTT gene are not only cytotoxic but also (mHTT) are unable to interact with other proteins involved in normal cellular processes. A perfect candidate for gene therapy is HD since it is a condition brought on by a single mutation and a single faulty protein.

The creation of HD cell models using gene editing techniques has been described in several studies[94–96] and can be used to verify the effectiveness of medication. An HD cell model was discovered to have abnormally high calcium influx[97] and ultrastructural synapses in prior studies.[98]

Furthermore, the amount of CAG repeats is correlated with the incidence of ultrastructural synapse abnormalities.[99]

In a different experiment, CRISPR/Cas9 was utilized to make HD140Q-KI mice lose their neuronal mHTT. The experimental group's motor dysfunction was improved as a result andreactive astrocytes significantly decreased.[100]

Another in vivo study that concentrated on the CAG repeat's first exon successfully inhibited HTT expression as well[101] (see Table 9.1). According to recent results, the HD phenotype can be successfully reduced by inhibiting CAG expression; cells that have undergone apoptosis, however, cannot be revived. After the success of the nonallele-specific CRISPR strategy in the PD animal model, two studies demonstrated the efficacy of allele-specific CRISPR.[102,103] CITP2 does more than just go after HTT mutations which were changed to interact with mutant huntingtin.[104] In addition, CAG expansion was frequently halted using ZFN and TALEN.[105,106]

9.4.4 ALS

A neurodegenerative disease with an adult-onset and deadly outcome is amyotrophic lateral sclerosis. Within 3–5 years following the commencement of symptoms, paralysis and death result from the gradual weakening as well as system-wide muscle atrophy due to increased loss of motor neurons (in the spinal cord, brain stem, and motor cortex). ALS is one of many NDDs that have progressed to an incurable state. C9orf72, SOD1,[107] FUS, TARDBP, and TBK1 are the main pathogenic genes for ALS. In light of the fact that most occurrences of ALS are sporadic, the disease's genetic foundation appears flimsy at best.

Several SOD1-specific cellular and animal models have been reported.[108,109] Mice with SOD1 damaged using adeno-associated virus (AAV)-driven CRISPR technology had less spinal cord protein expression and less muscle atrophy. The average mouse survival time rose by 28–30 days as motor function improved.[110] Other animal experiments with SOD1 deletion revealed similar positive outcomes.[111,112] Table 9.1 compiles a variety of in vivo experiments.

A recently identified pathogenic component in C9orf72 is the G4C2 hexanucleotide repeat.[113,114] Its pathogenic mechanism could be complex.

According to research,[115] the loss of C9orf72 exacerbated the axonal abnormalities and hence enhanced cell death. While recent research suggests that the CRISPR/Cas system can entirely correct this pathogenic expansion,[116] the effectiveness of DSB repair and gene editing have both been shown to be impacted by C9orf72 expression.[117] Editing the RNA at the GluA Q/R location may be interfered with, and mitochondrial Ca2+ absorption may be hampered, to generate the pathogenic impact.[118–120] Numerous potential dangers have been highlighted, and these include, for example, a link between KIF5A and cytoskeletal abnormalities in ALS.[121] Nevertheless, additional comprehensive research on these GWAS-identified locations is currently lacking.

9.5 GENE THERAPY FOR NEUROLOGICAL DISEASE: A CLINICAL STUDY

AAV vectors' efficacy in treating neurodegenerative illnesses has been the subject of more than 20 clinical trials to date.[122–124] Table 9.2 displays developments in gene therapy clinical trials for multiple neurological diseases. In animal models, AAV9 is a terrific vector since it can be delivered directly into the brain to cause extensive manifestation in the brain and spinal cord following peripheral systemic administration.[124–125]

9.6 CHALLENGES AND PROMISES

The potential to "create a durable treatment" and the capacity to address the etiology[138] have always served as the foundation for the promise in the field of gene therapy. However, most peripherally administered agents are either unable to cross the blood-brain barrier or only do so poorly,

Clinical Studies of Gene Therapy

TABLE 9.1 Preclinical Study of Gene Therapy for Neurological Disorders.

Gene editing software	Vector	Disorder	Target	Animal study	Injection	Result
Cas9 and CRISPR	px330 plasmid	AD	App 3 0-UTR	NL-G-F mice	Protomouse embryos were microinjected	In the App KI mice, deletion of the App 30 Aβ-UTR reduced the A pathology.
CRISPR and Cas9	px330 plasmid	PD	p13 exon1	C57BL/6J mice	Pronuclear-stage egg injections	In the substantia nigra, heterozygous p13 knockdown protects against motor impairments and the loss of dopaminergic neurons.
CRISPR/Cas9	AAV	HD	CAG-flanking region	HD 140Q-KI mice	Striatum injections	Targeted suppression of the CAG repeat has been shown to ameliorate neuropathological and behavioral problems in adult mice.
CRISPR/SaCas 9	AAV	HD	HTT exon 1	HD 140Q-KI mice	Injections into the striatum	Disruption on HTT lowered mHTT protein, enhanced longevity, and protected neurons from death; however, lost cells were not restored.
CRISPR/Cas9	AAV	ALS	SODI1	G93A-SOD1 mice	Administered intravenously into the facial vein	Mutant SOD1 disruption increases spinal cord motor neuron survival, enhances motor performance, and lengthens life.
Cytidine base editors	Dual AAV	ALS	SODI1	G93A-SOD1 mice	Placed in the subarachnoid space of the lower back	Survival rates were enhanced, motor neurons and neuromuscular connections were protected, the disease's course was halted, and muscle denervation was minimized thanks to these base editor systems.
CRISPR/Cas9	AAV	ALS	SODI1	G93A-SOD1 mice	ICV injection	SOD1 deletion increased lifespan and postponed motor neuron degeneration and illness onset.

TABLE 9.2   Gene Therapy for Neurological Disease: A Clinical Study.

Neurological disorder	Methods of gene therapy	Administration route	Phase	References
Alzheimer's disease	NGF-AAV2	Basal forebrain	Phase 1 and 2	[126]
	AAVrh.10hAPOE2	Administration through the intrasternal route	Stage 1	[127]
	AAV-hTERT	Intravenous and intrathecal	Phase 1	[128]
Parkinson's disease	LV-AADC	Putamen	Stage 1	[129]
	AAV2-GAD	Nucleus subthalamic	Phase 2 was later discontinued.	[130]
	AAV2-hAADC 2	Striatum	Phase 2	[131]
	AAV2-hAADC	Putamen	Phase 1/2	[132]
	AAV2- NTN	Substantia nigra	Phase 2	[133]
Amyotrophic lateral sclerosis	ASO (SOD1)	Intrathecal	Phase 1	[134]
	ASO (C9orf72)	Intrathecal	Phase 1	[135]
Huntington's disease	AAV5-miHTT	Striatum	Phase 1/2	[136]
	ASOs to miHTT premessenger RNA	Intrathecal	Phase 1	[137]

making the allure of a single, long-lasting intervention (one and done) especially appealing for diseases of the central nervous system (CNS), where repeated doses can easily achieve effective therapeutic concentrations. Some encouraging results have been seen with the use of the monoclonal antibody BAN2401 in the treatment of Alzheimer's disease (AD), although its concentration in human CSF is incredibly low—just 0.04%.[139] Although gene therapy has not been completely successful in curing neurological disorders, most clinical trials still rely on smaller molecules like drugs and antibodies. The traditional idea of gene therapy is that it can cure, while gene therapy has been shown to be effective in treating diseases with a single genetic cause, such as some forms of childhood cancer, its utility in treating diseases with several causes, such as neurodegenerative disorders, has been called into question. But nearly every treatment method focuses on a single target, whether or not it is based on genes. For instance, amyloid-(A) or tau has been the main focus of nearly all AD trials.[140] Additionally, as will be discussed later, gene-based therapies are utilized to treat sporadic neurodegenerative disorders by altering the amounts of genes, proteins, or other physiological properties of endogenous proteins. The long-term effects of some gene-based medications are both a benefit and a risk. Genetic modifications would be permanent once they were introduced into the DNA, especially in mature neurons. Additionally, there will be a unique set of side effects for each gene treatment set of drawbacks, such as the lingering effects of foreign proteins like bacterial Cas9 and unintended effects from DNA or RNA editing. Their therapeutic usefulness will probably be decided by a comprehensive assessment of the risk-benefit ratio, similar to other somewhat permanent therapies like operations, etc. It is still difficult to transfer gene products effectively and safely to the brain and spinal cord. The efficiency of nonviral delivery techniques for penetrating the CNS, including nanoparticles and ribonucleoprotein complexes, is still being studied.[141] Due to their strong neuronal attraction, wide accessibility, wide-ranging species distribution, and high safety records across the board, even in nonhuman primates (NHPs), AAV vectors are the undisputed leader in this field. There are certain restrictions, though, and they will be discussed in the part after this. Another rapidly progressing area is the modification of AAV capsids to promote neurotropism, an evolving topic.[142] The exogenous transgene used in many CNS gene treatments must be injected regularly for the rest of the patient's life to be well-adapted for this, in contrast to mitotically active cells where transduced AAVs eventually disappear because they cannot. The expression of AAVs can be maintained for decades in postmitotic cells like neurons because they have the potential to integrate into the host genome.[143] But how it all works on a fundamental level is still a mystery. The paucity of biomarkers and the difficulties associated with accessing brain tissue limit the ability to detect transgenic expression in living individuals. Even though AAVs have been utilized in over 200 human studies involving thousands of patients[144] and are generally regarded as safe, there are still some concerns. A number of cautions have also been raised, the majority of which are related to the viral proteins' capacity to instigate host immune responses. First, neutralizing host antibodies are created because similarities exist between the capsid proteins of recombinant AAV particles and those of common human pathogens. This can lessen the efficiency of transduction.[145] After being screened, one patient out of 16 was removed from the initial AVXS-101 trial for high levels of anti-AAV9 antibodies (>1:50).[146] Capsids for adeno-associated viruses that were not produced in the host cell have the potential to induce humoral immunity, which results in the production of neutralizing antibodies that block continued delivery,[147] or they can potentially transduce activating cytotoxic T lymphocytes that allow for the destruction of cells.[148] The serotypes AAV1 and AAV5 of adeno-associated virus (AAV) were discovered to ameliorate adaptive immune responses and have a strong affinity for antigen-presenting cells.[149] Another problem with AAVs is the detection of the capsid or vector genome by the activation of toll-like receptors that set off the innate immune response and the release of inflammatory cytokines.[150] If the transgene introduced into the host encodes a foreign protein—either a nonhuman protein or a replacement protein in a null genetic background—the injection may evoke both neutralizing antibodies and cytotoxic T cells.[151] Myotubular myopathy patients who received AAV-based gene therapy saw improvement in 60% who ultimately perished, while positive outcomes were noted in patients who received lower doses.[151] The alarming possibility that intravenous or intrathecal injections of AAVs could cause dorsal root ganglion illness, which does not seem to be connected to immune responses, has also come to light recently.[152] Research is being done in-depth on both preventative interventions and the interplay between vector adeno-associated viruses and host immune responses.[153]

KEYWORDS

- clinical trial
- Alzheimer's disease
- Parkinson's disease
- Huntington's disease
- ALS

REFERENCES

1. Weinberg, M. S.; Samulski, R. J.; McCown, T. J. Adeno-Associated Virus (AAV) Gene Therapy for Neurological Disease. *Neuropharmacology* **2013,** *69,* 82–88. https://doi.org/10.1016/j.neuropharm. 2012.03.004.
2. O'Connor, D. M.; Boulis, N. M. Gene Therapy for Neurodegenerative Diseases. *Trends Mol. Med.* **2015,** *21,* 504–512. https://doi.org/ 10.1016/j.molmed.2015.06.001.
3. Martier, R.; Konstantinova, P. Gene Therapy for Neurodegenerative Diseases: Slowing Down the Ticking Clock. *Front. Neurosci.* **2020,** *14,* 1002.
4. Harilal, S.; Jose, J.; Kumar, R.; Unnikrishnan, M. K.; Uddin, M. S.; Mathew, G. E.; Pratap, R.; Marathakam, A. et al. Revisiting the Blood-Brain Barrier: A Hard Nut to Crack in the Transportation of Drug Molecules. *Brain Res. Bull.* **2020,** *160,* 121–140.
5. Holt, C. E.; Martin, K. C.; Schuman, E. M. Local Translation in Neurons: Visualization and Function. *Nat. Struct. Mol. Biol.* **2019,** *26,* 557–566.
6. Richardson, R. M.; Varenika, V.; Forsayeth, J. R.; Bankiewicz, K. S. Future Applications: Gene Therapy. *Neurosurg. Clin. N. Am.* **2009,** *20,* 205–210. https://doi. org/10.1016/j.nec.2009.04.004.
7. Van Horn, J. D.; Pelphrey, K. A. Neuroimaging of the Developing Brain. *Brain Imaging Behav.* **2015,** *9,* 1–4. https://doi.org/10.1007/ s11682-015-9365-9.
8. Deverman, B. E.; Ravina, B. M.; Bankiewicz, K. S.; Paul, S. M.; Sah, D. W. Gene Therapy for Neurological Disorders: Progress and Prospects. *Nat. Rev. Drug. Discov.* **2018,** *17,* 641–659.
9. Simonato, M.; Bennett, J.; Boulis, N. M.; Castro, M. G.; Fink, D. J.; Goins, W. F.; Gray, S. J.; Lowenstein, P. R. et al. Progress in Gene Therapy for Neurological Disorders. *Nat. Rev. Neurol.* **2013,** *9,* 277–291. https://doi.org/10.1038/nrneurol.2013.56.
10. Ginn, S. L.; Amaya, A. K.; Alexander, I. E.; Edelstein, M.; Abedi, M. R. Gene Therapy Clinical Trials Worldwide to 2017: An Update. *J. Gene Med.* **2018,** *20,* e3015.
11. Sudhakar, V.; Richardson, R. M. Gene Therapy for Neurodegenerative Diseases. *Neurother. J. Am. Soc. Exp. Neurother.* **2019,** *16,* 166–175. https://doi.org/10.1007/ s13311-018-00694-0.
12. Sidorova, Y. A.; Saarma, M. Can Growth Factors Cure Parkinson's Disease? *Trends Pharmacol. Sci.* **2020,** *41* (12), 909–922.

13. Akhtar, A. A.; Gowing, G.; Kobritz, N.; Savinof, S. E.; Garcia, L.; Saxon, D.; Cho, N.; Kim, G. et al. Inducible Expression of GDNF in Transplanted IPSC-Derived Neural Progenitor Cells. *Stem Cell Rep.* **2018**, *10*, 1696–1704.
14. Gantner, C. W.; de Luzy, I. R.; Kauhausen, J. A.; Moriarty, N.; Niclis, J. C.; Bye, C. R.; Penna, V.; Hunt, C. P. et al. Viral Delivery of GDNF Promotes Functional Integration of Human Stem Cell Grafts in Parkinson's Disease. *Cell Stem Cell* **2020**, *26*, 511–526.
15. Gowing, G.; Svendsen, S.; Svendsen, C. N. Ex Vivo Gene Therapy for the Treatment of Neurological Disorders. *Prog. Brain Res.* **2017**, *230*, 99–132.
16. Savić, N.; Schwank, G. Advances in Therapeutic CRISPR/ Cas9 Genome Editing. *Transl. Res.* **2016**, *168*, 15–21.
17. Behrstock, S.; Ebert, A.; McHugh, J.; Vosberg, S.; Moore, J.; Schneider, B.; Capowski, E.; Hei, D. et al. Human Neural Progenitors Deliver Glial Cell Line-Derived Neurotrophic Factor to Parkinsonian Rodents and Aged Primates. *Gene Ther.* **2006**, *13*, 379–388.
18. Klein, S. M.; Behrstock, S.; McHugh, J.; Hofmann, K.; Wallace, K.; Suzuki, M.; Aebischer, P.; Svendsen, C. N. GDNF Delivery Using Human Neural Progenitor Cells in a Rat Model of ALS. *Hum. Gene Ther.* **2005**, *16*, 509–521.
19. Naldini, L. Ex Vivo Gene Transfer and Correction for Cell-Based Therapies. *Nat. Rev. Genet.* **2011**, *12*. 301–315.
20. Mingozzi, F.; High, K. A. Therapeutic In Vivo Gene Transfer for Genetic Disease Using AAV: Progress and Challenges. *Nat. Rev. Genet.* **2011**, *12*, 341–355.
21. Liu, Y.; Wang, D.-A. Viral Vector-Mediated Transgenic Cell Therapy in Regenerative Medicine: Safety of the Process. *Exp. Opin. Biol. Ther.* **2015**, *15*, 559–567.
22. Barrett, R.; Ornelas, L.; Yeager, N.; Mandefro, B.; Sahabian, A.; Lenaeus, L.; Targan, S. R.; Svendsen, C. N. et al. Reliable Generation of Induced Pluripotent Stem Cells from Human Lymphoblastoid Cell Lines. *Stem Cells Transl. Med.* **2014**, *3*, 1429–1434.
23. Vierbuchen, T.; Ostermeier, A.; Pang, Z. P.; Kokubu, Y.; Südhof, T. C.; Wernig, M. Direct Conversion of Fibroblasts to Functional Neurons by Defined Factors. *Nature* **2010**, *463*, 1035–1041.
24. Kawaja, M. D.; Rosenberg, M. B.; Yoshida, K.; Gage, F. H. Somatic Gene Transfer of Nerve Growth Factor Promotes the Survival of Axotomized Septal Neurons and the Regeneration of Their Axons in Adult Rats. *J. Neurosci.* **1992**, *12*, 2849–2864.
25. Tuszynski, M.; Roberts, J.; Senut, M.; U, H. S.; Gage, F. Gene Therapy in the Adult Primate Brain: Intraparenchymal Grafts of Cells Genetically Modified to Produce Nerve Growth Factor Prevent Cholinergic Neuronal Degeneration. *Gene Ther.* **1996**, *3* (4), 305–314.
26. Sorrentino, A.; Ferracin, M.; Castelli, G.; Bifoni, M.; Tomaselli, G.; Baiocchi, M.; Fatica, A.; Negrini, M. et al. Isolation and Characterization of CD146+ Multipotent Mesenchymal Stromal Cells. *Exp. Hematol.* **2008**, *36*, 1035–1046.
27. Amemori, T.; Jendelova, P.; Ruzicka, J.; Urdzikova, L. M.; Sykova, E. Alzheimer's Disease: Mechanism and Approach to Cell Therapy. *Int. J. Mol. Sci.* **2015**, *16*, 26417–26451.
28. Tanna, T.; Sachan, V. Mesenchymal Stem Cells: Potential in Treatment of Neurodegenerative Diseases. *Curr. Stem Cell Res. Ther.* **2014**, *9*, 513–521.

Clinical Studies of Gene Therapy

29. Svendsen, C. N.; ter Borg, M. G.; Armstrong, R. J.; Rosser, A. E.; Chandran, S.; Ostenfeld, T.; Caldwell, M. A. A New Method for the Rapid and Long Term Growth of Human Neural Precursor Cells. *J. Neurosci. Methods* **1998,** *85,* 141–152.

30. Seaberg, R. M.; van der Kooy, D. Stem and Progenitor Cells: The Premature Desertion of Rigorous Defnitions. *Trends Neurosci.* **2003,** *26,* 125–131.

31. Thomson, J. A.; Itskovitz-Eldor, J.; Shapiro, S. S.; Waknitz, M. A.; Swiergiel, J. J.; Marshall, V. S.; Jones, J. M. Embryonic Stem Cell Lines Derived from Human Blastocysts. *Science* **1998,** *282,* 11145–11147.

32. de Miguel-Beriain, I. The Ethics of Stem Cells Revisited. *Adv. Drug Deliv. Rev.* **2015,** *82,* 176–180.

33. Morizane, A.; Doi, D.; Kikuchi, T.; Okita, K.; Hotta, A.; Kawasaki, T.; Hayashi, T.; Onoe, H. et al. Direct Comparison of Autologous and Allogeneic Transplantation of IPSC-Derived Neural Cells in the Brain of a Nonhuman Primate. *Stem Cell Rep.* **2013,** *1,* 283–292.

34. Svendsen, C. N. Back to the Future: How Human Induced Pluripotent Stem Cells Will Transform Regenerative Medicine. *Hum. Mol. Genet.* **2013,** *22,* R32–R38.

35. Mirzaei, H.; Sahebkar, A.; Jaafari, M. R.; Hadjati, J.; Javanmard, S. H.; Mirzaei, H. R.; Salehi, R. PiggyBac as a Novel Vector in Cancer Gene Therapy: Current Perspective. *Cancer Gene Ther.* **2016,** *23,* 45–47.

36. Woodard, L. E.; Wilson, M. H. PiggyBac-Ing Models and New Therapeutic Strategies. *Trends Biotechnol.* **2015,** *33,* 525–533.

37. Eid, A.; Mahfouz, M. M. Genome Editing: The Road of CRISPR/Cas9 from Bench to Clinic. *Exp. Mol. Med.* **2016,** *48,* e265–e265.

38. Park C-Y, Lee, D. R.; Sung, J. J.; Kim D-W Genome-Editing Technologies for Gene Correction of Hemophilia. *Hum. Genet.* **2016,** *135,* 977–981.

39. Tsai, S. Q.; Joung, J. K. Defining and Improving the Genome-Wide Specificities of CRISPR–Cas9 Nucleases. *Nat. Rev. Genet.* **2016,** *17,* 300–312.

40. Im, W.; Moon, J.; Kim, M. Applications of CRISPR/Cas9 for Gene Editing in Hereditary Movement Disorders. *J. Mov. Disord.* **2016,** *9,* 136.

41. Kay, M. A.; Liu, D.; Hoogerbrugge, P. M. Gene Therapy. *Proc. Natl. Acad. Sci.* **1997,** *94,* 12744LP–12746. https://doi.org/10.1073/ pnas.94.24.12744.

42. Ingusci, S.; Verlengia, G.; Soukupova, M.; Zucchini, S.; Simonato, M. Gene Therapy Tools for Brain Diseases. *Front. Pharmacol.* **2019,** *10,* 724.

43. Shillitoe, E. J. Gene Therapy: The End of the Rainbow? *Head Neck Oncol.* **2009,** *1,* 7. https://doi.org/10.1186/1758-3284-1-7.

44. Teschemacher, A. G.; Wang, S.; Lonergan, T.; Duale, H.; Waki, H.; Paton JFR, Kasparov, S. Targeting Specific Neuronal Populations Using Adeno- and Lentiviral Vectors: Applications for Imaging and Studies of Cell Function. *Exp. Physiol.* **2005,** *90,* 61–69. https://doi.org/ 10.1113/expphysiol.2004.028191.

45. Bourdenx, M.; Dutheil, N.; Bezard, E.; Dehay, B. Systemic Gene Delivery to the Central Nervous System Using Adeno-Associated Virus. *Front. Mol. Neurosci.* **2014,** *7,* 50.

46. Artusi, S.; Miyagawa, Y.; Goins, W. F.; Cohen, J. B.; Glorioso, J. C. Herpes Simplex Virus Vectors for Gene Transfer to the Central Nervous System. *Dis. Basel Switz.* **2018,** *6,* 74. https://doi.org/10.3390/ diseases6030074.

47. Davidson, B. L.; Stein, C. S.; Heth, J. A.; Martins, I.; Kotin, R. M.; Derksen, T. A.; Zabner, J.; Ghodsi, A. et al. Recombinant Adeno-Associated Virus Type 2, 4, and 5 Vectors: Transduction of Variant Cell Types and Regions in the Mammalian Central Nervous System. *Proc. Natl. Acad. Sci. USA* **2000**, *97*, 3428–3432. https:// doi.org/10.1073/ pnas.050581197.

48. Kremer, E. J.; Perricaudet, M. Adenovirus and Adeno-Associated Virus-Mediated Gene Transfer. *Br. Med. Bull.* **1995**, *51*, 31–44. https://doi.org/10.1093/oxfordjournals. bmb.a072951.

49. Slack, R. S.; Miller, F. D. Viral Vectors for Modulating Gene Expression in Neurons. *Curr. Opin. Neurobiol.* **1996**, *6*, 576–583. https://doi.org/10.1016/S0959-4388 (96) 80088-2.

50. Strecker, J.; Ladha, A.; Gardner, Z.; Schmid-Burgk, J. L.; Makarova, K. S.; Koonin, E. V. et al. RNA-Guided DNA Insertion with CRISPR-Associated Transposases. *Science* **2019**, *365*, 48–53. DOI: 10.1126/science.aax9181

51. Klompe, S. E.; Vo, P. L. H.; Halpin-Healy, T. S.; Sternberg, S. H. Transposon-Encoded CRISPR-Cas Systems Direct RNA-Guided DNA Integration. *Nature* **2019**, *571*, 219–225. DOI: 10.1038/s41586-019-1323-z

52. Peters, J. E.; Makarova, K. S.; Shmakov, S.; Koonin, E. V. Recruitment of CRISPR-Cas Systems by Tn7-Like Transposons. *Proc. Natl. Acad. Sci. USA* **2017**, *114*, E7358–E7366. DOI: 10.1073/pnas.1709035114

53. Hou, Z.; Zhang, Y. Inserting DNA with CRISPR. *Science* **2019**, *365*, 25–26. DOI: 10.1126/science.aay2056

54. McKhann, G. M.; Knopman, D. S.; Chertkow, H.; Hyman, B. T.; Jack, C. R. Jr.; Kawas, C. H. et al. The Diagnosis of Dementia Due to Alzheimer's Disease: Recommendations from the National Institute on Aging-Alzheimer's Association Workgroups on Diagnostic Guidelines for Alzheimer's Disease. *Alzheimers Dement.* **2011**, *7*, 263–269. DOI: 10.1016/j.jalz.2011.03.005

55. Goate, A.; Chartier-Harlin, M. C.; Mullan, M.; Brown, J.; Crawford, F.; Fidani, L. et al. Segregation of a missense mutation in the amyloid precursor protein gene with familial Alzheimer's disease. Nature 349, 704–706. doi: 10. 1038/349704a0

56. Sherrington, R.; Rogaev, E. I.; Liang, Y.; Rogaeva, E. A.; Levesque, G.; Ikeda, M. et al. Cloning of a Gene Bearing Missense Mutations in Early-Onset Familial Alzheimer's Disease. *Nature* **1995**, *375*, 754–760. DOI: 10.1038/375754a0

57. Levy-Lahad, E.; Wijsman, E. M.; Nemens, E.; Anderson, L.; Goddard, K. A.; Weber, J. L. et al. A Familial Alzheimer's Disease Locus on Chromosome 1. *Science* **1995**, *269*, 970–973. DOI: 10.1126/science.7638621

58. Lambert, J. C.; Ibrahim-Verbaas, C. A.; Harold, D.; Naj, A. C.; Sims, R.; Bellenguez, C. et al. Meta-Analysis of 74,046 Individuals Identifies 11 New Susceptibility Loci for Alzheimer's Disease. *Nat. Genet.* **2013**, *45*, 1452–1458. DOI: 10.1038/ng.2802

59. Kunkle, B. W.; Grenier-Boley, B.; Sims, R.; Bis, J. C.; Damotte, V.; Naj, A. C. et al. Genetic Meta-Analysis of Diagnosed Alzheimer's Disease Identifies New Risk Loci and Implicates Aβ, Tau, Immunity and Lipid Processing. *Nat. Genet.* **2019**, *51*, 414–430. DOI: 10.1038/s41588-019-0358-352

60. Vacher, M.; Porter, T.; Villemagne, V. L.; Milicic, L.; Peretti, M.; Fowler, C. et al. Validation of a Priori Candidate Alzheimer's Disease SNPs with Brain Amyloid-Beta Deposition. *Sci. Rep.* **2019**, *9*, 17069. DOI: 10.1038/s41598-019-53604- 53605

Clinical Studies of Gene Therapy

61. Kunkle, B. W.; Schmidt, M.; Klein, H. U.; Naj, A. C.; Hamilton-Nelson, K. L.; Larson, E. B. et al. Novel Alzheimer Disease Risk Loci and Pathways in African American Individuals Using the African Genome Resources Panel: A Meta-Analysis. *JAMA Neurol.* **2021,** *78,* 102–113. DOI: 10.1001/jamaneurol.2020.3536

62. Burnham, S. C.; Laws, S. M.; Budgeon, C. A.; Doré, V.; Porter, T.; Bourgeat, P. et al. Impact of APOE-ε4 Carriage on the Onset and Rates of Neocortical Aβ-Amyloid Deposition. *Neurobiol. Aging* **2020,** *95,* 46–55. DOI: 10.1016/j.neurobiolaging.2020. 06.001

63. Belloy, M. E.; Napolioni, V.; Han, S. S.; Le Guen, Y.; and Greicius, M. D. Association of Klotho-VS Heterozygosity with Risk of Alzheimer Disease in Individuals Who Carry APOE4. *JAMA Neurol.* **2020,** *77,* 849–862. DOI: 10.1001/jamaneurol.2020.0414

64. Porter, T.; Burnham, S. C.; Milicic, L.; Savage, G.; Maruff, P.; Lim, Y. Y. et al. Klotho Allele Status Is Not Associated with Aβ and APOE ε4-Related Cognitive Decline in Preclinical Alzheimer's Disease. *Neurobiol. Aging* **2019,** *76,* 162–165. DOI: 10.1016/j.neurobiolaging.2018.12.014

65. Meyer, K.; Feldman, H. M.; Lu, T.; Drake, D.; Lim, E. T.; Ling, K. H. et al. REST and Neural Gene Network Dysregulation in iPSC Models of Alzheimer's Disease. *Cell Rep.* **2019,** *26,* 1112–1127.e9. DOI: 10.1016/j.celrep.2019.01.023

66. Arnold, M.; Nho, K.; Kueider-Paisley, A.; Massaro, T.; Huynh, K.; Brauner, B. et al. Sex and APOE ε4 Genotype Modify the Alzheimer's Disease Serum Metabolome. *Nat. Commun.* **2020,** *11,* 1148. DOI: 10.1038/s41467-020-14959-w

67. Guo, Y.; Wei, X.; Yan, H.; Qin, Y.; Yan, S.; Liu, J. et al. TREM2 Deficiency Aggravates α-Synuclein-Induced Neurodegeneration and Neuroinflammation in Parkinson's Disease Models. *FASEB J.* **2019,** *33,* 12164–12174. DOI: 10.1096/fj.201900992R

68. Nagata, K.; Takahashi, M.; Matsuba, Y.; Okuyama-Uchimura, F.; Sato, K.; Hashimoto, S. et al. Generation of App Knock-in Mice Reveals Deletion Mutations Protective Against Alzheimer's Disease-Like Pathology. *Nat. Commun.* **2018,** *9,* 1800. DOI: 10.1038/s41467-018-04238-4230

69. Szigeti, K.; Ihnatovych, I.; Birkaya, B.; Chen, Z.; Ouf, A.; Indurthi, D. C. et al. CHRFAM7A: A Human Specific Fusion Gene, Accounts for the Translational Gap for Cholinergic Strategies in Alzheimer's Disease. *EBioMedicine* **2020,** *59,* 102892. DOI: 10.1016/j.ebiom.2020.102892

70. Lessard, C. B.; Rodriguez, E.; Ladd, T. B.; Minter, L. M.; Osborne, B. A.; Miele, L. et al. Individual and Combined Presenilin 1 and 2 Knockouts Reveal That Both Have Highly Overlapping Functions in HEK293T Cells. *J. Biol. Chem.* **2019,** *294,* 11276–11285. DOI: 10.1074/jbc.RA119.008041

71. Sun, J.; Carlson-Stevermer, J.; Das, U.; Shen, M.; Delenclos, M.; Snead, A. M. et al. CRISPR/Cas9 Editing of APP C-Terminus Attenuates β-Cleavage and Promotes α-Cleavage. *Nat. Commun.* **2019,** *10,* 53. DOI: 10.1038/s41467-018-07971- 7978

72. Ittner, A.; Asih, P. R.; Tan, A. R. P.; Prikas, E.; Bertz, J.; Stefanoska, K. et al. Reduction of Advanced Tau-Mediated Memory Deficits by the MAP Kinase p38γ. *Acta Neuropathol.* **2020,** *140,* 279–294. DOI: 10.1007/s00401-020-02191-2191

73. Guha, S.; Fischer, S.; Johnson, G. V. W.; Nehrke, K. Tauopathy-Associated Tau Modifications Selectively Impact Neurodegeneration and Mitophagy in a Novel C. Elegans Single-Copy Transgenic Model. *Mol. Neurodegener.* **2020,** *15,* 65. DOI: 10.1186/s13024-020-00410-417

74. Gerring, Z. F.; Lupton, M. K.; Edey, D.; Gamazon, E. R.; Derks, E. M. An Analysis of Genetically Regulated Gene Expression Across Multiple Tissues Implicates Novel Gene Candidates in Alzheimer's Disease. *Alzheimers Res. Ther.* **2020,** *12,* 43. DOI: 10.1186/s13195-020-00611-618

75. Sundal, C.; Fujioka, S.; Uitti, R. J.; and Wszolek, Z. K. Autosomal Dominant Parkinson's Disease. *Parkinsonism Relat. Disord.* **2012,** *18* (Suppl. 1), S7–S10. DOI: 10.1016/s1353-8020 (11)70005-70000

76. Ferreira, M.; Massano, J. An Updated Review of Parkinson's Disease Genetics and Clinicopathological Correlations. *Acta Neurol. Scand.* **2017,** *135,* 273–284. DOI: 10.1111/ane.12616

77. Chen, V.; Moncalvo, M.; Tringali, D.; Tagliafierro, L.; Shriskanda, A.; Ilich, E. et al. The Mechanistic Role of Alpha-Synuclein in the Nucleus: Impaired Nuclear Function Caused by Familial Parkinson's Disease SNCA Mutations. *Hum. Mol. Genet.* **2020,** *29,* 3107–3121. DOI: 10.1093/hmg/ddaa183

78. Barbuti, P.; Antony, P.; Santos, B.; Massart, F.; Cruciani, G.; Dording, C. et al. Using High-Content Screening to Generate Single-Cell Genecorrected Patient-Derived iPS Clones Reveals Excess Alpha-Synuclein with Familial Parkinson's Disease Point Mutation A30P. *Cells* **2020,** *9,* 2065. DOI: 10.3390/ cells9092065

79. Jiang, Z.; Huang, Y.; Zhang, P.; Han, C.; Lu, Y.; Mo, Z. et al. Characterization of a Pathogenic Variant in GBA for Parkinson's Disease with Mild Cognitive Impairment Patients. *Mol. Brain* **2020,** *13,* 102. DOI: 10.1186/s13041- 020-00637-x

80. Arias-Fuenzalida, J.; Jarazo, J.; Qing, X.; Walter, J.; Gomez-Giro, G.; Nickels, S. L. et al. FACS-Assisted CRISPR-Cas9 Genome Editing Facilitates Parkinson's disease Modeling. *Stem Cell Rep.* **2017,** *9,* 1423–1431. DOI: 10.1016/j. stemcr.2017.08.026

81. Kantor, B.; Tagliafierro, L.; Gu, J.; Zamora, M. E.; Ilich, E.; Grenier, C. et al. Downregulation of SNCA Expression by Targeted Editing of DNA Methylation: A Potential Strategy for Precision Therapy in PD. *Mol. Ther.* **2018,** 26, 2638–2649. DOI: 10.1016/j.ymthe.2018.08.019

82. Chen, X.; Xie, C.; Tian, W.; Sun, L.; Zheng, W.; Hawes, S. et al. Parkinson's Disease-Related Leucine-Rich Repeat Kinase 2 Modulates Nuclear Morphology and Genomic Stability in Striatal Projection Neurons During Aging. *Mol. Neurodegener.* **2020,** *15,* 12. DOI: 10.1186/s13024-020-00360-360

83. Suda, Y.; Kuzumaki, N.; Sone, T.; Narita, M.; Tanaka, K.; Hamada, Y. et al. Down-Regulation of Ghrelin Receptors on Dopaminergic Neurons in the Substantia Nigra Contributes to Parkinson's Disease-Like Motor Dysfunction. *Mol. Brain* **2018,** *11,* 6. DOI: 10.1186/s13041-018-0349-348

84. Inoue, N.; Ogura, S.; Kasai, A.; Nakazawa, T.; Ikeda, K.; Higashi, S. et al. Knockdown of the Mitochondria-Localized Protein p13 Protects Against Experimental Parkinsonism. *EMBO Rep.* **2018,** *19,* e44860. DOI: 10.15252/embr. 201744860.

85. Vetchinova, A. S.; Simonova, V. V.; Novosadova, E. V.; Manuilova, E. S.; Nenasheva, V. V.; Tarantul, V. Z. et al. Cytogenetic Analysis of the Results of Genome Editing on the Cell Model of Parkinson's Disease. *Bull. Exp. Biol. Med.* **2018,** *165,* 378–381. DOI: 10.1007/s10517-018-4174-y

86. Ohta, E.; Sone, T.; Ukai, H.; Hisamatsu, T.; Kitagawa, T.; Ishikawa, M. et al. Generation of Gene-Corrected iPSCs Line (KEIUi001-A) from a PARK8 Patient

Clinical Studies of Gene Therapy   211

iPSCs with Familial Parkinson's Disease Carrying the I2020T Mutation in LRRK2. *Stem Cell Res.* **2020**, *49*, 102073. DOI: 10.1016/j.scr.2020.102073

87. Ahfeldt, T.; Ordureau, A.; Bell, C.; Sarrafha, L.; Sun, C.; Piccinotti, S. et al. Pathogenic Pathways in Early-Onset Autosomal Recessive Parkinson's Disease Discovered Using Isogenic Human Dopaminergic Neurons. *Stem Cell Rep.* **2020**, *14*, 75–90. DOI: 10.1016/j.stemcr.2019.12.005

88. Wulansari, N.; Darsono, W. H. W.; Woo, H. J.; Chang, M. Y.; Kim, J.; Bae, E. J. et al. Neurodevelopmental Defects and Neurodegenerative Phenotypes in Human Brain Organoids Carrying Parkinson's Disease-Linked DNAJC6 Mutations. *Sci. Adv.* **2021**, *7*, eabb1540. DOI: 10. 1126/sciadv.abb1540

89. Chang, M. Y.; Oh, B.; Choi, J. E.; Sulistio, Y. A.; Woo, H. J.; Jo, A. et al. LIN28A Loss of Function Is Associated with Parkinson's Disease Pathogenesis. *EMBO J.* **2019**, *38*, e101196. DOI: 10.15252/embj.2018101196

90. Chang, D.; Nalls, M. A.; Hallgrímsdóttir, I. B.; Hunkapiller, J.; van der Brug, M.; Cai, F. et al. A Meta-Analysis of Genome-Wide Association Studies Identifies 17 New Parkinson's Disease Risk Loci. *Nat. Genet.* **2017**, *49*, 1511–1516. DOI: 10.1038/ng. 3955

91. Nabais, M. F.; Laws, S. M.; Lin, T.; Vallerga, C. L.; Armstrong, N. J.; Blair, I. P. et al. Meta-Analysis of Genome-Wide DNA Methylation Identifies Shared Associations Across Neurodegenerative Disorders. *Genome Biol.* **2021**, *22*, 90. DOI: 10.1186/s13059-021-02275-2275

92. Horvath, S.; Langfelder, P.; Kwak, S.; Aaronson, J.; Rosinski, J.; Vogt, T. F. et al. Huntington's Disease Accelerates Epigenetic Aging of Human Brain and Disrupts DNA Methylation Levels. *Aging* **2016**, *8*, 1485–1512. DOI: 10.18632/aging.101005

93. McColgan, P.; Tabrizi, S. J. Huntington's Disease: A Clinical Review. *Eur. J. Neurol.* **2018**, *25*, 24–34. DOI: 10.1111/ene.13413

94. An, M. C.; Zhang, N.; Scott, G.; Montoro, D.; Wittkop, T.; Mooney, S. et al. Genetic Correction of Huntington's Disease Phenotypes in Induced Pluripotent Stem Cells. *Cell Stem Cell* **2012**, *11*, 253–263. DOI: 10. 1016/j.stem.2012.04.026

95. Xu, X.; Tay, Y.; Sim, B.; Yoon, S. I.; Huang, Y.; Ooi, J. et al. Reversal of Phenotypic Abnormalities by CRISPR/Cas9-Mediated Gene Correction in Huntington Disease Patient-Derived Induced Pluripotent Stem Cells. *Stem Cell Rep.* **2017**, *8*, 619–633. DOI: 10.1016/j.stemcr.2017.01.022

96. Dunbar, G. L.; Koneru, S.; Kolli, N.; Sandstrom, M.; Maiti, P.; Rossignol, J. Silencing of the Mutant Huntingtin Gene Through CRISPR-Cas9 Improves the Mitochondrial Biomarkers in an In Vitro Model of Huntington's Disease. *Cell Transplant* **2019**, *28*, 460–463. DOI: 10.1177/0963689719840662

97. Vigont, V. A.; Grekhnev, D. A.; Lebedeva, O. S.; Gusev, K. O.; Volovikov, E. A.; Skopin, A. Y. et al. STIM2 Mediates Excessive Store-Operated Calcium Entry in Patient-Specific iPSC-Derived Neurons Modeling a Juvenile form of Huntington's Disease. *Front. Cell Dev. Biol.* **2021**, *9*, 625231. DOI: 10.3389/fcell.2021. 625231

98. Malankhanova, T.; Suldina, L.; Grigor'eva, E.; Medvedev, S.; Minina, J.; Morozova, K. et al. A Human Induced Pluripotent Stem Cell-Derived Isogenic Model of Huntington's Disease Based on Neuronal Cells Has Several Relevant Phenotypic Abnormalities. *J. Pers. Med.* **2020**, *10*, 215. DOI: 10.3390/jpm10040215

99. Morozova, K. N.; Suldina, L. A.; Malankhanova, T. B.; Grigor'eva, E. V.; Zakian, S. M.; Kiseleva, E. et al. Introducing an Expanded CAG Tract into the Huntingtin Gene Causes a Wide Spectrum of Ultrastructural Defects in Cultured Human Cells. *PLoS One* **2018**, *13*, e0204735. DOI: 10.1371/journal.pone.0204735

100. Yang, S.; Chang, R.; Yang, H.; Zhao, T.; Hong, Y.; Kong, H. E. et al. CRISPR/Cas9-Mediated Gene Editing Ameliorates Neurotoxicity in Mouse Model of Huntington's Disease. *J. Clin. Invest.* **2017**, *127*, 2719–2724. DOI: 10. 1172/jci92087

101. Ekman, F. K.; Ojala, D. S.; Adil, M. M.; Lopez, P. A.; Schaffer, D. V.; Gaj, T. CRISPR-Cas9-Mediated Genome Editing Increases Lifespan and Improves Motor Deficits in a Huntington's Disease Mouse Model. *Mol. Ther. Nucleic Acids* **2019**, *17*, 829–839. DOI: 10.1016/j.omtn.2019.07.009

102. Shin, J. W.; Kim, K. H.; Chao, M. J.; Atwal, R. S.; Gillis, T.; MacDonald, M. E. et al. Permanent Inactivation of Huntington's Disease Mutation by Personalized Allele-Specific CRISPR/Cas9. *Hum. Mol. Genet.* **2016**, *25*, 4566–4576. DOI: 10.1093/hmg/ddw286

103. Monteys, A. M.; Ebanks, S. A.; Keiser, M. S.; Davidson, B. L. CRISPR/Cas9 Editing of the Mutant Huntingtin Allele In Vitro and In Vivo. *Mol. Ther.* **2017**, *25*, 12–23. DOI: 10.1016/j.ymthe.2016.11.010

104. Fjodorova, M.; Louessard, M.; Li, Z.; De La Fuente, D. C.; Dyke, E.; Brooks, S. P. et al. CTIP2-Regulated Reduction in PKA-Dependent DARPP32 Phosphorylation in Human Medium Spiny Neurons: Implications for Huntington Disease. *Stem Cell Rep.* **2019**, *13*, 448–457. DOI: 10.1016/j.stemcr.2019.07. 015

105. Fink, K. D.; Deng, P.; Gutierrez, J.; Anderson, J. S.; Torrest, A.; Komarla, A. et al. Allele-Specific Reduction of the Mutant Huntingtin Allele Using Transcription Activator-Like Effectors in Human Huntington's Disease Fibroblasts. *Cell Transplant* **2016**, *25*, 677–686. DOI: 10.3727/096368916x690863

106. Zeitler, B.; Froelich, S.; Marlen, K.; Shivak, D. A.; Yu, Q.; Li, D. et al. Allele-Selective Transcriptional Repression of Mutant HTT for the Treatment of Huntington's Disease. *Nat. Med.* **2019**, *25*, 1131–1142. DOI: 10.1038/s41591-019-0478- 473

107. Rosen, D. R.; Siddique, T.; Patterson, D.; Figlewicz, D. A.; Sapp, P.; Hentati, A. et al. Mutations in Cu/Zn Superoxide Dismutase Gene Are Associated with Familial Amyotrophic Lateral Sclerosis. *Nature* **1993**, *362*, 59–62. DOI: 10.1038/ 362059a0

108. Müller, K.; Brenner, D.; Weydt, P.; Meyer, T.; Grehl, T.; Petri, S. et al. Comprehensive Analysis of the Mutation Spectrum in 301 German ALS Families. *J. Neurol. Neurosurg. Psychiatry* **2018**, *89*, 817–827. DOI: 10.1136/jnnp-2017-317611

109. Gaj, T.; Ojala, D. S.; Ekman, F. K.; Byrne, L. C.; Limsirichai, P.; Schaffer, D. V. In Vivo Genome Editing Improves Motor Function and Extends Survival in a Mouse Model of ALS. *Sci Adv.* **2017**, *3*, eaar3952. DOI: 10.1126/sciadv.aar3952

110. Kim, B. W.; Ryu, J.; Jeong, Y. E.; Kim, J.; and Martin, L. J. Human Motor Neurons with SOD1-G93A Mutation Generated from CRISPR/Cas9 Gene-Edited iPSCs Develop Pathological Features of Amyotrophic Lateral Sclerosis. *Front. Cell Neurosci.* **2020**, *14*, 604171. DOI: 10.3389/fncel.2020.604171

111. Duan, W.; Guo, M.; Yi, L.; Liu, Y.; Li, Z.; Ma, Y. et al. The Deletion of Mutant SOD1 via CRISPR/Cas9/sgRNA Prolongs Survival in an Amyotrophic Lateral Sclerosis Mouse Model. *Gene Ther.* **2020**, *27*, 157–169. DOI: 10.1038/s41434-019-0116-111

Clinical Studies of Gene Therapy

213

112. Lim, C. K. W.; Gapinske, M.; Brooks, A. K.; Woods, W. S.; Powell, J. E.; Zeballos, C. M. et al. Treatment of a Mouse Model of ALS by In Vivo Base Editing. *Mol. Ther.* **2020,** *28,* 1177–1189. DOI: 10.1016/j.ymthe.2020.01.005

113. DeJesus-Hernandez, M.; Mackenzie, I. R.; Boeve, B. F.; Boxer, A. L.; Baker, M.; Rutherford, N. J. et al. Expanded GGGGCC Hexanucleotide Repeat in Noncoding Region of C9ORF72 Causes Chromosome 9p-Linked FTD and ALS. *Neuron 72,* 245–256. DOI: 10.1016/j.neuron.2011.09.011

114. Renton, A. E.; Majounie, E.; Waite, A.; Simón-Sánchez, J.; Rollinson, S.; Gibbs, J. R. et al. A Hexanucleotide Repeat Expansion in C9ORF72 Is the Cause of Chromosome 9p21-Linked ALS-FTD. *Neuron* **2011,** *72,* 257–268. DOI: 10.1016/j. neuron.2011.09.010

115. Abo-Rady, M.; Kalmbach, N.; Pal, A.; Schludi, C.; Janosch, A.; Richter, T. et al. Knocking out C9ORF72 Exacerbates Axonal Trafficking Defects Associated with Hexanucleotide Repeat Expansion and Reduces Levels of Heat Shock Proteins. *Stem Cell Rep.* **2020,** *14,* 390–405. DOI: 10.1016/j.stemcr.2020.01.010

116. Ababneh, N. A.; Scaber, J.; Flynn, R.; Douglas, A.; Barbagallo, P.; Candalija, A. et al. Correction of Amyotrophic Lateral Sclerosis Related Phenotypes in Induced Pluripotent Stem Cell-Derived Motor Neurons Carrying a Hexanucleotide Expansion Mutation in C9orf72 by CRISPR/Cas9 Genome Editing Using Homology-Directed Repair. *Hum. Mol. Genet.* **2020,** *29,* 2200–2217. DOI: 10.1093/hmg/ ddaa106

117. Moore, S.; Alsop, E.; Lorenzini, I.; Starr, A.; Rabichow, B. E.; Mendez, E. et al. ADAR2 Mislocalization and Widespread RNA Editing Aberrations in C9orf72-Mediated ALS/ FTD. *Acta Neuropathol.* **2019,** *138,* 49–65. DOI: 10.1007/ s00401-019-01999-w

118. Andrade, N. S.; Ramic, M.; Esanov, R.; Liu, W.; Rybin, M. J.; Gaidosh, G. et al. Dipeptide Repeat Proteins Inhibit Homology-Directed DNA Double Strand Break Repair in C9ORF72 ALS/FTD. *Mol. Neurodegener.* **2020,** *15,* 13. DOI: 10.1186/ s13024-020-00365-369

119. Konen, L. M.; Wright, A. L.; Royle, G. A.; Morris, G. P.; Lau, B. K.; Seow, P. W. et al. A New Mouse Line with Reduced GluA2 Q/R Site RNA Editing Exhibits Loss of Dendritic Spines, Hippocampal CA1-Neuron Loss, Learning and Memory Impairments and NMDA Receptor-Independent Seizure Vulnerability. *Mol. Brain* **2020,** *13,* 27. DOI: 10.1186/s13041-020-0545-541

120. Dafinca, R.; Barbagallo, P.; Farrimond, L.; Candalija, A.; Scaber, J.; Ababneh, N. A. et al. Impairment of Mitochondrial Calcium Buffering Links Mutations in C9ORF72 and TARDBP in iPS-Derived Motor Neurons from Patients with ALS/FTD. *Stem Cell Rep.* **2020,** *14,* 892–908. DOI: 10.1016/j.stemcr.2020.03.023

121. Nicolas, A.; Kenna, K. P.; Renton, A. E.; Ticozzi, N.; Faghri, F.; Chia, R. et al. Genome-Wide Analyses Identify KIF5A as a Novel ALS Gene. *Neuron* **2018,** *97,* 1268–1283.e6. DOI: 10.1016/j.neuron.2018.02.027

122. Jain, K. K. Gene Therapy of Neurological Disorders. In: *Applications of Biotechnology in Neurology*; Springer: Berlin, 2013; pp 383–476.

123. Ortolano, S.; Spuch, C.; Navarro, C. Present and Future of Adeno Associated Virus Based Gene Therapy Approaches. *Recent Pat. Endocr. Metab. Immune Drug Discov.* **2012,** *6,* 47–66.

124. Naso, M. F.; Tomkowicz, B.; Perry, W. L.; Strohl, W. R. Adeno Associated Virus (AAV) as a Vector for Gene Therapy. *BioDrugs* **2017,** *31,* 317–334.

125. Dayton, R. D.; Wang, D. B.; Klein, R. L. The Advent of AAV9 Expands Applications for Brain and Spinal Cord Gene Delivery. *Exp. Opin. Biol. Ther.* **2012**, *12*, 757–766.
126. https://clinicaltrials.gov/ct2/show/NCT00876863 (assessed on 12 Jan 2023).
127. https://clinicaltrials.gov/ct2/show/NCT03634007 (assessed on 12 and 13 Jan 2023)
128. https://clinicaltrials.gov/ct2/show/NCT04133454 (assessed on 13 Jan 2023).
129. https://clinicaltrials.gov/ct2/show/NCT01856439 (assessed on 12 Jan 2023).
130. https://clinicaltrials.gov/ct2/show/NCT00643890 (assessed on 12 Jan 2023).
131. https://clinicaltrials.gov/ct2/show/NCT03562494 (assessed on 12 Jan 2023).
132. https://clinicaltrials.gov/ct2/show/NCT02418598 (assessed on 13 Jan 2023).
133. https://clinicaltrials.gov/ct2/show/NCT00985517 (assessed on 13 Jan 2023).
134. https://clinicaltrials.gov/ct2/show/NCT01041222 (assessed on 12 Jan 2023).
135. https://clinicaltrials.gov/ct2/show/NCT03626012 (assessed on 13 Jan 2023).
136. https://clinicaltrials.gov/ct2/show/NCT04120493 (assessed on 13 Jan 2023).
137. https://clinicaltrials.gov/ct2/show/NCT03225833 (assessed on 13 January 2023).
138. Keeler, C. E. Gene Therapy. *J. Hered.* **1947**, *38*, 294–298.
139. Logovinsky, V. et al. Safety and Tolerability of BAN2401—A Clinical Study in Alzheimer's Disease with a Protofbril Selective Aβ Antibody. *Alzheimers Res. Ter.* **2016**, *8*, 14.
140. Doudna, J. A. Te Promise and Challenge of Therapeutic Genome Editing. *Nature* **2020**, *578*, 229–236.
141. Huang, L. K.; Chao, S. P.; Hu, C. J. Clinical Trials of New Drugs for Alzheimer Disease. *J. Biomed. Sci.* **2020**, *27*, 18.
142. Bedbrook, C. N.; Deverman, B. E.; Gradinaru, V. Viral Strategies for Targeting the Central and Peripheral Nervous Systems. *Annu. Rev. Neurosci.* **2018**. https://doi.org/10.1146/annurev-neuro-080317-062048.
143. Leone, P. et al. Long-Term Follow-Up After Gene Therapy for Canavan Disease. *Sci. Transl. Med.* **2012**, *4*, 165ra163.
144. Ginn, S. L.; Amaya, A. K.; Alexander, I. E.; Edelstein, M.; Abedi, M. R. Gene Therapy Clinical Trials Worldwide to 2017: An Update. *J. Gene Med.* **2018**, *20*, e3015.
145. Calcedo, R.; Vandenberghe, L. H.; Gao, G.; Lin, J.; Wilson, J. M. Worldwide Epidemiology of Neutralizing Antibodies to Adeno-Associated Viruses. *J. Infect. Dis.* **2009**, *199*, 381–390..
146. Mingozzi, F. et al. CD8+ T-Cell Responses to Adeno-Associated Virus Capsid in Humans. *Nat. Med.* **2007**, *13*, 419–422.
147. Petry, H. et al. Efect of Viral Dose on Neutralizing Antibody Response and Transgene Expression After AAV1 Vector Re-administration in Mice. *Gene Ter.* **2008**, *15*, 54–60.
148. Lu, Y.; Song, S. Distinct Immune Responses to Transgene Products from rAAV1 and rAAV8 Vectors. *Proc. Natl Acad. Sci. USA* **2009**, *106*, 17158–17162.
149. Ashley, S. N.; Somanathan, S.; Giles, A. R. & Wilson, J. M. TLR9 signaling mediates adaptive immunity following systemic AAV gene therapy. Cell Immunol. 346, 103997 (2019).
150. Mendell, J. R. et al. Dystrophin Immunity in Duchenne's Muscular Dystrophy. *N. Engl. J. Med.* **2010**, *363*, 1429–1437.
151. Wilson, J. M. & Flotte, T. R. Moving Forward After Two Deaths in a Gene Therapy Trial of Myotubular Myopathy. *Hum. Gene Ter.* **2020**, *31*, 695–696.

Clinical Studies of Gene Therapy

152. Hinderer, C. et al. Severe toxicity in nonhuman primates and piglets following high-dose intravenous administration of an Adeno-Associated Virus Vector Expressing Human SMN. *Hum. Gene Ter.* **2018,** *29,* 285–298.

153. Nidetz, N. F. et al. Adeno-Associated Viral Vector-Mediated Immune Responses: Understanding Barriers to Gene Delivery. *Pharmacol. Ter.* **2020,** *207,* 107453.

Index

A

Adeno-associated virus (AAV), 90–93
Adenovirus (Ad), 89–90
Aggregated proteins, 40
Alzheimer's disease (AD)
  mechanism of action, 4–5
  pathophysiology, 3–4
  pharmacotherapy, 5–8
Amyloid, 176
  ApoE acts, 177
  astrocyte-conditioned medium (ACM), 178
  low-density lipoprotein receptor (LDLR), 177
  low-density lipoprotein receptor-related protein 1 (LRP1), 177
  proteolysis, 178
  very low-density lipoprotein receptor (VLDLR), 177
Amyloid precursor protein (APP), 166
Amyotrophic lateral sclerosis (ALS), 11–12, 59
Artificial chromosomes, 138–140
Astrocyte-conditioned medium (ACM), 178
Astrocytes
  Alzheimer's disease (AD), 173–175
  amyloid, 176
    ApoE acts, 177
    astrocyte-conditioned medium (ACM), 178
    low-density lipoprotein receptor (LDLR), 177
    low-density lipoprotein receptor-related protein 1 (LRP1), 177
    proteolysis, 178
    very low-density lipoprotein receptor (VLDLR), 177
  blood brain barrier (BBB)
    and lymphatic borders, 169–171
  central nervous system (CNS)
    chondroitin sulfate proteoglycans (CSPGs), 172

glial fibrillary acidic protein (GFAP), 171
microglia, 173
in disease and health
  blood brain barrier (BBB), 168
  star-shaped cells, 167
neuron symbiosis
  and multilateral synapse, 168–169
tenderness
  nonsteroidal anti-inflammatory drugs (NSAIDs), 176
  targeted cell sorting calls, 175
  tumor necrosis factor (TNF), 175–176

B

Blood brain barrier (BBB), 168
  and lymphatic borders, 169–171

C

Central nervous system (CNS)
  chondroitin sulfate proteoglycans (CSPGs), 172
  glial fibrillary acidic protein (GFAP), 171
  microglia, 173
Cerebrospinal fluid (CSF), 42
Chondroitin sulfate proteoglycans (CSPGs), 172
Clinical studies
  ALS, 199–200
  Alzheimer's disease (AD), 196–197
  challenges and promises, 200, 203–204
  gene therapy, 193–194, 200
  gene treatment, 194–195
  glial cell line-derived neurotrophic factor (GDNF), 193
  Huntington's disease gene (HTT), 198–199
  Parkinson's disease (PD), 197–198
  in vivo study, 195
Complementary DNA (cDNA), 130
Creutzfeldt Jacob's disease (CJD), 60
Creutzfeldt–Jakob disease (CJD), 29

218   *Index*

E

Embryonic stem cells (ESCs), 16–17

F

False of junk genes, 131–133

G

Gene therapy
  adeno-associated virus (AAV), 90–93
  adenovirus (Ad), 89–90
  artificial chromosomes, 138–140
  DNA methylation and histone
    modification, 133–135
  DNA transposons, 95–96
  false of junk genes, 131–133
  Herpes simplex virus type 1 (HSV1),
    137–138
  modes, 98–100
  nanoparticles, 93–95
    rhodopsin knockout (RKO) animals,
      141
    untranslated regions (UTRs), 140
  nonviral vectors, 93
  optogenetics, 98
  regulatory mechanisms, 97
  retrovirus/lentivirus, 86–89
  transgene expression control, 97
  transgenic animals, 135–137
  viral vectors, 84–86
Genomic DNA (gDNA), 130
Gerstmann–Straussler–Scheinker
  syndrome, 31
Glial cell line-derived neurotrophic factor
  (GDNF), 193
Glial fibrillary acidic protein (GFAP), 171

H

Herpes simplex virus (HSV), 130
Herpes simplex virus type 1 (HSV1), 137–138
Human therapeutic studies, 167
Huntington (HD) prions, 67–68
Huntington's disease (HD)
  amyotrophic lateral sclerosis (ALS), 11–12
  brain tumors, 13
  spinal cord injury (SCI), 12
  stroke, 12–13
Huntington's disease gene (HTT), 198–199

I

Induced pluripotent stem cells (iPSCs), 17

K

Koch's postulates, 54–56

L

Low-density lipoprotein receptor (LDLR),
  177
Low-density lipoprotein receptor-related
  protein 1 (LRP1), 177
Lymphocytic choriomeningitis virus
  (LCMV), 151

M

Massive varicosities, 166
Mesenchymal stem cells (MSCs), 18, 117
Microglia, 173
Microtubule-associate protein tau
  (MAPT), 34
Molecule-based clues, 34
  aggregation-prone peptides, 35
  degenerative diseases, 38
  dopaminergic neurons, 37
  infectious forms, 35
  mutant Htt (mHtt), 37
  pathogenic organism, 36
  tau gene (MAPT), 36
Mouse brain (MOK-G), 151
Mutant Htt (mHtt), 37

N

Nanoparticles, 93–95
  rhodopsin knockout (RKO) animals, 141
  untranslated regions (UTRs), 140
Neural stem cells (NSCs), 15–16, 116
Neurodegenerative, 149
Neurodegenerative disorders (NDs), 1
  Alzheimer's disease (AD)
    mechanism of action, 4–5
    pathophysiology, 3–4
    pharmacotherapy, 5–8
  bacterial infection and biomedical
    presentation, 30
    Gerstmann–Straussler–Scheinker
      syndrome, 31

Index

219

blood–brain barrier (BBB), 2, 3
blood–cerebrospinal fluid, 3
cellular disease, theory, 31, 33
  superoxide dismutase 1 (SOD1), 32
clinical studies
  ALS, 199–200
  Alzheimer's disease (AD), 196–197
  challenges and promises, 200,
      203–204
  gene therapy, 193–194, 200
  gene treatment, 194–195
  glial cell line-derived neurotrophic
      factor (GDNF), 193
  Huntington's disease gene (HTT),
      198–199
  Parkinson's disease (PD), 197–198
  in vivo study, 195
concepts and disputes
  aggregated proteins, 40
  protein aggregation, 39
  transsynaptic processes, 38
  trans-synaptic propagation, 39
diseases and prions, 69–70
genetics
  microtubule-associate protein tau
      (MAPT), 34
  presenilin, 33
Huntington's disease (HD)
  amyotrophic lateral sclerosis (ALS),
      11–12
  brain tumors, 13
  spinal cord injury (SCI), 12
  stroke, 12–13
molecule-based clues, 34
  aggregation-prone peptides, 35
  degenerative diseases, 38
  dopaminergic neurons, 37
  infectious forms, 35
  mutant Htt (mHtt), 37
  pathogenic organism, 36
  tau gene (MAPT), 36
Parkinson's disease (PD)
  pathophysiology, 8–9
  pharmacotherapy, 9–10
prion disease
  pomegranate seed oil (PSO), 10
prion proteins
  amyloid-β prions, 61–63

Creutzfeldt Jacob's disease (CJD), 60
  functional characteristics, 68–69
  huntington (HD) prions, 67–68
  pathogenic characteristics, 68–69
  physical characteristics, 68–69
  α-synuclein prions, 65–66
  tau prion proteins, 63–65
stem cell therapy
  embryonic stem cells (ESCs), 16–17
  induced pluripotent stem cells
      (iPSCs), 17
  integrative medicine, 18–19
  mesenchymal stem cells (MSCs), 18
  neural stem cells (NSCs), 15–16
stem-cell-employed gene therapy
  cellular carriers, 115
  multiple mechanisms, 116
symptoms, 40
  cerebrospinal fluid (CSF), 42
  natural human macromolecules, 41
  neurodegenerative illnesses, 42
therapeutic gene expression
  Alzheimer's disease (AD), 120
  applications, 117
  brain tumor, 118–119
  clinical trials, 121
  mesenchymal stem cells (MSCs), 117
  neural stem cells (NSCs), 116
  regulations, 121–122
  spinal cord damage, 119–120
  stroke, 119
transport and cell-to-cell diversion
    mechanisms
  diagnostic strategies, 71–72
  transmission, 70–71
treatment strategy
  gene therapy, 13–14
Neuron symbiosis
  and multilateral synapse, 168–169
Neurons, 28
Nonsteroidal anti-inflammatory drugs
    (NSAIDs), 176

P

Parkinson's disease (PD), 197–198
  pathophysiology, 8–9
  pharmacotherapy, 9–10

220   *Index*

Polyethylene glycol (PEG), 131
Pomegranate seed oil (PSO), 10
Positron emission tomography (PET), 166
Prion disease
   amyloid-β prions, 61–63
   Creutzfeldt Jacob's disease (CJD), 60
   functional characteristics, 68–69
   huntington (HD) prions, 67–68
   pathogenic characteristics, 68–69
   physical characteristics, 68–69
   pomegranate seed oil (PSO), 10
   α-synuclein prions, 65–66
   tau prion proteins, 63–65
Prion-like features
   amyotrophic lateral sclerosis (ALS), 59
   cell transplantation, 59
   fetal cells, 59, 60
   Koch's postulates, 54–56
   seeds of infectiousness, 56–59
   Southwest German Psychiatrists
     (SWGP), 56
Progressive neurodegenerative disorders, 54
Protein aggregation, 39
Proteotoxicity, 29

R

Rhodopsin knockout (RKO) animals, 141
RNAi-based technologies, 154–156

S

Southwest German Psychiatrists (SWGP),
  56
Spinal cord damage, 119–120
Spinal cord injury (SCI), 12
Stem cell therapy
   embryonic stem cells (ESCs), 16–17
   induced pluripotent stem cells (iPSCs),
    17
   integrative medicine, 18–19
   mesenchymal stem cells (MSCs), 18
   neural stem cells (NSCs), 15–16
Stem-cell-employed gene therapy
   cellular carriers, 115
   multiple mechanisms, 116
Superoxide dismutase 1 (SOD1), 32
α-Synuclein prions 65–66

T

Targeted cell sorting calls, 175
Targeting oligodendrocytes
   adeno-associated virus (AAV), 151
   adeno-associated virus serotype 2
    (AAV2), 150
   affect cellular tropism, 153
   artificial miRNA, 156–157
   glialspecific promoters and retargeting
    AAV vector approaches, 151–153
   lentiviral vectors, 150
   lymphocytic choriomeningitis virus
    (LCMV), 151
   mouse brain (MOK-G), 151
   RNAi-based technologies, 154–156
   transcribed-direct synthesis, 157–158
   virus G envelope protein (VSV-G)
    pseudotypes, 150–151
Tau gene (MAPT), 36
Therapeutic gene expression
   Alzheimer's disease (AD), 120
   applications, 117
   brain tumor, 118–119
   mesenchymal stem cells (MSCs), 117
   neural stem cells (NSCs), 116
   regulations, 121–122
   spinal cord damage, 119–120
   stroke, 119
Transmissible spongiform
   encephalopathies (TSEs), 53
   prion-like features
    amyotrophic lateral sclerosis (ALS),
     59
    cell transplantation, 59
    fetal cells, 59, 60
    Koch's postulates, 54–56
    seeds of infectiousness, 56–59
    Southwest German Psychiatrists
     (SWGP), 56
   progressive neurodegenerative
    disorders, 54
Transport and cell-to-cell diversion
   mechanisms
   diagnostic strategies, 71–72
   transmission, 70–71
Transsynaptic processes, 38

Index

221

Trans-synaptic propagation, 39
Treatment strategy
  gene therapy, 13–14
Tumor necrosis factor (TNF), 175–176

U

Untranslated regions (UTRs), 140

V

Very low-density lipoprotein receptor
  (VLDLR), 177
Viral vectors, 84–86
Virus G envelope protein (VSV-G)
  pseudotypes, 150–151

9781774916780